Nursing and Midwifery: A Public Health Perspective

Nursing and Midwifery: A Public Health Perspective

Edited by Selina Douglas

hayle medical

New York

Hayle Medical,
750 Third Avenue, 9th Floor,
New York, NY 10017, USA

Visit us on the World Wide Web at:
www.haylemedical.com

ISBN: 978-1-63241-853-1

The publisher's policy is to use permanent paper from mills that operate a sustainable forestry policy. Furthermore, the publisher ensures that the text paper and cover boards used have met acceptable environmental accreditation standards.

Printed in China.

Cataloging-in-Publication Data

Nursing and midwifery : a public health perspective / edited by Selina Douglas.
p. cm.
Includes bibliographical references and index.
ISBN 978-1-63241-853-1
1. Nursing. 2. Midwifery. 3. Public health. I. Douglas, Selina.
RT42 .N87 2020
610.73--dc21

Table of Contents

Preface

This book has been a concerted effort by a group of academicians, researchers and scientists, who have contributed their research works for the realization of the book. This book has materialized in the wake of emerging advancements and innovations in this field. Therefore, the need of the hour was to compile all the required researches and disseminate the knowledge to a broad spectrum of people comprising of students, researchers and specialists of the field.

Nursing is concerned with the prevention of illness, promotion of health, and care of the ill, disabled and dying. Midwifery is a health profession concerned with the provision of healthcare in childbirth, pregnancy, the postpartum period and care of the newborn. Nursing has a wide scope in terms of its reach in diverse areas, such as women's health, neonatal care, pediatrics, adult gerontology, etc. Midwifery-led care has been associated with fewer episiotomies, reduction in the use of epidurals and a decreased risk of losing the baby before 24 weeks of gestation. However, it has also been associated with increased mean length of labor. A midwife is responsible for conducting routine checkups, tests and examinations during the three trimesters of pregnancy, informing a mother about birthing options, assisting with childbirth, and infant and mother assessment. This book aims to shed light on some of the unexplored aspects of nursing and midwifery and the recent researches in these domains. The various studies that are constantly contributing towards advancing technologies and evolution of these fields are examined in detail. It aims to equip students and experts with the advanced topics and upcoming concepts in these disciplines.

At the end of the preface, I would like to thank the authors for their brilliant chapters and the publisher for guiding us all-through the making of the book till its final stage. Also, I would like to thank my family for providing the support and encouragement throughout my academic career and research projects.

Editor

Prevalence and predictors of antenatal depressive symptoms among women attending Adama Hospital Antenatal Clinic, Adama, Ethiopia

Martha Assefa Sahile[1], Mesfin Tafa Segni[2]*, Tadese Awoke[3] and Dessalegn Bekele[4]

[1]Department of Nursing, College of Health Science, Arsi University, Assela, Ethiopia.
[2]Department of Public Health, College of Health Science, Arsi University, Assela, Ethiopia.
[3]Department of Epidemiology and Biostatistics, Institute of Public Health, University of Gondar, Gondar, Ethiopia.
[4]Department of Psychiatry, Amanuel Specialized Hospital, Addis Ababa, Ethiopia.

Antenatal depressive disorders are serious health problems and pose multiple dangers to both the mother and her fetus, however, not given due attention. They are found with significantly higher prevalence rates in low income countries and associated with socio-economic and socio-cultural factors predominantly. The main objective of this study was to assess the prevalence of antenatal depressive disorders and associated factors among Adama Hospital Antenatal clinic attendants. A hospital based cross sectional study was conducted from March 1st to April 21st, 2011 at Adama Hospital, Adama, Ethiopia. About 231 pregnant women were interviewed using systematic sampling method. Pretested Beck Depression Inventory (BDI) structured questionnaire was used to collect data. The presence of depressive disorders was explained by the sum of BDI items scored 21 and above. And, data entry was done by SPSS version 15 and analyzed using logistic regression. The mean age was 26.32±0.24. About 56.7% were in third trimester and 45% were nulliparous. Regarding pattern of current pregnancy, unwanted pregnancy accounted 42%. Prevalence rate of antenatal depressive disorders was found to be 31.2%. Previous abortion [AOR=2.86, CI (1.13, 7.24)], fear of pregnancy complications [AOR=3.49, CI (2.21, 22.17)], economic problem [AOR=9.52, CI (2.68, 33.78)] and unwanted pregnancy [AOR=6.99, CI (2.21, 22.17) and marital conflict [AOR=22.68, CI(3.61, 142.33] were found to have strong association with depressive disorders. The prevalence of antenatal depressive disorders was high at the study area. Psychosocial factors, economic problems and obstetric features were significantly associated with maternal depressive disorder. Adama Hospital should integrate mental health service with existing antenatal clinic service. In addition, screening of antenatal care (ANC) attendants for potential risk factors of antenatal depressive disorders could be crucial to hamper the impending dangers through early detection.

Key word: Antenatal depressive disorders, pregnant women, Adama hospital, beck depression inventory.

INTRODUCTION

Antenatal depressive disorders are significant health problems; especially in low and middle income countries (Das, 1994). Though reports on prevalence rates lack consistency, substantial higher rates are from developing countries (Felice et al., 2008).

A systemic review of 15 counties reported 32.2%

prevalence rate of antenatal depressive disorders. This may even be higher among high risk groups; within the range of 38 to 50 % (Bennettt et al., 2004; Nasreen et al., 2010). Standard survey was carried out on ten Michigan Obstetric units and the report viewed 20% prevalence rate (Marcus et al., 2003). Another study conducted among rural and urban pregnant women at Ankara antenatal settings found prevalence of 33.1% (Senturk et al., 2011). And also; a hospital based study in Hong Kong took the samples at the antenatal clinic and revealed 37% prevalence of depressive symptoms (Lee et al., 2007).

Unlike the commonly reported findings from developing countries, a recent community based study in Nigeria showed prevalence rate of 8%. However; there is paucity of information on antenatal depressive disorders from Africa. And, no available studies were carried out at health institutions (Adewuya et al., 2007).

Antenatal depressive disorders were found in association with some factors; marital conflict, economic problems, poor support from husband, unwanted pregnancy, previous abortion and past obstetric complications (Adewuya et al., 2007; Kaaya et al., 2010; Dayan et al., 2010). History of past psychiatric disorders, chronic medical illness and poor antenatal care were also reported (Rubertsson et al., 2005; Pereira et al., 2009); however, controversies in the data exist (Hartley et al., 2011; Nasreen et al., 2011; Sawyer et al., 2010).

Pregnant women with antenatal depressive disorders are at risk for recurrent spontaneous abortions, obstetric complications, postnatal depressive disorders and poor child rearing capacity. Babies are also at increased danger for intrauterine growth retardation, preterm delivery, impaired postnatal growth and frequent infant diarrheal diseases (Stewart et al., 2010; Deyessa et al., 2010). Moreover; such women are in danger of troubled social functioning and immune related disease states (Hart and Mahon, 2006; Stein et al., 1991).

Assessment of psychosocial problems and mental health is an integral part of antenatal services to ensure safe pregnancy and delivery. But developing countries lack such antenatal care (ANC) services; and even if available, lack coverage, quality or support from stake holders. In accordance with this fact, a study at Nottingham University notified that WHO has formulated a focused ANC guideline including women's mental health package to be used during ANC assessment (Menon et al., 2010).

In addition to lack of available reports both at national and local study area of this study, higher prevalence rate of antenatal depressive disorders occur at health care settings; therefore, the purpose of this study was to assess the magnitude of antenatal depressive disorders and identify predictors of Antenatal Depressive symptoms among Adama Hospital antenatal clinic attendants.

METHODOLOGY

Study design

Institutional based cross-sectional study design was used.

Study area and period

Adama Hospital is found in Adama town; East Shoa, about 99 km away from Addis Ababa. The Hospital is used for practical teaching of accelerated health officers, clinical nurses, and midwifery, laboratory and pharmacy students at BSc and diploma level besides serving the community. Antenatal care is one of the hospital services organized under health promotion case team. All pregnant mothers who visited the clinic were given appointment for re-visit accordingly. Pregnant mothers were allowed to come back to the clinic at any time on working days and hours for perceived emergency signs and symptoms of pregnancy complications. There was only one midwifery nurse carrying out the ANC services.

The ANC service is organized since establishment of the hospital. There was one psychiatry outpatient department. The system for mental health has no link with antenatal clinic; hence no access of integrated activities for pregnant ladies suffering from mental problems. The study was conducted from March 1st to April 21, 2011.

Study population

Pregnant women attending antenatal clinic within the study period, whose pregnancy was at least 16 weeks (4 months) and below 37 weeks.

Exclusion criteria

1. Those previously diagnosed for depressive disorders
2. Critically ill ones
3. Who were on treatment for mental disorders

Sample size determination and sampling procedures

Single population formula was used with the assumption of 95% confidence interval, precision (d) of 0.03, proportion 8% from the study done in Nigeria and adding 10% non-response rate, 243 women were participated in the study. Systematic sampling procedure was used to interview the study subjects. Every third pregnant woman was approached for the interview during follow up period until the required sample size fulfilled.

Study variables

1. Dependent variable: Antenatal depressive disorders

*Corresponding author. E-mail: mesfintafa2011@gmail.com.

2. Independent variable: Age, educational level, occupation, marital status, level of monthly income, marital conflict, history of abortion, unplanned pregnancy, fear of pregnancy complications, poor husband support, number of live children, perceived poor antenatal care.

Operational definition

Depressive disorders

The presence of depressive disorders was explained by the sum of BDI items scored 21 and above.

Data collection method and quality assurance

Data was collected by interview technique using standardized and validated Beck Depression Inventory (BDI) and structured questionnaire after translated in to Amharic.

BDI was developed and revised to reflect the revision in the current DSM-IV-TR and had been extensively tested for content validity. BDI was composed of 21 questions, each with four possible responses. Each response was assigned a score ranging from zero to three, indicating severity of a symptom. Two BSc nurses supervisor and three diploma clinical nurses data collectors were recruited. Training was given for data collectors and supervisors before data collection and then pretest was done to avoid errors during the actual data collection period. The data was checked daily by supervisors.

Data analysis

All returned questionnaires were checked for completeness and consistency. Data was coded and then entered, cleaned, stored and analyzed using SPSS 15. Descriptive analysis was used to depict frequency and percentages of variables. Logistic regression was used to find out association between depressive disorders and suggested related factors and strength of association was evaluated using odds ratio at 95% confidence interval and P-values 0.05 was considered to declare significant associations.

Ethical consideration

Ethical approval was obtained from Adama Hospital ethical committee after having authorized letter from University of Gondar and Amanuel Specialized Mental Hospital. All antenatal clinic attending mothers were approached and subjects who gave written consent were interviewed. The interview was conducted in a single separate room around the antenatal clinic. Confidentiality was maintained through no registration of personal identification. Subjects identified with depressive disorders were advised to visit the psychiatric clinic and given referral.

RESULTS

A total of 231 pregnant women were interviewed and has 95% response rate. The mean age was 26.32 $\pm$ 0.24. Regarding their level of education; unable to read and write was 7.8%, read and write to primary school were 30.8%, secondary school was 44.2% while higher education constituted 17.7%. Majority (82.3%) was married and house wife (58%). Prevalence rate of antenatal depressive disorders was found to be 31.2%. About 56.7% were in third trimester and 45% were nulipara. A total of 37.8% had history of abortion. Unwanted pregnancy accounted 42% (Table 1).

Overall, 55% stated pregnancy is not joyful for them and 16.9% respondents explored they have poor husband support. About 16% reported their husbands are not happy on the occurrence of current pregnancy (Table 2).

Participants were made to indicate or choose factors at which they mostly worry about through the current pregnancy. Accordingly; fear of pregnancy complications 27.7%, unwanted pregnancy 22.5% and economic problem 20% were more frequent (Table 3).

About 98.3% reported their happiness on services of the antenatal clinic; however 66.7% stated lack of enough information regarding possible outcomes of pregnancy and expected labor. Moreover, 97% complained their ANC visit did not help for psychosocial problems.

Association of covariates with antenatal depressive disorders

From logistic regression, there was statistically significant association between antenatal depressive disorder and previous abortion history [AOR=2.86, 95%CI=(1.13, 7.24)], unwanted pregnancy [AOR=6.99, 95%CI=(2.68, 33.78)], marital conflict (AOR=22.68 CI (3.61, 142.33)], economic problem [AOR=9.52, 95%CI=(2.21, 22.17)] and fear of pregnancy complications [AOR=3.49,95%CI=(1.45, 8.41)]. However, there was no statistically significant association between socio demographic variables and antenatal depressive disorder (Table 4).

DISCUSSION

This hospital based study attempted to assess the magnitude of antenatal depressive disorders and associated factors among Adama hospital antenatal clinic attendants. The screening material for prevalence rate was the standard BDI. Beck depression inventory was considered because it is revised recently in considering the DSM IV TR which is currently in use for psychiatric evaluation. Moreover, psychosocial factors, obstetric information, health and ANC related factors were recognized to assess associated factors.

Prevalence rate of antenatal depressive disorders in this study was 31.2%; within the range of previous reports at clinical settings. A report at Michigan Obstetric Clinics showed 20% and there was 33.1% prevalence rate at Ankara antenatal clinic (Mohammed and Gamble, 2011). Generally, considerable higher prevalence rates have been seen with screenings at health care facilities than community based studies. This could be due to effects of study designs, sample size, types of instrument and different cut-off points (Hart and Mahon, 2006; Stein

Table 1. Frequency distribution of obstetric and other health related features among women attending Adama hospital antenatal clinic, Adama, Ethiopia (n=231).

Characteristics	Frequency	Percentage
Trimester		
Second	100	43.3
Third	131	56.
Parity		
Nulliparous	104	45
Multipara	127	55
Number of live children		
≤ 2	89	70.1
≥ 3	7	5.5
Zero	31	24.4
History of pregnancy complications		
Yes	15	11.8
No	112	88.2
History of complicated labour		
Yes	24	18.9
No	103	81.1
History of abortion		
Yes	48	37.8
No	79	62.2
Pattern of previous abortion		
Spontaneous	8	37.5
Induced	30	62.2
Pattern of current pregnancy		
Planned	134	58
Unwanted	97	42
Presence of Chronic illness		
Yes	20	8.7
No	211	91.3

et al., 1991).

Socio-demographic characteristics of participants were explained by age, educational status, income level, marital status and occupation. None of socio demographic features show association. This is analogous with a previous systemic review in Africa (Mohammed and Gamble, 2011).

There was discrepancy observed between influence of monthly income and economic problems on presence of antenatal depressive disorders. About 20.8% of subjects reported that economic problems were something that caused frequent stress. Similarly, pregnant women having economic problems were found to be 9.52 times prone to antenatal depressive disorders than financially stable ones. Conversely, monthly income was not found as an association. This may attributed women having less economic power and an unbalanced share on the financial management of family income. Furthermore, more than half of the participants were housewives who reported monthly income of their husbands.

Presence of bad obstetric history (complications of pregnancy and/or labour), number of live children, parity and age of pregnancy were not found in association with presence of antenatal depressive disorders. This was supported by a systemic review done in Africa (Mohammed and Gamble, 2011). But, opposite to previous report from rural Malawi (Rubertsson et al., 2005). Unwanted pregnancy indicated 6.99 times increased risk [AOR= 6.99 CI (2.21, 22.17)]; similar to a study in Brazil (Pereira et al., 2005). However; it was in contrast to findings at Cape Town (Kaaya et al., 2010). This could be due to the difference in sample size, inclusion exclusion criteria and used instruments. Fear of pregnancy complications [AOR=3.49, CI (1.45, 8.41)] and previous abortion [AOR=2.86, CI (1.13, 7.24)] showed strong association; analogous with a prior report in Africa (Lee et al., 2007).

A positive relationship between presence of chronic illness and antenatal depressive disorders was seen prior to controlling confounders but no longer existed; opposite to previous findings (Senturk et al., 2011). This might be explained by the variation in sample size and instruments.

Table 2. Frequency distribution of information on psychosocial factors among Women attending ANC clinic at Adama Hospital, Adama, Ethiopia (n=231).

Factors	Percentage
Extra joy due to pregnancy	
Yes	55
No	45
Husbands feeling on pregnancy	
Happy	84
Unhappy	16
Husbands support	
Good	83.1
Poor	16.9
Perceived community care	
Good	93.5
Poor	6.5
Pregnancy disclosure	
Easy	56.7
Difficult	43.3
Burden of social responsibilities	
Yes	6.9
No	93.1
Extra care from husband	
Yes	77.1
No	22.9

Table 3. Frequency distribution of emotionally disturbing factors through the current pregnancy as indicated among Women attending ANC clinic at Adama Hospital, Adama, Ethiopia (n=231).

Characteristics	Frequency (%)	
	Yes	No
Lack of family support	14.3	85.7
Burden of household duties	7.8	92.2
Economic problems	20.8	79.2
Fear of pregnancy complications	27.7	72.3
Lack of access to health care	0.4	99.6
Unwanted pregnancy	22.5	77.5
Previous mishandling by health professionals	0.4	99.6
Previous mishandling by health professionals	0.4	99.6
History of induced abortions	4.3	95.7
Fear of being unable to care the new born baby	13	87
Marital conflict	14.7	85.3
Uncertainty on the quality of hospital delivery service	2.2	97.8
Pregnancy related disorders	3	97

About 98.7% participants were happy on ANC service. Contrary to this, 68.8% of the study subjects and 97.2% of those having depressive disorders witnessed no enough information was provided at ANC about possible outcomes and expected delivery of the current pregnancy. This was found in line with the positive relationship between fear of pregnancy complications and antenatal depressive disorders [AOR=3.17, CI (1.45, 8.41)]. Moreover; 97% affirmed no benefit of ANC visits for their psychosocial problems. These all showed discrepancy to service satisfaction obtained from participants suggesting that perhaps participants did not

Table 4. Logistic regression analysis of selected variables of pregnant women towards antenatal depressive disorders at Adama Hospital antenatal clinic, Adama, Ethiopia (n=231).

Variable	Depressive disorders		Crude OR at 95% CI	Adjusted OR at 95% CI
	Yes	No		
Occupation				
Employee	27	36	1.07(.46, 2.50)	1.22(.36, 4.16)
Housewife	31	107	.43(.19, .95)	.40(.13, 1.28)
Own business	14	20	1	1
Previous abortion				
Yes	23	25	2.52(1.31, 4.84)	**2.86(1.13, 7.24)***
No	49	134	1	1
Chronic illness				
Yes	12	8	3.77(1.47, 9.70)	1.04(.23, 4.68)
No	60	151	1	1
Marital conflict				
Yes	31	3	39.32(11.45, 135.02)	**22.68(3.61, 142.33)***
No	41	156	1	1
Economic problem				
Yes	39	9	19.70(8.70, 44.58)	**9.52(2.21, 22.17)***
No	33	150	1	1
Husband support				
Good	44	146	1	1
Poor	28	13	6.30(3.0, 13.26)	.38 (.05, 2.87)
Fear of pregnancy complications				
Yes	32	32	3.17(1.73, 5.82)	**3.49 (1.45, 8.41)***
No	40	127	1	1
Unwanted pregnancy				
Yes	41	11	17.79(8.24, 38.43)	**6.99 (2.68, 33.78)***
No	31	148	1	1
Unwanted pregnancy by husbands				
Yes	28	150	10.61(4.66, 24.15)	2.04(.29, 14.46)
No	44	9	1	1

feel comfortable reporting dissatisfaction because the survey took place at the hospital.

Marital conflict was associated to antenatal depressive disorders [AOR=22.68, CI (3.61, 142.33)] and this was similar to other studies (Pereira et al., 2009; Hartley et al., 2011). Opposite to societal values about pregnancy as joyful period for women, about 45% of study subjects declared pregnancy did not brought extra joy. This was also in line with other studies (Bennettt et al., 2004).

As limitation of this, it prone to demerits of the study design nature being cross sectional. The other limitation could be information bias may be introduced while using the measurement of BDI.

Conclusion

The prevalence of antenatal depressive disorder was high among Adama Hospital antenatal clinic attendants. It could be because this study is inclusive to all types of depressive disorders likely to occur at antenatal period. The effects of previous abortion, fear of pregnancy complications, economic problems, unwanted pregnancy and marital conflict have significant association with the development of antenatal depressive disorders. There should be consideration of integration of mental health service to antenatal clinic services by the hospital. Moreover; refreshment of the Hospital health professionals on antenatal depressive disorders, including common mental disorders within the contents of health education and early screening of pregnant women may help more.

CONFLICT OF INTERESTS

The authors have not declared any conflict of interests.

ACKNOWLEDGEMENTS

The authors would like to thank Amanuel Specialized

Mental Hospital for financial support which made this study possible. They also would like to thank the study participants who volunteered to participate in the study and the hospital officials for their cooperation during data collection and other processes during the study. They also pass out gratitude for the data collectors for their tolerance and collaboration during data collection period.

REFERENCES

Adewuya AO, Ola BA, Aloba OO, Dada AO, Fasoto OO (2007). Prevalence and correlates of depression in late pregnancy among Nigerian women. Depress. Anxiety 24(1):15-21.

Bennett HA, Einorson A, Taddio A (2004). Prevalence of depression during pregnancy: systemic review. Obstet. Gynecol. 103(4):698-709.

Das V (1994). Moral orientations to suffering: Legitimation, power and healing. In: health and social change in international perspective; Chen L, Kleinman A and Ware N (eds,). pp. 139-170.

Dayan J, Creveuil C, Dreyfus M, Herlicoviez M, Baleyte JM, O'Keane V (2010). Developmental Model of Depression Applied to Prenatal Depression: Role of Present and Past Life Events, Past Emotional Disorders and Pregnancy Stress. PLoS One 5(9):e12942.

Deyessa N, Berhane Y, Emmelin M, Ellsberg MC, Kullgren G, Högberg U (2010). Joint effect of maternal depression and intimate partner violence on increased child death in rural Ethiopia. Arch. Dis. Child 95(10):771-775.

Felice E, Saliba J, Grech V, Cox J (2008). Prevalence rates and psychosocial characteristics associated with depression in pregnancy and postpartum in Maltese women. J. Affect. Disord. 82(2):297-301.

Hart R, McMahon CA (2006). Mood state and psychological adjustment to pregnancy. Arch. Womens Ment. Health 9(6):329-337.

Hartley M, Tomlinson M, Greco E, Comulada WS, Stewart J, Le Roux I, Mbewu N, Rotheram-Borus MJ (2011). Depressed mood in pregnancy: prevalence and correlates in two Cape Town peri-urban settlements. Reprod. Health 8(1):9.

Kaaya SF, Mbwambo JK, Kilonzo GP, Van Den Borne H, Leshabari MT, Fawzi MC, Schaalma H (2010). Socio-economic and partner relationship factors associated with antenatal depressive morbidity among pregnant women in Dares Salaam, Tanzania. Tanzan. J. Health Res. 12(1):23-35.

Lee AM, Lam SK, Lau SM, Chong CS, Chui HW, Fong DY (2007). Prevalence, course, risk factors for antenatal anxiety and depression. J. Obstet. Gynaecol. 110:1102-1112.

Marcus SM, Flynn HA, Blow FC, Barry KL (2003). Depressive symptoms among pregnant women screened in obstetrics settings. J. Women's Health 12(4):373-380.

Menon JA, Musonda VCT, Glazebrook C (2010). Perception of care in Zambian women attending community antenatal clinics. Educ. Res. 1(9):356-362.

Mohammad KI, Gamble J, Creedy DK (2011). Prevalence and factors associated with the development of antenatal and postnatal depression among Jordanian women. Midwifery 27(6):e238-45.

Nasreen HE, Kabir ZN, Forsell Y, Edhborg M (2010). Low birth weight in offspring of women with depressive and anxiety symptoms during pregnancy: results from a population based study in Bangladesh. BMC Public Health 10(1):515.

Nasreen HE, Kabir ZN, Forsell Y, Edhborg M (2011). Prevalence and associated factors of depressive and anxiety symptoms during pregnancy: A population based study in rural Bangladesh. BMC Womens Health 11:22.

Pereira PK, Lovisi GM, Pilowsky DL, Lima LA, Legay LF (2005). Depression during pregnancy: prevalence and risk factors among women attending a public health clinic in Rio de Janeiro, Brazil. Cad Saude Pub. 25(12):2725-2736.

Rubertsson C, Wickberg B, Gustavsson P, Rådestad I (2005). Depressive symptoms in early pregnancy, two months and one year postpartum-prevalence and psychosocial risk factors in a national Swedish sample. Arch. Womens Ment. Health 8(2):97-104.

Sawyer A, Ayers S, Smith H (2010). Pre and post natal psychological well-being in Africa: A systemic review. J. Affect. Disord. 123(1-3):17-29.

Senturk V, Abas M, Berksun O, Stewart R (2011). Social support and antenatal depression in extended and nuclear family environments in Turkey: a cross-sectional survey. BMC Psychiatry 11(1):48.

Stein M, Miller AH, Trestman RL (1991). Depression, the immune system, and health and illness: findings in search of meaning. Arch. Gen. Psychiatry 48(2):171-177.

Stewart RC, Bunn J, Vokhiwa M, Umar E, Kauye F, Fitzgerald M, Tomenson B, Rahman A, Creed F (2010). Common mental disorders and associated factors among women with young infants in rural Malawi. Soc Psychiatry Psychiatr. Epidemiol. 45(5):551-559.

Comparative study of general with Spinal Anesthesia on maternal outcomes for caesarean delivery among preeclamptic women at Tikur Anbessa Specialized Hospital, Addis Ababa, Ethiopia

Tsehay Terefe[1*], Yohannes Tekalegn[2] and Abraham Irena[1]

[1]Tikur Anbessa Specialized Hospital, College of Health Sciences, Addis Ababa University, Ethiopia.
[2]Gobba Referral Hospital, College of Health Sciences, Madda Walabu University, Ethiopia.

Anesthetic management of preeclamptic patients remains a challenge. Although general anesthesia can be used safely in pre-eclamptic women, it is fraught with greater maternal morbidity and mortality. The added risks associated with general anesthesia include airway difficulties due to edema (often aggravated by tracheal intubation) and the pressure response to laryngoscope and intubation. However, several studies support the use of spinal anesthesia as first choice reasoning less post-operative morbidity and mortality. To compare maternal outcome among preeclamptic women after caesarian delivery under general and spinal anesthesia in Tikur Anbessa Specialized Hospital, Addis Ababa, Ethiopia. Hospital based retrospective comparative cross sectional study was used to compare maternal outcomes. All preeclamptic mothers that underwent Caesarian Section in Obstetrics and Gynecology Ward, Tikur Anbessa Specialized Hospital from October 2014 to October 2016 was included in the study. Data collection was carried out by using structured questionnaire. Data entry and analysis was done on SPSS version 20. Independent sample T-test and logistic regression was conducted to compare the outcome in both groups of spinal and general anesthesia, 95% confidence interval (CI) and p value < 0.05 is set as cut off point for statistical significance. The mean age of study subjects were 28.18 years and SD= ± 4.66 years, the median age is 28 years (IQR: 25-30 years). Majority 152 (91%) of the cesarean sections (C/S) was emergency C/S and the rest 15 (9%) were elective C/S. 78 (46.7%) of parturient operated under general anesthesia, and 89 (53.3%) were operated under spinal anesthesia. None of the mothers developed post-op complication, and none of the maternal death were documented until discharge from the hospital in both groups of parturient. The present finding shows that statistically significant higher intra operative blood pressure and pulse rate was observed among GA group when compared with SA group. In conclusion, SA is safer than GA in terms of stable intra operative vital signs among preeclamptic women.

Key words: Preeclampsia, caesarean section, general anesthesia, spinal anesthesia, Ethiopia.

INTRODUCTION

Preeclampsia is a multi-systemic disorder characterized by hypertension and new-onset of proteinuria which develops after the 20th week of pregnancy in previously normo-tensive women. It is a common cause of maternal and perinatal morbidity and mortality in both developed and developing countries affecting 2 to 8% of pregnancies (World Health Organization (WHO), 1988). WHO estimates that the incidence of preeclampsia is 7 times higher in low- and middle-income countries than in high-income countries, and From 10 to 25% of these cases will result in maternal death (Engender Health, 2007; Dolea and AbouZahr, 2003). Pre-eclampsia/Eclampsia is responsible for an estimated 16% of global maternal mortality (63,000 maternal deaths) annually (Khan et al., 2006).

Rates from African countries such as South Africa, Egypt, Tanzania, and Ethiopia vary from 1.8 to 7.1% (Kimbally et al., 2007; Mahaba et al., 2001; Thiam et al., 2003; Teklu and Gaym, 2006). According to WHO report, an estimated 350 women per 100,000 live births were dying of pregnancy and related causes in Ethiopia. The Ethiopian National Emergency Obstetric and Newborn Care (EMONC) survey showed that preeclampsia contributed to the complication of approximately 1% of all deliveries and 5% of all pregnancies. Moreover, 16% of direct maternal mortality and 10% of all maternal mortality (direct and in direct) was due to preeclampsia/eclampsia (Gaym et al., 2011). A maternal mortality trend analysis showed an increasing trend of preeclampsia in Ethiopia (Abdella, 2010). Caesarean section is one of the lifesaving surgical interventions attributed to the decrease of maternal and perinatal mortality and morbidity. The frequency of cesarean section births continues to steadily rise worldwide (Gori et al., 2007). According to Demographic Health Survey (1990 to 2014), the global cesarean section rate is 18.6%. The average cesarean section rate in Africa is 7.3%, the highest Egypt (51.8%) and 0.6% for Ethiopia which is very low. But the national cesarean section rate in Ethiopia varies from 2 to 27% (Betrán et al., 2016).

Cesarean anesthesia has gained importance as the cesarean birth rates have increased. Even though the cesarean procedure has become very safe over the years, it is still associated with maternal and perinatal mortality and morbidity (Liu et al., 2007). The overall postoperative morbidity rate associated with cesarean births is 35.7%. The higher mortality and morbidity rates might be attributable not only to the surgical procedure but also to the anesthetic technique preferred (Saygıl et al., 2015).

This study aimed to compare outcomes of preeclamptic parturient following caesarean delivery under either general or spinal anesthesia.

MATERIALS AND METHODS

Study area and setting

A hospital based retrospective cross sectional study was used to compare maternal outcomes following caesarian delivery in preeclamptic women under general and spinal anesthesia in Tikur Anbessa Specialized Hospital Addis Ababa, Ethiopia; from November to December, 2016. Addis Ababa is the capital city of Ethiopia. It is the largest city with a population of 3,384,569 according to the 2007 population census. It lays at an altitude of 7,546 ft (2,300 m) above sea level in the southern periphery, the city rises to over 9,800 ft (3,000 m) in the north. It has 11 government hospitals and 86 health centers in the city. Tikur Anbessa Specialized Hospital is tertiary referral, teaching governmental hospital and the largest of all public hospitals in Ethiopia. The hospital has a total of 800 beds, 80 of which are currently being used in obstetrics and gynecology ward. About 3000 deliveries are attended each year and 60% of these are operative deliveries (Aya et al., 2003).

Inclusion and exclusion criteria

Inclusion criteria

All preeclamptic mothers admitted in obstetrics and gynecology ward of Tikur Anbessa Specialized Hospital from October 2014 to October 2016 and underwent CS was included in the study.

Exclusion criteria

Mothers who also do not have complete records on their charts like operation sheet, anesthesia sheet, and socio demographic characteristics data were excluded from the study.

Sample size determination

All preeclamptic mothers that underwent CS in obstetrics and gynecology ward, Tikur Anbessa Specialized Hospital from October 2014 to October 2016 were included in the study.

Sampling procedures

First, all mothers with preeclampsia undergone CS for delivery with either GA or SA were selected by the principal investigator from CS registration book by counting cases that were enrolled between October 2014 and October 2016. Then all eligible patients' card was collected from card room to conduct data collection.

Data collection procedures

Medical records were reviewed for all preeclamptic patients who had CS from October, 2014 to October, 2016. Data was collected from patients' medical records by using checklists. Five nurses and two anesthetic nurses with experience of data collection and supervision was involved as data collectors and supervisors, respectively, after taking training for one day on how to collect records and fill on the format prepared. Socio demographic, reproductive health characteristics, pre-operative, intra-operative and post-operative data were collected after taking the selected parturient card from card store.

*Corresponding author. E-mail: tsehayterefe484@gmail.com.

Data analysis procedures

The collected data were cleaned, coded, entered into SPSS version 20 statistical software for analysis. Data were checked for completeness and consistency. Frequency tables and graphs were used to describe the study variables. Independent sample T-test was applied to see whether there is significant difference between continuous independent variables and outcome variables. And logistic regression was applied for testing association between categorical independent variables and outcome variables. The significant level is declared at P-value < 0.05.

Data quality control

For data quality control, data collection tools were adopted from existing literatures and pretest of the questionnaire was carried out. Prior to data collection, one day training was provided for data collectors and supervisors on how to review records from the selected patient's card and fill on the prepared format after taking 5% of the sample size from card room for pretest. Supervisors were assigned to supervise the data collectors and monitor the data collection process. The principal investigator role was to coordinate over all activities of the data collection process. There was meeting and discussion between data collectors, supervisor and the principal investigator after the end of data collection daily to ensure completeness and consistency.

Operational definitions

Maternal outcomes

The incidence of pre and post-operative morbidity (elevated blood pressure, hypotension, intra operative aspiration, peri-operative maternal death, peri-operative infection, length of hospital stay, peri-operative maternal death and admission in ICU) was collected.

General anesthesia

After pre oxygenation, thiopental 4 to 5 mg/kg and succinylcholine 1 to 2 mg/kg were administered and they were intubated under sellicke's maneuver. Maintenance of anesthesia was achieved with 100% oxygen and 0.5 to 1% halothane. Blood pressure and heart rate were monitored in the ward before induction after intubation and at 5 min interval till completion of the operation.

Spinal anesthesia

For spinal anesthesia (SA), isobaric bupivacaine (0.5%), 10 to 15 mg was given intrathecally at level of L3/L4 and 500 ml of normal saline given before induction and bilateral IV line secured to give crystalloid fluids and analgesics as required. Patients received 2 to 3 L/min oxygen from nasal prong throughout surgery. Blood pressure and heart rate were monitored at ward, before SA and after spinal anesthesia and at 5 min interval till completion of the operation.

Severe preeclampsia

Is the development of hypertension characterized by systolic blood pressure exceeding 160 mmHg and/or diastolic blood pressure exceeding 110 mmHg, together with proteinuria (>5 g/24 h) after 20 weeks of gestation (Leeman and Fontaine, 2008).

Ethical statement

Ethical clearance was obtained from Research Ethical Review Board of Addis Ababa University (AAU), permission to conduct the study was obtained from the clinical service director of Tikur Anbessa Specialized hospital prior to data collection. Participant records were treated anonymously and only accessed by research team; hence, confidentiality of participants' records and privacy of the health facility were secured.

RESULTS

Socio demographic characteristics of respondents

A total of 170 patients' document was reviewed based on the eligibility criteria and availability of the documents. The mean age of the study subjects were 28.18 years and SD= ±4.66 years, the median age is 28 years (IQR: 25-30). Majority of the cases 129 (78.7%) were from urban and the rest 34 (20.7%) are from rural areas. Regarding marital status, 153 (96.8%) were married and 5 (3.2%) were unmarried (Tables 1 and 2).

Obstetric characteristics

Clinical characteristics

Majority 152 (91%) of the cesarean sections (C/S) were emergency C/S and the rest 15 (9%) were elective C/S. 78 (46.7%) of the parturient were operated under general anesthesia and 89 (53.3%) were under spinal anesthesia. 130 (83.9%) of operators were resident (GP) and the rest 25 (16.1%) were senior gynecology and obstetrics surgeons.

Comparison of the maternal outcomes under either spinal or general anesthesia

Out of the total study subjects, 78 (46.7%) were operated under general anesthesia and 89 (53.3%) were under spinal anesthesia. Mean age of mothers was 28.2±4.5 vs. 28.1±4.8 years in general and spinal anesthesia groups, respectively. None of the patients had post operative complication in both groups. Mean days of hospital stay after C/S in both groups is comparable. None of the mothers died after C/S in both groups. There is no significant difference between GA and SA groups in terms of post operative complication, days of hospital stay, and death (Tables 3 and 4).

Comparison of maternal vital signs under GA vs. SA

Comparison of pulse rate

The mean pulse rate of mothers at ward and before

Table 1. Socio demographic characteristics of preeclamptic women underwent C/S at Tikur Anbessa Specialized Hospital, Addis Ababa, Ethiopia, from 2014 to 2016.

Variable		GA (%)	SA (%)	P-value
Marital status	Married	67 (44.7)	83 (55.3)	1
	Unmarried	4 (80)	1 (20)	0.1
Age	<20	1 (50)	1 (50)	1
	20-34	70 (47.3)	78 (52.7)	0.9
	≥35	7 (41.2)	10 (58.8)	0.8
Residence	Urban	55 (44)	70 (56)	1
	Rural	17 (50)	17 (50)	0.5

Table 2. Comparison of obstetric characteristics of preeclamptic women underwent C/S At Tikur Anbessa Specialized Hospital, Addis Ababa, Ethiopia, From 2014 To 2016.

Obstetric history		GA (%)	SA (%)	P-value
Parity	Nullipara	35 (46.7)	40 (53.3)	1
	1-4	38 (46.3)	44 (53.7)	0.93
	≥5	1 (50)	1 (50)	1
Gestational age	<37 weeks	10 (71.4)	4 (28.6)	1
	37-40 weeks	67 (44.7)	83 (55.3)	0.38
ANC follow up	Yes	59 (47.2)	66 (52.8)	1
	No	13 (41.9)	18 (58.1)	0.68
Referred from another health institution	Yes	22 (55)	18 (45)	1
	No	54 (44.6)	67 (55.4)	0.42
Had Previous history of C/S	Yes	8 (44.4)	10 (55.6)	1
	No	146	89	0.47

Table 3. Comparison of clinical characteristics of preeclamptic women underwent C/S at Tikur Anbessa Specialized hospital, Addis Ababa, Ethiopia, from 2014 to 2016.

Clinical characteristics		GA	SA	P-value
Type of C/S	Elective	4 (26.7)	11 (73.3)	0.098
	Emergency	74 (49)	77 (51)	1
Operator status	Senior	12 (50)	12 (50)	1
	Resident(GP)	58 (45.3)	70 (54.7)	0.67
Anti-hypertensive treatment used for preeclampsia	Hydralazine	44 (48.4)	47 (51.6)	0.94
	Labetalol	0 (0)	2 (100)	0.99
	Nifedipine	0 (0)	5 (100)	0.99
	Methyldopa	2 (50)	2 (50)	1
Anti convulsant treatment used for preeclampsia	Magnesium sulfate	25 (52.1)	23 (47.9)	0.53
	Diazepam	1 (33.3)	2 (66.7)	1

Table 4. Comparison of maternal outcome, among preeclamptic women underwent C/S, under GA and SA, at Tikur Anbessa Specialized Hospital, Addis Ababa, Ethiopia, from 2014 to 2016.

Variable		Type of anesthesia		
		General (%), n=78	Spinal (%), n=89	P-value
Mean age		28.2+4.5	28.1+4.8	0.86
Post-operative complication	Yes	0 (0)	0 (0)	1
	No	78 (100)	89 (100)	0.39
Days of hospital stay	4-7 days	57 (75)	64 (73.6)	1
	≥7 days	1 (1.3)	0 (0)	0.6
Maternal outcome at discharge from hospital	Alive	78 (100)	89 (100)	1
	Dead	0 (0)	0 (0)	0.39

induction in GA vs. SA groups had no statistically significant difference. The mean pulse rate after induction and throughout intra operative period is significantly higher among GA group when compared with SA (Table 5).

Comparison of blood pressure

Despite the mean blood pressure of mothers at ward and before induction in GA vs. SA groups, there was no significant difference; the mean blood pressure after induction and throughout intra operative period is significantly higher among GA group than SA group (Table 5).

DISCUSSION

This study aimed to compare the outcome of preeclamptic women who gave birth through cesarean section, under either general or spinal anesthesia.

In the present study, 89 patients were administered spinal anesthesia and 78 patients received general anesthesia for cesarean section with a diagnosis of severe preeclampsia.

The present finding shows that both general and spinal anesthesia has no difference in terms of maternal survival status at discharge from the hospital. This finding is in line with previous studies study conducted in Jordan that there is no significant difference among both spinal and general anesthesia in terms of maternal outcome (Qublan et al., 2001). This finding is contrary to the retrospective study in Pakistan which found higher maternal mortality among GA group than SA group (Ahsan-Ul-Haq, 2004). This variation could be explained by the fact that there is no reported death in both groups of patients in our the present retrospective study during the study period and pertaining to morbidity might be less reported as they are not recorded on the patient documented and there may be trends of reporting less morbidity report.

The mean pulse rate, mean systolic blood pressure, and mean diastolic blood pressure of parturient before induction of anesthesia had no statistically significant difference (p>0.05). This result revealed homogeneity of hemodynamic status in both groups; this could be very favorable to compare the effect of both anesthesia types on the vital signs of patients.

The mean pulse rate, mean systolic blood pressure, and mean diastolic blood pressure after induction and throughout intra operative period is significantly higher for patients that underwent caesarean delivery under general anesthesia when compared with those operated under spinal anesthesia (p<0.05). This result shows GA groups had relatively elevated pulse rate and blood pressure when compared with SA group. This finding is in line with prospective study conducted in India, retrospective study conducted in Pakistan and randomized controlled study conducted in India which found prevalence of uncontrolled hypertension and tachycardia to be higher among GA group when compared with SA group (Ahsan-Ul-Haq, 2004; Chattopadhyay et al., 2014; Denu et al., 2015). This result could be explained by the exaggerated response of patients' to laryngoscopy after intubation of endotracheal tube. Hypotension was treated with conventional treatment using IV fluid therapy and hypertension was controlled with hydralazin or nifedipine. It was observed that although intra operative haemodynamic changes during SA and GA had statistically significant difference but clinically these were acceptable and manageable and did not have any deleterious effect on the patients of both groups.

Conclusion

The present study revealed that maternal outcomes such

Table 5. Comparison of maternal vital signs, among preeclamptic women underwent C/S, under GA and SA, at Tikur Anbessa Specialized hospital, Addis Ababa, Ethiopia, from 2014 to 2016.

Variable		General	Spinal	95% CI of mean difference	p-value
Pulse rate	Mean Base line pulse rate at ward	97.04±9.14	93.78±11.85	3.25 (-0.038-6.52)	0.053
	Mean Pulse rate before induction	98.97±7.45	95.66±8.85	3.32 (-0.64-7.28)	0.09
	Mean Pulse rate after induction/SA	103.19±10.55	92.83±12.32	10.36 (4.1-16.6)	0.002*
	Mean 10th minute pulse rate	99.66±9.63	88.93±9.69	10.73 (7.70-13.76)	<0.001*
	Mean 15th minute pulse rate	89.74±5.62	73.64±8.72	16.1 (10.89-21.3)	<0.001*
	Mean 20th minute pulse rate	96±8.5	84±9.2	11.53 (8.7-14.3)	<0.001*
	Mean 25th minute pulse rate	95.75±8.5	78.5±9.2	17.2 (12.2-22.2)	<0.001*
	Mean 60th minute pulse rate	90.05±5.7	82.67±6.9	7.38 (5.4-9.36)	<0.001*
	Mean 30th minute pulse rate	93.12±6.88	82.62±8.66	7.9 (5.9-10.04)	<0.001*
	Mean 60th minute pulse rate	90.05±5.78	82.67±6.98	7.38 (5.4-9.36)	<0.001*
Systolic blood pressure	Mean Baseline systolic BP at ward	153.68±12.26	149.76±13.85	3.92 (-0.12-7.9)	0.057
	Mean Systolic BP before induction	154.54±19.34	151.23±12.38	3.31 (-0.410.7)	0.37
	Mean Systolic BP after induction	162.27±12.34	144.93±12.76	17.33 (10.53-24.1)	<0.001*
	Mean systolic BP 5th minute	162.7±14	147.6±15.7	15.1 (5.92-24.29)	0.002*
	Mean systolic BP 10th minute	157.8+12.7	137.7+13.3	20 (16-24.17)	<0.001*
	Mean systolic BP 15th minute	150.5+16.8	131.1+17	19.36 (8.8-29.9)	<0.001*
	Mean systolic BP 20th minute	148.9+11.3	127.6+12.6	21.38 (17.6-25.12)	<0.001*
	Mean systolic BP 30th minute	141.5+11.9	119.6+13	21.88 (17.9-25.7)	<0.001*
	Mean systolic BP 60th minute	134.7+9.6	122.7+10.5	12 (8.9-15.1)	<0.001*
Diastolic blood pressure	Mean Baseline diastolic BP at ward	93.18±8.3	91.61±8.37	1.57 (-0.9-4.1)	0.22
	Mean Diastolic BP before induction	97.64±7.67	92.54±9.24	5.1 (1.33-8.86)	0.009*
	Mean Diastolic BP after induction	96.54±18.72	88.76±8.84	7.78 (-0.006-15.5)	0.05
	Mean 10th minute diastolic BP	92.77±12.74	81.4±8.9	11.37 (8.74-14.00)	<0.001*
	Mean 20th minute diastolic BP	86.5±6.3	73.07±8.6	13.49 (11.09-15.88)	<0.001*
	Mean 30th minute diastolic BP	82.18±9.71	67.63±8.43	14.55 (11.74-17.35)	<0.001*
	Mean 60th minute diastolic BP	78.24±11.2	71.64±11.28	6.60 (3.13-10.06)	<0.001*

*Significant at p<0.05.

as post operative complication, days of hospital stay, and maternal survival at discharge, have no statistically significant difference in both spinal and general anesthesia groups. General as well as spinal anesthetic techniques are acceptable for caesarean delivery in pregnancies complicated by severe preeclampsia if steps are taken to ensure a careful approach to either method. Spinal anesthesia could be considered as first choice for severe preeclamptic patients, associated with less intraoperative hypertension.

RECOMMENDATION

This study is recommended with strong design to be conducted in the area to come up with strong evidences.

CONFLICT OF INTERESTS

The authors have not declared any conflict of interests.

Abbreviations:

AAU, Addis Ababa University; **CI,** confidence interval; **CS,** caesarian section; **DBP,** diastolic blood pressure; **EDHS,** Ethiopia demographic and health survey; **EMONC,** Ethiopian emergency obstetric and newborn care; **GA,** general anesthesia; **HELLP,** hemolysis elevated liver enzymes and low platelet count; **ICU,** intensive care unit; **MCH,** maternal and child health; **SA,** spinal anesthesia; **SBP,** systolic blood pressure; **SNNPR,** South Nation Nationality People Region; **SPSS,** statistical package for social science; **WHO,** World Health Organization.

ACKNOWLEDGEMENT

The authors are grateful to Addis Ababa University for the financial and technical support.

REFERENCES

Abdella A (2010). Maternal mortality trend in Ethiopia. Ethiop. J. Health Dev. 24(1):115-22.

Ahsan-Ul-Haq MM (2004). Analysis of outcome of general versus spinal anesthesia for caesarean delivery in severe pre-eclampsia with foetal compromise. J. Biomed. 20:1-8.

Betrán AP, Ye J, Moller AB, Zhang J, Gülmezoglu AM, Torloni MR (2016). The Increasing Trend in Caesarean Section Rates: Global, Regional and National Estimates: 1990-2014. PLoS One 11(2):e0148343.

Chattopadhyay S, Das A, Pahari S (2014). Feto maternal Outcome in Severe Preeclamptic Women Undergoing Emergency Cesarean Section under either General or Spinal Anesthesia. J. Pregnancy 2014:1-10.

Denu ZA, Awoke T, Melkie TB, Adefris M (2015). Trends in Obstetrics Anesthesia at Gondar University Hospital. EC Anaesthesia. Available at: https://www.ecronicon.com/ecan/pdf/ECAN-02-000017.pdf

Dolea C, AbouZahr C (2003). Global Burden of Hypertensive Disorders of Pregnancy in the year 2000. World health organization working paper, Geneva. Available at: http://www.who.int/healthinfo/statistics/bod_hypertensivedisordersofpregnancy.pdf

Engender Health (2007). Balancing the scales. Expanding treatment for pregnant women with life-threatening hypertensive conditions in developing countries. A report on barriers and solutions to treat pre-eclampsia and eclampsia. Available at: http://www.srhr-ask-us.org/publication/balancing-scales-expanding-treatment-pregnant-women-life-threatening-hypertensive-conditions-developing-countries-report-barriers-solutions-treat-pre-eclampsia-eclamps/

Gaym A, Bailey P, BLuwei P, Admasu K, Gebrehiwot Y (2011). Disease burden due to preeclampsia/eclampsia and the Ethiopian health system's response. Int. J. Gynecol. Obstet.115:112-116.

Gori F, Pasqualucci A, Corradetti F, Milli M, Peduto VA (2007). Maternal and neonatal outcome after cesarean section: the impact of anesthesia. J. Matern. Fetal Neonatal Med. 20(1):53-57.

Khan KS, Wojdyla D, Say L, Gülmezoglu AM, Van Look PF (2006). World health organization (WHO) analysis of causes of maternal death. A systematic review. Lancet 367(9516):1066-1074.

Kimbally KG, Barassoumbi H, Buambo SF, Gombet T, Kibeke P, Monabeka HG, Iloki LH, Ekoundzola JR (2007). Arterial hypertension epidemiological aspects and risk factors on pregnant and delivered woman. Dakar Med. J. 52(2):148-152.

Leeman L, Fontaine P (2008). Hypertensive disorders of pregnancy. Am. Fam. Phys. 78(1):93-100.

Liu S, Liston RM, Joseph KS, Heaman M, Sauve R, Kramer MS (2007). Maternal mortality and severe associated with low-risk planned cesarean delivery versus planned vaginal delivery at term. CMAJ 176(4):455-460.

Mahaba HM, Ismail NA, El Damaty SI, Kamel HA (2001). Pre-eclampsia: epidemiology and outcome of 995 cases. J. Egyptian Public Health Assoc. 76(5-6):357-368.

Qublan HS, Merhej A, Dabbas MA, Hindawi IM (2001). Spinal versus general anesthesia for elective c/s delivery a prospective comparative study. Clin. Exp. Obstet. Gynecol. 28(4):246-248.

Saygıl A, Özdamar O, Gün I, Emirkad H, Müngen E, Akpak YK (2015). Comparison of maternal and fetal outcomes among patients undergoing cesarean section under general and spinal anesthesia: a randomized clinical trial. Sao Paulo Med. J. 133(3):227-234.

Aya AG, Mangin R, Vialles N, Ferrer JM, Robert C, Ripart J, de La Coussaye JE (2003). Patients with severe preeclampsia experience less hypotension during spinal anesthesia for elective cesarean delivery than healthy parturient. Anesth. Analg. 97(3):867-872.

Teklu S, Gaym A (2006). Prevalence and clinical correlates of the hypertensive disorders of pregnancy at Tikur Anbessa Hospital, Addis Ababa, Ethiopia. Ethiop. Med. J. 44(1):17-26.

Thiam M, Goumbala M, Gning SB, Fall PD, Cellier C, Perret JL (2003). Maternal and fetal prognosis of hypertension and pregnancy in Africa (Senegal). J. Gynecol. Obstet. Biol. Reprod. 32(1):35-38.

World Health Organization (WHO) (1988). International Collaborative Study of Hypertensive Disorders of Pregnancy. Geographic variation in the incidence of hypertension in pregnancy. Am. J. Obstet. Gynecol, 158(1):80-83.

3

Uterine balloon tamponade for the management of uncontrolled postpartum hemorrhage by midwives and family physicians

Zaid Altawil[1,2*], Emily de Redon[2], Hao Dinh[2], Daniela Suarez-Rebling[2] and Thomas F. Burke[2,3,4]

[1]Department of Emergency Medicine, Boston Medical Center, Boston, MA 02118, USA.
[2]Division of Global Health and Human Rights, Department of Emergency Medicine, Massachusetts General Hospital, Boston, MA 02114, USA.
[3]Harvard Medical School, Boston, MA 02115, USA.
[4]Harvard T.H. Chan School of Public Health, Boston, MA, 02115, USA.

Postpartum hemorrhage (PPH) is the leading cause of maternal morbidity and mortality world-wide. Although declining globally, maternal mortality is on the rise in the United States. Since uterine balloon tamponade (UBT) has been shown to be safe as well as highly effective in arresting PPH and halting shock progression, this study sought to clarify the practice and perceptions of UBT use among midwives and family physicians in the United States. A cross-sectional 12-item survey on the practice, experiences and perceptions of uterine balloon tamponade utilization for PPH management was conducted among midwives and family physicians that perform deliveries in the United States. The survey settings were one family medicine and two midwifery national conferences in the United States. One hundred and ninety-seven midwives (164; 83.2%) and family physicians (33; 16.8%) completed the surveys. The 197 providers had previously cared for a mean of 6.0 (SD= 18.8) uncontrolled PPH cases each, over the course of their career till date. Eighty (40.6%) of the 197 respondents had been involved with at least one hemorrhaging woman in which a UBT was placed, but only 13 (7.9%) of the 164 midwives and 6 (18.2%) of the 33 family physicians had ever placed a UBT device themselves. One hundred and thirty-one (73.6%) of 178 providers desired training on use of UBT. Midwives and family physicians in the United States care for women with uncontrolled PPH, however, infrequently place a UBT device. Most midwives and family physicians would like training on uterine balloon tamponade.

Key words: Uterine balloon tamponade, post-partum hemorrhage, maternal hemorrhage, emergency obstetric care.

INTRODUCTION

Postpartum hemorrhage (PPH) is the leading cause of maternal morbidity and mortality worldwide. It is estimated that PPH is responsible for 130,000 deaths and 2.6 million injured women across the globe annually (AbouZahr, 2003; World Health Organization, 2012; MacDorman et al., 2013). While many low and middle-income countries have made considerable strides to reduce their maternal mortality ratios (MMR) over the past two decades, the MMR in the United States has worsened by 136% over the past 20 years (World Health Organization, 2014). The incidence of PPH in the United States has increased by over 30% since 2004 and today it is estimated to occur in 2.9% of deliveries (Bateman et al., 2010). It is notable that one in ten women with PPH will fail first line therapies and are thus classified as having uncontrolled PPH (Ononge et al., 2016).

The most common cause of PPH is uterine atony. First-line treatment options for PPH from uterine atony include uterine massage, uterus and bladder emptying and uterotonic agents such as oxytocin, ergometrine, misoprostol and prostaglandin F2a (PGF2a) (World Health Organization, 2012). When first-line interventions are unsuccessful, PPH is called "uncontrolled". Interventions that target uncontrolled PPH from atonic uterus include aortic compression, intravenous tranexamic acid (Collaborators, 2017), uterine balloon tamponade, uterine artery embolization, and fluid, blood and blood product resuscitation once hemorrhage control has been gained (World Health Organization, 2012). Surgical approaches to uncontrolled postpartum hemorrhage include internal iliac artery ligation, uterine compression sutures and emergency hysterectomy (El Senoun et al., 2011).

Over the past seven years, the authors have studied the impact of uterine balloon tamponade in resource-limited settings by studying efficacy, safety, cost-effectiveness, barriers and facilitators to optimal use, as well as models for scale (Natarajan et al., 2016; Burke et al., 2016). During this time, UBT use for uncontrolled PPH has been endorsed by the WHO, the International Federation of Obstetrics and Gynecology, the American College of Obstetrics and Gynecology, the Royal College of Obstetrics and Gynecology and the International Confederation of Midwives, among others, as the best evidence clinical intervention (World Health Organization, 2012; Doumouchtsis et al., 2007; Tindell et al., 2013; Lalonde et al., 2006; Mavrides et al., 2016).

The authors' work has shown that if applied in a timely fashion, uterine balloon tamponade arrests hemorrhage, halts shock progression (Burke et al., 2017), averts nearly all deaths and emergency hysterectomies (Pendleton et al., 2016; Burke et al., 2017), is "safe" and "highly cost-effective" (Mvundura et al., 2017), and can be placed successfully by any cadre, including illiterate front-line health workers (Natarajan et al., 2016). Deploying a UBT device involves placing a balloon within the uterine cavity and inflating it until hemorrhage ceases. A variety of uterine balloon devices are available, including the Sengstaken-Blakemore tube, Bakri balloon, Rusch balloon, Ebb (Belfort-Didley), and the condom catheter balloon (Pendleton et al., 2016; Dildy et al., 2014).

The authors believe that lessons learned in low- and middle-income countries may inform opportunities for improving health outcomes in highly resourced settings, such as the United States and elsewhere (Tindell et al., 2013; Pendleton et al., 2016; Burke et al., 2016). The purpose of this study was to clarify the practice and perceptions of UBT use in the United States among midwives and family physicians.

MATERIALS AND METHODS

Ethical approval was obtained from the Partners Human Research Committee (Massachusetts General Hospital, Boston, MA, USA). A cross-sectional 12-item survey on the practice, experiences, and perceptions of uterine balloon tamponade utilization for PPH management was developed by the authors through an iterative process. Uncontrolled PPH was defined as hemorrhage unresponsive to a first dose of treatment uterotonics. Appropriate utilization of uterine balloon tamponade was defined as uterine placement of a UBT in each case of uncontrolled post-partum hemorrhage. Respondent credentials, location and years spent in practice, number of deliveries attended per month, number of uncontrolled PPH cases cared for and experience with uterine balloon tamponade were recorded.

Setting

The survey instrument was administered among midwives and family physicians in the United States at three national conferences: the American College of Nurse Midwives 60th Annual Meeting and Exhibition (Washington, DC, June 27, 2015); the American Academy of Family Physicians Family Medicine Experience (Denver, CO, September 29, 2015); and the Midwives Alliance of North America Annual Convention (Albuquerque, NM, October 15, 2015).

Study population

Conference regulations did not allow solicitation beyond the authors' exhibitor booth; therefore, the study participants were among those that voluntarily approached the booth. Providers were queried as to whether they provided obstetric delivery care. If the response was positive, the provider was invited to participate in the study and complete a survey. Oral consent was obtained and all surveys remained anonymous.

Inclusion and exclusion criteria

All providers that approached the authors' exhibitor booth were potential study participants. Exclusion criteria included health cadres other than midwives or family physicians, providers who did not practice obstetrics, students, providers who had less than one year of clinical experience and providers who primarily practiced outside United States.

Data analysis

Each of the 12 questions was analyzed individually. If no answer was provided to a question, the individual data point was removed

*Corresponding author. E-mail: zaidaltawil@gmail.com.

Table 1. Interventions in the 198 described cases of uncontrolled PPH[a].

Intervention	Total (N=198) n(%)
B-lynch sutures	24 (12.1)
Uterine balloon tamponade	80 (40.4)
Uterine artery ligation	29 (14.6)
Hysterectomy	53 (26.8)
Dilation and curettage	9 (4.5)
Unspecified surgical intervention	3 (1.5)

[a]Respondents could choose multiple answers; one, more than one, or none of the above interventions.

from both the numerator and the denominator. The registry was built using Microsoft Excel 2007 (Seattle, Washington, USA) and critically examined using standard descriptive analysis in Stata 13 (College station, Texas, USA).

RESULTS

Respondent characteristics

One hundred and ninety-seven providers met the inclusion criteria and completed the surveys. One hundred and sixty-four (83.3%) were midwives and 33 (16.7%), family physicians. The mean years of clinical practice of the 197 providers was 15.6 years (range: 1 to 45). One hundred and fifteen (70.1%) of the 164 midwives provided details of their training. Sixty (52.2%) of the 115 midwives were certified nurse midwives (CNM), 25 (21.7%) were certified professional midwives (CPM), and 18 (15.7%) were dual CPM and lay midwife (LM) certified. Among the 33 family physicians, five (15.2%) had pursued additional fellowship training in obstetric care and three (9.1%) were certified Advanced Life Support in Obstetrics (ALSO) providers. Of the 193 providers that described their practice location(s), 110 (57.0%) performed deliveries exclusively in hospitals, 63 (32.6%) in non-hospital settings (independent birthing centers and private homes) and 12 (6.2%) in both.

Experience with postpartum hemorrhage

One hundred and eighty-two (92.4%) of the 197 providers estimated the number of uncontrolled PPH cases they had cared for over the course of their career. The mean number of uncontrolled PPH cases per provider over the course of their career was 6.0 (SD= 18.8). In response to a request for a narrative on each of the provider's two most recent cases of uncontrolled PPH, 182 providers described a total of 198 women hemorrhaging uncontrollably (Table 1). Respondents provided information on one, two or no cases. A UBT device was placed in 80 (40.4%) of the 198 women with uncontrolled PPH. Seventy-six (38.4%) of the 198 cases of uncontrolled PPH directly underwent surgical intervention without an attempt at a UBT device placement.

Nineteen (9.6%) of the 197 respondents had placed at least one UBT device at some point in their career. The 19 included 13 (7.9%) of the 164 midwives and 6 (18.2%) of the 33 family physicians. Two midwives reported having improvised a UBT device with a condom and Foley catheter.

Seventy-one of 110 (64.5%) respondents reported that the Bakri balloon was the most common uterine balloon at their facility. The next most common uterine balloon devices reported were the Foley catheter (8.2%) and the condom catheter (1.8%), followed by the Sengsten-Blakemore tube (0.9%), the Ebb balloon (0.9%) and the Rusch balloon (0.9%). One hundred and thirty-one (73.6%) of the 178 providers who responded that they had never placed a UBT device, wished to become trained on it in the future.

DISCUSSION

The 197 midwives and family physicians that participated in the survey collectively cared for almost 1,200 women with uncontrolled postpartum hemorrhage over the course of their careers. Although, UBT is widely endorsed by leading maternal health and obstetric physician organizations, only 9.6% of the surveyed providers had ever placed at least one. The surveyed providers reported that, in their experience, 38.4% of hemorrhaging women proceeded directly to emergency surgery with no UBT placement attempts. Most (73.5%) of the surveyed providers expressed a desire to become trained on UBT use.

Although, uterine balloon tamponade has been shown to be highly effective in the hands of all levels of healthcare providers (Tindell et al., 2013), very few had ever placed a UBT among this cohort of midwife and family physician obstetric providers despite considerable experience with women suffering from uncontrolled PPH. While this study was not designed to uncover barriers to appropriate use of uterine balloon tamponade, lack of knowledge and training were likely contributors to suboptimal use. Since many of the interviewed providers performed deliveries outside the hospitals and since it is well known that early UBT placement leads to improved outcomes (Burke et al., 2017), it appears that there may be considerable untapped opportunity for strengthening the policies and clinical pathways for the emergency care of uncontrolled PPH.

During the course of the authors' research, it was inspiring to observe the near elimination of PPH deaths and emergency hysterectomies in major medical centers across several low-income countries, yet it is surprising and unsettling to learn about the significant number (38.4%) of hemorrhaging women reported by this cohort of providers, who were taken directly to emergency surgery without attempting uterine balloon placement. Previous research by the authors has clearly demonstrated that uterine balloon tamponade can both avert hysterectomies and other surgical interventions as well as arrest hemorrhage and shock progression (Pendleton et al., 2016; Burke et al., 2017). It appears there may have been numerous missed opportunities to avert emergency surgical intervention among those surveyed in this study.

The main limitations of this study were: being restricted to surveying only providers that were attracted to, and chose to visit the authors' exhibitor booth. Despite the sample size of 197 obstetric midwife and family practice providers, the surveyed providers collectively had considerable experience with uncontrolled PPH. While providers that were attracted to the booth related to the topic on PPH were more likely to be more knowledgeable on PPH, the findings demonstrated a striking lack of awareness and training on uterine balloon tamponade.

Conclusion

There may be considerable opportunity to improve appropriate use of uterine balloon tamponade across multiple levels of obstetric delivery providers in the United States.

CONFLICT OF INTERESTS

The authors have not declared any conflict of interests.

ACKNOWLEDGEMENT

This research was supported by the Ujenzi Charitable Trust.

REFERENCES

AbouZahr C (2003). Global burden of maternal death and disability. Br. Med. Bull. 67(1):1-11.

Bateman BT, Berman MF, Riley LE, Leffert LR (2010). The epidemiology of postpartum hemorrhage in a large, nationwide sample of deliveries. Anesthesia Analg. 110(5):1368-1373.

Burke, TF, Ahn R, Nelson BD, Hines R, Kamara J, Oguttu M, Dulo L, Achieng E, B Achieng, Natarajan A, Maua J, Kargbo SAS, Altawil Z, Tester K, de Redon E, Niang M, Abdalla K, Eckardt MJ (2016). A postpartum haemorrhage package with condom uterine balloon tamponade: a prospective multi-centre case series in Kenya, Sierra Leone, Senegal, and Nepal. BJOG 123(9):1532-1540.

Burke TF, Danso-Bamfo S, Guha M, Oguttu M, Tarimo V, Nelson BD (2017). Shock progression and survival after use of a condom uterine balloon tamponade package in women with uncontrolled postpartum hemorrhage. Int. J. Gynecol. Obstet. doi: 10.1002/ijgo.12251

Collaborators WT (2017). Effect of early tranexamic acid administration on mortality, hysterectomy, and other morbidities in women with post-partum haemorrhage (WOMAN): an international, randomised, double-blind, placebo-controlled trial. Lancet 389(10084):2105-2116.

Dildy GA, Belfort MA, Adair CD, Destefano K, Robinson D, Lam G, Strong TH, Polon C, Massaro R, Bukkapatnam J, Van Hook JW (2014). Initial experience with a dual-balloon catheter for the management of postpartum hemorrhage. Am. J. Obstet. Gynecol. 210(2)136-e1.

Doumouchtsis SK, Papageorghiou AT, Arulkumaran S (2007). Systematic review of conservative management of postpartum hemorrhage: what to do when medical treatment fails. Obstet. Gynecol. Surv. 62(8):540-547.

El Senoun GA, Singh M, Mousa HA, Alfirevic Z (2011). Update on the new modalities on the prevention and management of postpartum haemorrhage. Fetal Matern. Med. Rev. 22(4):247-264.

Lalonde A, Daviss BA, Acosta A, Herschderfer K (2006). Postpartum hemorrhage today: ICM/FIGO initiative 2004-2006. Int. J. Gynecol. Obstet. 94(3):243-253.

Likis FE, Sathe NA, Morgans AK, Hartmann KE, Young JL, Carlson-Bremer D, Schorn M, Surawicz T, Andrews J (2015). Management of Postpartum Hemorrhage. Comparative Effectiveness Review No. 151. Agency for Healthcare Research and Quality. PMID: 26020092

MacDorman MF, Declerq E, Matthews TJ (2013). Recent trends in out-of- hospital births in the United States. J. Midwifery Womens Health 58(5):494-501.

Mavrides E, Allard S, Chandraharan E, Collins P, Green L, Hunt BJ, Riris S, Thomson AJ (2016). Prevention and management of postpartum haemorrhage. BJOG 124:e106-e149.

Mvundura M, Kokonya D, Abu-Haydar E, Okoth E, Herrick T, Mukabi J, Carlson L, Oguttu M, Burke, T (2017). Cost-effectiveness of condom uterine balloon tamponade to control severe postpartum hemorrhage in Kenya. Int. J. Gynecol. Obstet. 137(2):185-191.

Natarajan A, Alaska Pendleton A, Nelson BD, Ahn R, Oguttu M, Dulo L, Eckardt MJ, Burke TF (2016). Provider experiences with improvised uterine balloon tamponade for the management of uncontrolled postpartum hemorrhage in Kenya. Int. J. Gynecol. Obstet. 135(2):210-213.

Ononge S, Mirembe F, Wandabwa J, Campbell OM (2016). Incidence and risk factors for postpartum hemorrhage in Uganda. Reprod. Health 13(1):38.

Pendleton AA, Natarajan A, Ahn R, Nelson BD, Eckardt MJ, Burke TF (2016). A qualitative assessment of the impact of a uterine balloon tamponade package on decisions regarding the role of emergency hysterectomy in women with uncontrolled postpartum haemorrhage in Kenya and Senegal. BMJ Open. 6(1):p.e010083.

Pendleton AA, Natarajan A, Ahn R, Nelson BD, Eckardt MJ, Burke TF (2016). Emergency hysterectomy for uncontrolled postpartum hemorrhage may be averted through uterine balloon tamponade in Kenya and Senegal. Int. J. Gynecol. Obstet. 133(1):124-124.

Tindell K, Garfinkel R, Abu-Haydar E, Ahn R, Burke TF, Conn K, Eckardt M (2013). Uterine balloon tamponade for the treatment of postpartum hemorrhage in resource-poor settings: a systematic review. BJOG 120(1):5-14.

World Health Organization (WHO) (2014). Trends in maternal mortality 1990 to 2013: estimates by WHO, UNICEF, UNFPA, The World Bank and the United Nations Population Division. ISBN 978 92 4 150722 6

World Health Organization (WHO) (2012). WHO recommendations for the prevention and treatment or postpartum haemorrhage: evidence base. Geneva: World Health Organization. Available at: http://apps.who.int/iris/bitstream/10665/75411/1/9789241548502_eng.pdf

4

Cultural competency of Saudi student nurses as rated by Filipino clinical instructors at the University of Ha'il, Kingdom of Saudi Arabia

Daisy Andal Vcencio[1], Bandar Saad Albagawi[1], Farhan Alshammari[1] and Hatim Ali Elsheikh[2*]

[1]College of Nursing, University of Ha'il, Kingdom of Saudi Arabia.
[2]Department of Clinical Pharmacology, College of Medicine, Taif University, Kingdom of Saudi Arabia.

Acquiring cultural competence is an ongoing process in which healthcare professionals strive continuously to achieve the ability to work effectively within the context of their client's culture. This study investigated clinical cultural competence of Saudi student nurses' behaviors at the University of Hail, Kingdom of Saudi Arabia. The Cultural Competence Clinical Evaluation Tool- Teacher Version was used to measure the different dimensions of Saudi student nurses' clinical cultural competence behaviors as rated by their clinical instructors. The student nurses level of clinical cultural competence behavior was rated as "average". The score of the Affective domain scored the highest mean, followed by the practical domain, with the cognitive domain being the lowest. There were significant differences in the clinical cultural competence behavior levels of the student nurses. These student nurses' average cultural competency, reflected their own cultural competence, because they viewed their instructors as role models, enabling the acquisition of learning via knowledge transfer; Clinical Instructors teach the student nurses in circumstances as similar as possible to those in which nursing laboratory simulation to actual hospital setting will be employed.

Key words: Cultural competence, clinical instructors, student nurses, cultural assessment.

INRODUCTION

The process of acquiring cultural competence is imperative for nurses, faculty and student nurses learning their profession (Montenery et al., 2013). Nurses spend more time in caring for their patients than any other healthcare professional. They have a unique opportunity to influence access to care, quality of care and patient outcomes, and their knowledge on the patients' culture, belief, and healthcare practices greatly influence their practice (Vicencio et al., 2015). Faculty and student nurses care for their patients in the same way. As the

*Corresponding author. E-mail: elsheikh59@yahoo.com.

faculty members mentor the students in their quest for knowledge, they spend most of their time at the bedside. This process requires cultural competence. According to Campinha-Bacote (2002), this is an ongoing process in which healthcare professionals continuously strive to achieve the ability to work effectively within the context of the client's culture. Culture is a factor that can make a difference in promoting wellness, preventing illness, restoring health, facilitating coping and enhancing the quality of life for all individuals, families and communities (Jeffreys, 2015). Cultural competence, when applied to educators, is the ability to successfully teach students who from cultures other than their own successfully, to develop certain personal and interpersonal awareness and sensitivities along with certain bodies of cultural knowledge, and involves mastering a set of skills. Taken together, these skills generate effective cross-cultural teaching. In addition, Jeffreys (2015) stated that nursing educators are empowered to make an immense difference by introducing, nurturing and modeling optimal cultural competence. On the other hand, Montenery et al. (2013) emphasized that nursing educators should work with the intention of empowering students to provide holistic and comprehensive care, with the concept that cultural competence is essential in the delivery of comprehensive patient-centered care. Cultural competence as earlier defined by Jeffreys (2015) is an ongoing, multidimensional learning process that integrates transcultural nursing skills in all three learning domains- cognitive, practical, and affective- involving transcultural self-efficacy (confidence) as a major influencing factor, and that aims to achieve culturally congruent care.

Both nursing educators and their students must demonstrate an understanding that people of diverse cultures and belief systems perceive health and illness according to their own view and respond differently to various symptoms, diseases and treatments. In addition, Douglas et al. (2014) elucidated that an individual's knowledge of the impact of culture on attitudes, values, traditions, and behaviors affects their health-seeking behaviors.

The Kingdom of Saudi Arabia (KSA), one of the Muslim countries in the Middle East, has its own unique culture, beliefs and health practices. For the Saudi family, considerable cultural clashes can arise when patients are hospitalized and receive care from health-care professionals who do not understand Saudi cultural beliefs and values. In addition, the Arab News network (www.arabnews.com; February 4, 2016) reported data from the Saudi Department of Statistics and Information that the population of the KSA comprises 21.1 million native Saudis and 10.4 million expatriates: nearly 33% of the total population. Of these, 75% are Indian, Pakistani, Egyptian, Bangladeshi and Filipino while the remaining 25% are Sri Lankan, Yemini, Jordanian/Palestinian, Indonesian, Sudanese, Syrian, Turkish, and Westerners. These data clearly show that the country has a very diverse population, which means that professional nurses, as well as clinical instructors and nursing students, are challenged with a wide variety of cultural, linguistic and health literacy barriers (Singleton and Krause 2009). Hence, cultural beliefs and practices concerning the health and illness in the Kingdom of Saudi Arabia can only be addressed by healthcare providers through advanced knowledge of the Saudi population culture (Johnson et al., 2017). According to Campinha-Bacote (2002), cultural awareness is the self-examination and in-depth exploration of one's own cultural and professional background. In this context, nursing educators and clinical instructors must be aware of their own biases, prejudices, and assumptions about individuals who are different from them culturally, so that they will not enforce their own cultural beliefs and patterns of behavior on the nursing students whom they supervise and teach. Bednarz et al. (2010) stressed that nursing educators serve as role models for their students through their own efforts to expand the scope and depth of cultural competence, and in demonstrating the ongoing quest for excellence that needs to be a part of professional nursing practice.

The Saudi nursing curriculum covers a five-year period (10 semesters) for a bachelor's degree, which is allocated to classes, laboratory work and clinical practice. Clinical practice is conducted on two to three days per week throughout the semester, wherein students are rotated to the different specialties of clinical practice (Mutair, 2015). Nursing students' clinical practice is supervised by an officially designated clinical instructor, who has a dual role in the accomplishment of their role, which includes patient safety in the hands of the student learner, and facilitating students' learning. Nursing students practice their skills directly on the patient, and that is why clinical instructors must be equipped with the knowledge and clinical competence required of a professional nurse along with their postgraduate degree and work experience to enrich knowledge and expertise. They are clinical teachers who are skilled, experienced nurses dedicated to maintaining and improving standards of patient care, and are concerned to help learners develop their potential as nurses. This is achieved through building good relationships, counseling, supporting, and advising, aside from demonstrating expertise in caring for patients because the patient's life - or certainly his/her well-being - could be at risk (Mutair, 2015). This process does not consist merely of passing on information or knowledge, but is also mainly an expression of values and attitudes. What teachers usually get back from their students is what they themselves have brought to the teaching-learning process (Thanasoulas, 2002). Therefore, the quality of student learning is dependent not only on the type of clinical experience but also on the characteristics and skills of the teacher who facilitates learning (Mutair, 2015).

University-based clinical instructors must be able to demonstrate cultural competency while teaching the students directly and giving indirect care to patients from different cultures. Cultural competence, according to Loftin et al. (2013), involves having the necessary attitudes, knowledge, and skills for the delivery of culturally appropriate care to a diverse patient population. According to Riyadh Arab News (www.alriyadh.com, dated June 13, 2014), there are 18,000 expatriate teachers in KSA universities, serving in various positions including professors, associate professors, assistant professors, lecturers and assistant lecturers. The University of Hail College of Nursing, located at Hail City, KSA, is one of those universities employing expatriate teachers. There are forty-five Filipino clinical instructors serving the college, both in the clinical and classroom settings. They were hired based on their relevant expertise.

The aim of this study was to determine the cultural competency of Saudi nursing students as rated by their clinical educators, who mentor and train them to become globally competitive, culturally aware professional nurses.

MATERIALS AND METHODS

This is a descriptive/evaluative study aimed at determining differences between the levels of cultural competency of Saudi student nurses from the perceptions of their clinical instructors. The study was conducted at the College of Nursing, Hail University, Kingdom of Saudi Arabia. Thirty full-time clinical instructors participated in this study out of the total population of thirty-six (83%). A purposive sampling technique was used, and the respondents were chosen because of their specific culture, skills and experience. The clinical instructor genders were equally distributed (50% female and 50% male), with the most common age range being 40 to 44 years (30%). Of these, 23 (76%) mostly worked at the medical surgical department, 28 (93%) were lecturer/nurse specialists, 27 (90%) with a Master's degree. Eleven (37%) of them had 16 to 20 years of work experience in the academic field but most of them (27; 90%) had less than 1 to 5 years of experience in this healthcare institution. Nineteen (63%) of them had undertaken no formal education in transcultural nursing, and 22 (73%) of the respondents were not studying relevant education units. The research questionnaire was prepared based on the Cultural Competence Education Resource (CCER) toolkit authored by Jeffreys and Dogan (2012). The following research instruments were used based on the CCER:

1. A Demographic Profile Questionnaire was designed based on the Demographic Data Sheet for Nurses (DDSN), but with some adjustment for the University's work position category, existing unit or department, and educational and work-experience requirement for employment.
2. The Cultural Competence Clinical Evaluation Tool-Teacher Version (CCCET-TV) comprised of 83-item questionnaire adapted from the Transcultural Self-Efficacy Tool (TSET), an instrument consisting of 83 items subdivided into three sections of cognitive, practical, and affective domains. This contained three subscales measuring different dimensions of students' clinical cultural competence behaviors as rated by the teacher or their preceptor: extent of culturally specific care (Subscale 1, Cognitive Scale); cultural assessment (Subscale 2, Practical Scale); culturally sensitive and professionally appropriate attitudes, values, or beliefs including awareness, acceptance, recognition, appreciation and advocacy necessary for providing culturally sensitive professional nursing care (Subscale 3, Affective Scale). These were evaluated utilizing a Likert-type scale, rating answers from 1 (low competence level) to 10 (high competence level). A low rating was assigned to scores of 1 or 2 on the Likert scale, an average level to scores of 3 to 8, and a high level of competence to responses with scores of 9 or 10. Specific answers to the following questions were drawn from the questionnaire:

1. How can the profiles of the Filipino Clinical Instructors be described in terms of the following factors? Age; gender; work setting; current work position, highest educational attainment, work experience in academic or health-care institutions; previous college courses in transcultural nursing; and continuing education units in transcultural nursing.
2. What is the level of Saudi student nurses' clinical cultural competence behavior in providing nursing care to patients from varied cultures? This evaluation included the extent of culturally specific care (cognitive scale), cultural assessment (practical scale), culturally sensitive and professionally appropriate attitudes, values, or beliefs in providing sensitive professional nursing care (affective scale) as rated by the clinical instructors.
3. Is there a significant difference among the level of Saudi student nurses' clinical cultural competence behavior in providing nursing care to patients from varied cultures? This was evaluated in terms of the extent of culturally specific care (cognitive scale); cultural assessment (practical scale), and culturally sensitive and professionally appropriate attitude, values, or beliefs in providing sensitive professional nursing care (affective scale) as rated by the clinical instructors when grouped by their own demographic profiles.

The study was approved by the Institutional Review Board (IRB) of the University of Hail. Thereafter, consent for participation was obtained from respondents after they were notified of the aims, methods, anticipated benefits and potential hazards of the research. They were informed that they had the right to terminate their participation at any time and that confidentiality would always be maintained in terms of their responses.

Statistical analysis

The obtained data were analyzed using analysis of variance (ANOVA) for comparisons between the various groups in terms of specific questionnaire factors. This was used to determine any significant differences among the levels of Saudi student nurses' clinical cultural competence, behavior in performing nursing care to the patients from varied cultures in terms of: the extent of culturally specific care, cultural assessment, culturally sensitive and professionally appropriate attitudes, values, or beliefs in providing sensitive professional nursing care, as rated by the clinical instructors and when grouped by their own demographic profiles. Differences between means were considered as significant at $P \leq 0.05$.

RESULTS

The mean score distributions for the level of Saudi student nurses' clinical cultural competence behavior in the extent of culturally specific care (Cognitive Scale), as rated by the Clinical Instructors are shown in Table 1. Among the 25 studied variables, safety had the highest mean score of 5.76, followed by relief of pain and discomfort with a total mean score of 5.66 and informed consent with a mean score of 5.31, while dealing with

Table 1. Mean score distribution of the level of Saudi student nurses' clinical cultural competence behavior in the extent of culturally specific care (cognitive scale), as rated by Filipino Clinical Instructors.

Rank	Mean	±SD	Cognitive scale
1	5.76	3.18	Safety
2	5.66	3.03	Pain relief and comfort
3	5.31	3.44	Informed consent
4	5.24	3.20	Health restoration
5	5.14	2.80	Health history and interview
6	5.14	3.17	Physical examination
7	5.14	3.51	Blood tests
8	5.14	3.18	Rest and sleep
9	5.00	3.00	Health maintenance
10	4.93	2.80	Patient teaching
11	4.79	2.87	Illness prevention
12	4.72	3.28	Diagnostic tests
13	4.62	2.74	Health promotion
14	4.55	3.04	Exercise and activity
15	4.48	3.11	Diet and nutrition
16	4.38	3.23	Life support and resuscitation
17	4.28	2.95	Hygiene
18	4.17	2.75	Anxiety and stress reduction
19	3.41	2.60	Grieving and loss
20	3.28	2.80	Aging
21	3.28	2.72	Dying and death
22	2.62	2.56	Pregnancy
23	2.59	2.50	Growth and development
24	2.31	2.55	Birth
25	1.72	1.33	Sexuality

sexuality had the lowest score of 1.72 along with birth at 2.35. On the other hand, the mean score distribution on the level of Saudi student nurses' clinical cultural competence behavior in the cultural assessment (Practical scale) as rated by Filipino Clinical Instructors is presented in Table 2. Socioeconomic background had the highest mean score of 6.59 followed by educational background and interest with a mean score of 4.66, and the third in rank is traditional health and illness beliefs with 4.66 mean score, while discrimination and bias experience had the lowest mean score of 3.41, acculturation with 3.48 and 3.52 for aging. While in Table 3, the mean score distribution on the level of Saudi student nurses' clinical cultural competence behavior in culturally sensitive and professionally appropriate attitude, values or belief (Affective scale) for providing culturally sensitive professional nursing care as rated by Filipino Clinical Instructor was shown. The results revealed that student nurses' clinical cultural competence behaviour in culturally sensitive and professionally appropriate attitude, values or belief (affective scale) falls on average level in all items mentioned at affective scale and were rated average on the level of competency scale by their clinical instructors. They are aware, they accept, appreciate, and recognize the importance of one's cultural values, and beliefs in the provision of nursing care. Moreover, awareness of his/her own cultural heritage and belief systems top the rank with a mean score of 6.14, followed by more aware of insensitive and prejudicial treatment with 6.10 mean score and the third one is: more readily recognizes the impact of roles on health care practices with a mean score of 5.52, while the "more appreciative of: Cultural sensitivity and awareness" obtained the lowest mean of 4.45, "More appreciative of: Client's world view" (philosophy of life) has a mean score of 4.52, and the "more readily recognize: Importance of home remedies and folk medicine" is 4.55 mean score presents the average mean score of the three scales of cognitive, practical and affective competency levels. It shows that affective scales got the highest average score of 5.04, followed by the cognitive scale with 4.31 average score and the practical scale got the lowest average of 4.08, which falls on the average level of cultural competency (Table 4). Table 5 presents the inferential statistics (ANOVA) results on the level of Saudi student nurses' clinical cultural competence behavior rating when

Table 2. Mean score distribution of the level of Saudi student nurses' clinical cultural competence behavior in cultural assessment (practical scale) as rated by Filipino Clinical Instructors.

Rank	Mean	Score ± SD	Practical scale
1	6.59	3.75	Socioeconomic background
2	4.66	2.86	Educational background and interests
3	4.66	2.53	Traditional health and illness beliefs
4	4.59	2.97	Religious practices and beliefs
5	4.48	2.94	Kinship ties
6	4.45	2.92	Gender role and responsibility
7	4.34	3.11	Language preference
8	4.28	2.40	Religious background and identity
9	4.17	2.45	Time perception and orientation
10	4.17	2.80	Folk medicine tradition and use
11	4.17	2.63	Role of family during illness24
12	4.07	2.37	Ethnic background and identity
13	4.00	2.80	Attitudes about health care technology
14	3.97	2.40	Racial background and identity
15	3.97	2.72	Ethnic food preferences
16	3.90	2.57	Meaning of nonverbal behaviors
17	3.86	2.66	Meanings of space and touch
18	3.86	2.52	Home environment
19	3.79	2.93	Financial concerns
20	3.72	2.68	World view (philosophy of life)
21	3.72	2.34	Acceptance sick role behaviors
22	3.69	2.52	Meaning if verbal communication patterns
23	3.66	2.54	Level of English comprehension
24	3.66	2.64	Role of children
25	3.55	2.64	Role of elders
26	3.52	2.46	Aging
27	3.48	2.65	Acculturation
28	3.41	2.29	Discrimination and bias experiences

grouped by Filipino Clinical Instructor's demographic profile. The results show that there are significant differences on the rated level of Saudi student nurses' clinical cultural competence behavior when grouped by Filipino Clinical instructor demographic profile ($p \leq 0.05$), this only shows that Filipino Clinical Instructors' method of rating the student nurses varies and affects student nurses' competency level.

DISCUSSION

The Saudi nursing students in the eyes of their clinical instructors had average cultural competency levels in the provision of safety, relief of pain and discomfort, as well as in eliciting informed consent to particular treatments. Informed consent, confidentiality, privacy, autonomy, safety, respect, treatment choice, refusal of treatment, and participating in an agreed treatment plan are specified in most patients' bills of rights (Habib and Al-Siber 2013), while patient safety is an essential and vital component of quality nursing care (Ballard, 2003). This shows that the Clinical Instructors could inculcate into their students, their knowledge on the patients' bill of rights and patient safety, which is vital in the provision of nursing care. This is in accord with the study of Alsulaimani et al. (2014) on the cognitive competency of Filipino nurses working at Taif City, wherein the provision of safety to patients was associated with education and training levels. Nurses are for the most part altruistic and strive to do what is morally right in the service of human beings and society (Roy and Jones, 2006). On the other hand, relieving patient from pain and discomfort is fundamental to nursing care. According to Kolcaba's Comfort Theory (2010), nursing is described as the process of assessing the patient's comfort needs, developing and implementing appropriate nursing interventions, and evaluating the patient's comfort needs following nursing interventions. In this study, the Clinical Instructors had clearly instilled basic knowledge in the minds of the Saudi nursing students on addressing the comfort needs of the sick patient upon initial encounter or

Table 3. Mean score distribution on the level of Saudi student nurses' clinical cultural competence behavior in culturally sensitive and professionally appropriate attitude, values or belief (affective scale) for providing culturally sensitive professional nursing care as rated by Filipino Clinical Instructor.

Rank	Score	± SD	Mean affective scale
1	6.14	2.90	Awareness of: His/her own cultural heritage and belief systems
2	6.10	9.63	More awareness of: Insensitive and prejudicial treatment
3	5.52	2.81	More readily recognizes: Impact of roles on health care practices
4	5.48	2.79	More committed advocate for: Client's decisions based on cultural beliefs
5	5.45	2.84	Awareness of: Difference within His/her cultural group
6	5.45	2.92	More aware of: Professional caring behaviors
7	5.41	2.80	More readily recognize: Impact of values on health care practices
8	5.38	2.68	Awareness of: His /her biases and limitations
9	5.21	2.92	More aware of: Interaction between nursing, folk, and professional systems
10	5.17	3.26	More appreciative of: Interaction with people of different cultures
11	5.03	2.99	More readily recognize: Impact of socioeconomic factors on health care practices
12	5.03	2.58	More readily recognize: Need of cultural care accommodation/negotiation
13	5.00	2.74	More readily recognize: Need of cultural care preservation/maintenance
14	4.97	2.53	More readily recognize: Need of cultural care repatterning/restructuring
15	4.93	2.51	More readily recognize: Impact of political factors on health care practices
16	4.90	2.97	More accepting of: Similarities between cultural groups
17	4.86	2.60	More readily recognize: Inadequacies in the Government health care system
18	4.86	2.84	More committed advocate for: Culture-specific care
19	4.83	2.65	More aware of: Differences in perceived role of the nurse
20	4.83	2.49	More readily recognize: Need to prevent ethnocentric views
21	4.79	2.80	More aware of: Comfort and discomfort felt when entering a culturally different world
22	4.79	2.92	More accepting of: Client's refusal of treatment based on beliefs
23	4.79	3.30	More appreciative of: Role of family in providing health care
24	4.76	2.92	More accepting of: Differences between cultural groups
25	4.72	2.64	More aware of: Traditional caring behaviors
26	4.72	2.59	More readily recognize Need to prevent cultural imposition
27	4.69	2.88	More appreciative of: Culture-specific health care
28	4.55	2.56	More readily recognize: Importance of home remedies and folk medicine
29	4.52	3.12	More appreciative of: Client's world view (philosophy of life)
30	4.45	2.63	More appreciative of: Cultural sensitivity and awareness

assessment. Thus, they were aware that a person in pain cannot respond readily to the assessment process, because the tendency of the patient in pain or in discomfort is avoidance (American Academy of Pediatrics, 2001). Informed consent is another tenet of "patient rights" wherein the patient has the right to be fully informed of any nursing or medical procedures to be provided as well as their diagnosis and treatment plan (Almoajel, 2012). However, these students had poor cultural competency levels in terms of dealing with sexuality. This can be attributed to language barriers, because the clinical instructors were not proficient in the Arabic language and found it difficult to ask questions of the patients in terms of sexuality and the birthing process, and vice versa. The patients also had difficulty in understanding the English language, so the nurse educators/clinical instructors could not discuss sexuality or birth processes in detail in front of the patient, while coaching the nursing students. This is consistent with the study by Karout et al. (2013) on Saudi Arabian women's experience and perception of maternal health services, that the biggest problem discussed by most women was that of linguistic diversity; not only the difference between the English and Arabic languages but extending to the accents of non-English speakers such as Indians, Filipinos and Pakistanis. In addition, the study conducted by Albagawi (2014) on examining barriers and facilitators to effective nurse-patient communication within the Saudi Arabian cultural context found that effective communication was not achieved because of many complex and overlapping personal, professional and organizational factors. Furthermore, according to Schyve (2007), differences in language and cultural differences are barriers to effective communication, resulting in low health literacy. Alsulaimani et al. (2014), in their study of cognitive competency of Filipino nurses working at some

Table 4. Average mean score distribution on the level of Saudi student nurses' clinical cultural competence behavior on the three domains of cognitive, affective and practical scale as rated by Filipino Clinical Instructors.

Cultural domain	Average mean score	Competency level
Provision of culturally specific care (cognitive domain)	4.31	Average
Cultural assessment (practical domain)	4.08	Average
Culturally sensitive and professionally appropriate attitude, values or belief (affective domain)	5.04	Average

Table 5. Inferential statistics (ANOVA) results of rated cultural competency level of Saudi nursing students when grouped by the respondents' profile.

Profile	1	2	3	4	5	6	7	8	9
Cognitive	0.4316	0.8248	0.4886	0.1226	0.1807	0.315	0.0141	0.0504	0.0791
Practical	0.5436	0.2723	0.3671	0.1769	0.4021	0.2926	0.0439	0.147	0.0272
Affective	0.225	0.6507	0.319	0.0789	0.1913	0.8171	0.2346	0.9424	0.583

1: Age; 2: Gender; 3: Work setting; 4: Current work position; 5: Highest educational attainment; 6: Work experience in the academe; 7: Work experience in Healthcare Institution; 8: Previous College course in transcultural nursing; 9: Continuing education in transcultural nursing. Level of significance of difference is p-value ≤ 0.05.

hospitals of Taif City, revealed that aside from language barriers, shyness and reluctance of Saudi patients to discuss sexuality and birth are factors to consider, because they are hesitant to disclose detailed information about themselves and their families. Being conservative, they can be embarrassed by questions on their sexual relationships and other personal matters. Karout et al. (2013) found in their study of Saudi Arabian women's experiences and perception of maternal health services that "the presence of non-Muslim service providers did not satisfy them because they believed that Muslim service providers will not look at their uncovered bodies especially their genitalia unless there is a need for that, and they will be conscious uncovering themselves". Thus, the Clinical Instructors found it difficult to create scenarios for the students to experience and participate in the learning process because of the patient's culture. Consequently, this lack of opportunity for the Saudi nursing students to perform the task expected of them decreased their self-efficacy. As Bandura (2006) stressed, "If a person sees someone similar to them succeed, it can increase their self-efficacy, and also, seeing someone fail can lower self-efficacy". Furthermore, according to Bandura (2006), "positive and negative experiences can influence the ability of an individual to perform a given task". This is one reason why the clinical instructors perceived Saudi nursing students' cultural competency level to be low in terms of discussing sexuality and birth as they have little knowledge in these particular concepts because of lack of the opportunity to perform in the practice care setting. This is in agreement with the study conducted by Lofmark and Wikblad (2001) that opportunities to practice different tasks and understanding the total picture facilitate the development of learning, while supervision that lacks continuity and lack of opportunities to practice hinders development of learning. In addition, a supportive clinical environment is one factor for enabling an effective clinical experience, which includes the atmosphere of a clinical placement unit, and the relationships shared with clinical staff supervisors and mentors (Lawal et al., 2016).

This study shows that, these Saudi student nurses had only average cultural competency, according to the ratings by the clinical instructors that reflected their own level of cultural competence. This was because nursing students view their clinical instructors as their role models and their learning acquisition was a result of knowledge transfer. These clinical instructors demonstrated competence in teaching and were able to role model cultural nursing even without previous knowledge or continuing education in transcultural nursing. Their academic preparation and expertise in the clinical area had significant impacts on student learning ability.

The role of clinical instructors in the learning development of nursing students is crucial as they greatly influence students' learning processes. Interactions with their clinical instructors, peers and patients contribute to the students' professional value systems. Therefore, provision of environments wherein the nursing students will experience all aspects of nursing roles will increase their self-confidence, professional values and clinical skills. The cultural competency of the nursing students will advance as they continuously provide nursing to culturally diverse patients. Clinical instructors must always emphasize to the students that "knowledge of the role of culture in health and illness" is essential for the development of culturally sensitive communication skills, while awareness of one's own cultural health beliefs and practices in the performance of nursing care will develop culturally congruent communication skills as well as the development of skills in identifying variations between and within cultures.

The findings suggest that all clinical instructors must be included as respondents in the same study at the same locale to measure the student nurses' clinical and cultural competence behavior aiming to establish a strong basis for transcultural nursing. This must be included in the curriculum, and self-evaluations of the student nurses and clinical instructors' cultural competence must also be studied. Continuous updating on transcultural nursing for all clinical instructors is recommended to enrich their knowledge and skills in this field.

CONFLICT OF INTERESTS

The authors have not declared any conflict of interests.

ACKNOWLEDGEMENTS

The authors express their appreciation to the Filipino Clinical Instructors working at the College of Nursing, University of Ha'il, for their cooperation and particiption in this study.

REFERENCES

Albagawi BS (2014). Examining barriers and facilitators to effective nurse-patient communication within a Saudi Arabic cultural context. Doctoral dissertation, RMIT University, Australia. Available at: https://researchbank.rmit.edu.au/view/rmit:160737

Almoajel AM (2012). Hospitalized patients' awareness of their rights in Saudi governmental hospital. Middle-East J. Sci. Res. 11(3):329-335.

American Academy of Pediatrics (2001). The assessment and management of acute pain in infants, children, and adolescents. Pediatrics 108(3):793-797.

Alsulaimani AA, Vicencio DA, Ruiz FB, Elsheikh HA (2014). Cognitive competency of Filipino nurses working in some hospitals of Taif City, Kingdom of Saudi Arabia. Egypt. J. Hosp. Med. 57:384-394.

Ballard KA (2003). Patient safety: a shared responsibility. Online J. Issues Nurs. 8(3):4.

Bandura A (2006). Guide for constructing self-efficacy scales. Self-efficacy beliefs of adolescents. pp. 307-337.

Bednarz H, Schim S, Doorenbos A (2010). Cultural diversity in nursing education: Perils, pitfalls, and pearls. J. Nurs. Educ. 49(5):253-260.

Campinha-Bacote J (2002). The process of cultural competence in the delivery of healthcare services: A model of care. J. Transcult. Nurs. 13(3):181-184.

Douglas MK, Rosenkoetter M, Pacquiao DF, Callister LC, Hattar-Pollara M, Lauderdale J, Milstead J, Nardi D, Purnell L (2014). Guidelines for implementing culturally competent nursing care. J. Transcult. Nurs. 24(2):109-121.

Habib FM, Al-Siber HS (2013). Assessment of Awareness and Source of Information of Patients' Rights: a Cross-sectional Survey in Riyadh Saudi Arabia. Am. J. Res. Comm. 1(2):1-9.

Jeffreys MR, Dogan E (2012). Evaluating the influence of cultural competence education on students' transcultural self-efficacy perceptions. J. Transcult. Nurs. 23(2):188-197.

Jeffreys MR (2015). Teaching cultural competence in nursing and health care: Inquiry, action, and innovation. 3rd Edn, Springer Publishing Company, New York, USA.

Johnson JM, MacDonald CD, Oliver L (2017). Recommendations for healthcare providers preparing to work in the Middle East: A Campinha-Bacote cultural competence model approach. J. Nurs. Educ. Pract. 7(2):25-30.

Karout N, Abdelaziz SH, Goda M, AlTuwaijri S, Almostafa N, Ashour R, Alradi H (2013). Cultural diversity: A qualitative study on Saudi Arabian women's experience and perception of maternal health services. J. Nurs. Educ. Pract. 3(11):172-182.

Kolcaba K (2010). An introduction to comfort theory. In the comfort line. Available at: http://currentnursing.com/nursing_theory/comfort_theory_Kathy_Kolcaba.html

Lawal J, Weaver S, Bryan, V, Lindo JL (2016). Factors that influence the clinical learning experience of nursing students at a Caribbean school of nursing. J. Nurs. Educ. Pract. 6(4):32-39.

Lofmark A, Wikblad K (2001). Facilitating and obstructing factors for development of learning in clinical practice: a student perspective. J. Adv. Nurs. 34(1):43-50.

Loftin C, Hartin V, Branson M, Reyes H (2013). Measures of cultural competence in nurses: An integrative review. Sci. World J. 1-10.

Montenery SM, Jones AD, Perry N, Ross D, Zoucha R (2013). Cultural competence in nursing faculty: A journey, not a destination. J. Prof. Nurs. 29(6):e51-e57.

Mutair AAl (2015). Clinical Nursing Teaching in Saudi Arabia Challenges and Suggested Solutions. J. Nurs Care S1:007.

Roy SC, Jones DA (2006). Nursing knowledge development and clinical practice: opportunities and directions. Springer Publishing Company, New York, USA.

Singleton K, Krause E (2009). Understanding cultural and linguistic barriers to health literacy. Online J. Issues Nurs. 14(3):4.

Schyve PM (2007). Language differences as a barrier to quality and safety in health care: The Joint Commission perspective. J. Gen. Int. Med. 22(2):360-361.

Thanasoulas D (2002). What do teachers bring to the teaching-learning process? Available at: http://www.tefl.net/esl-articles/teaching-learning.htm

Vicencio DA, Alsulaimani AA, Ruiz FB, Elsheikh HA (2015). Affective competency of Filipino nurses working in the hospitals of Taif City Kingdom of Saudi Arabia. Int. J. Nurs. Midwifery 7(4):46-53.

Health care seeking behaviour on neonatal danger signs among mothers in Tenta District, Northeast Ethiopia

Gebeyaw Molla[1*], Alemayehu Gonie[2], Tefera Belachew[3] and Bitiya Admasu[3]

[1]Amara Regional Private Health Facility and Professional Association, Bahirdar, Ethiopia
[2]College of Medicine and Health Sciences; Maddawalabu University, Robe, Ethiopia.
[3]College of Medicine and Health Sciences; Jimma University, Jimma, Ethiopia.

Health care seeking behaviour is any action undertaken by individuals who perceive to have a health problem or to be ill for finding an appropriate remedy. It involves recognition of symptoms, perceived nature of illness, followed initially by appropriate home care and monitoring. In Ethiopia, little is known about mother's health care seeking behaviour on neonatal danger signs. Therefore, this study assessed the health care seeking behaviour on neonatal danger signs among mothers in Tenta district, Northeast Ethiopia. Community based cross-sectional study was conducted from October 23 to November 17, 2015. The study district was stratified into urban and rural kebeles. From each stratum, 1 out of 3 urban and 7 out of 25 rural kebeles were selected by simple random sampling technique. A total of 527 mothers were interviewed using structured and pre-tested questionnaire. The data were checked for missing values and outliers, and analysed using SPSS version 20.0. Logistic regression analyses were employed to see the association between dependent and independent variables. Mothers who sought medical care for neonatal danger signs were 167 (41.3%). Mothers' secondary educational level (AOR=4.64, 95% CI=1.1-19.81), have given birth in health center (AOR=3.35, 95% CI=1.31-8.56), practicing optimal thermal care (AOR=2.52, 95% CI=1.08-5.85), and having higher decision-making abilities in seeking neonatal health care (AOR=11.28, 95% CI=4.36-29.22) were significant predictors of mother's health seeking behaviour towards neonatal danger signs. Long distance of the residence from health facility, experiencing less serious neonatal danger signs, and beliefs that some danger signs were caused by evil spirits were the most common reasons cited by mothers who did not seek neonatal medical care. In this study, more than half of mother's did not seek medical care for neonatal danger signs. Maternal education and improving their decision-making abilities, and promoting institutional delivery are the recommended interventions to improve mother's health care seeking for neonatal illness. Health facilities should integrate essential neonatal care service during ANC and PNC follow up to improve the quality of health information about neonatal danger signs. At the community level, health extension workers should educate mothers about newborn care practices and neonatal danger signs.

Key words: Mothers' health care seeking behaviour, neonatal danger signs, Tenta district.

INTRODUCTION

Worldwide, in 2012, 2.9 million babies died within 28 days of life. About two-thirds of neonatal deaths occur in the African and southeast-Asian regions (Save the Children, 2014). Sub-Saharan Africa generally has higher rates of neonatal mortality (Mrisho et al., 2012). Ethiopia has made notable progress in decreasing infant mortality ratio from 97 deaths per 1,000 live births to 59 deaths per 1,000 live births in 2011, and to 48 deaths per 1,000 live births in 2016 (EDHS, 2016).

The largest proportion of neonatal deaths occur at home, where a few families sought medical care for signs of new-born illness and nearly no neonates were taken to health facilities when they were sick. Delayed health care seeking can contribute neonatal mortality (Herbert et al., 2012). Understanding the care-seeking behaviour minimize potential delays and effectively improve new-borns health (Mrisho et al., 2012).

Health care seeking behaviour is any action undertaken by individuals who perceive to have a health problem or to be ill for finding an appropriate remedy. It involves recognition of symptoms, perceived nature of illness, followed initially by appropriate home care and monitoring. Health care seeking behaviour is not only a matter of knowledge about the cause and treatment of the disease, but also of perceived seriousness and duration, cultural practices and socio-economic status (Anyanwu and Okeke, 2014).

Millions of mothers and their new-borns throughout the world are living in a social environment that does not encourage health care seeking behaviour (Herbert et al., 2012). Thus, many mothers did not generally seek formal healthcare during pregnancy, childbirth and puerperium, which have a major impacts on health care seeking for mothers and survival of their new-borns (Gelaw et al., 2014).

Many new-borns are often dying due to delay in recognizing danger signs, delay in deciding to get medical care and delay in reaching a health worker or facility (Awasthi et al., 2009). Behaviourally, modifiable factors such as poor recognition of neonatal danger signs, local illness beliefs, use of traditional/home remedies, and inability of mothers to identify health providers delayed the health care-seeking behaviour of mothers for their new-borns (Beck et al., 2004). Delayed health care seeking behaviour for ill neonates contribute to high infant mortality rates (Sandberg et al., 2014; Syed et al., 2006). The vast majority of neonates (73%) died at home due to mothers who did not seek care during the neonatal period (Dongre et al., 2009). Early detection of neonatal illness and increasing facility births improve care-seeking behaviour for neonatal illness (Marsh et al., 2002; Dongre et al., 2009).

Different studies showed that prompt health care seeking behaviour for neonatal danger signs serve as backbone in reducing neonatal mortality (Sandberg et al., 2014; Chandwani and Pandor, 2015). However, a variety of cultural barriers, norms of poor hygiene and isolation impeded neonatal health care seeking behaviour of mothers (Mrisho et al., 2012). Herbert et al. (2012) reported that 47.5 present of neonates who were ill or suspected to be ill were taken to health facility.

In Peri-Urban of Wardha, India, about 37.5% of newborn with danger signs were taken to the doctor and only two mothers consulted faith healer for treatment (Dongre et al., 2009). Another study conducted in Rural Wardha, India, only 41.8% of such sick newborn got treatment from either government or private hospitals and 46.1% of sick babies received no treatment. The reasons for not seeking neonatal danger signs were ignorance of parents, lack of money, faith in supernatural causes, non-availability of transport, home remedy, and absence of responsible person at home (Dongre et al., 2009). In Gujarat, India, joint family structure, mass media exposure, literacy status, and socioeconomic status of mothers were found to be associated significantly with the health care seeking behaviour of the mothers (Chandwani and Pandor, 2015).

In Yemen, 51.42% of caregivers sought medical care for their sick babies. Mothers who attended secondary education were 5.8 times more likely to seek neonatal medical care for their sick neonate (Webair and Bin-Gouth, 2013). Knowledge of at least one WHO recognized danger sign were found to be significant factors for health care seeking behaviour for neonatal illness in Enugu State, Southeast Nigeria (Ekwochi et al., 2015). Yenagoa Metropolis reported that self-medication and the use of home remedies delayed health care seeking behaviour for neonatal illness. The commonest reason for not timely consultation was lack of money (Alex-Hart et al., 2014). In rural Southern Tanzania, mothers who delivered at health facilities were more likely to seek neonatal care than those who delivered at home (Mwifadhi Mrisho et al., 2012). In rural western Kenya, 32.4% of the mothers purchased and administered drugs to their sick children without seeking medical attention. The most commonly reported reasons for this behaviour were: distance of government health facilities, poor and inability to afford services at the private hospitals and clinics (Mbagaya et al., 2005).

In study conducted in Bure district, Ethiopia, marital status, completion of health extension package, and sex of child were significantly associated with health care

*Corresponding author. E-mail: gebeyawmolla48@gmail.com.

seeking behaviour of urban mothers. Similarly, age of child, occupation of mothers, educational level of fathers, wealth quintile, and type of reported illness were significantly associated with rural mothers. For health care seeking behaviour (Gelaw et al., 2014). In Bihar Dar, Ethiopia (Ababa, 2008) mother's decision-making level had significant effect on health seeking behaviours for child health services. Another study in Jabitenan district, Ethiopia, mothers who delivered at health facilities were more likely to seek neonatal care than those who delivered at home (Workineh and Hailu, 2014).

Generally, early determination of health care seeking behaviours of mothers on neonatal danger signs could save the new-borns during life threatening complications. Therefore, understanding the factors related to health care seeking behaviour for neonatal danger signs are critical for countries like Ethiopia with alarmingly high neonatal mortality. Despite the fact that health-seeking behaviour plays a critical role in reducing neonatal morbidity and mortality, studies on the area are limited and inconsistent. Therefore, this study assessed the health care seeking behaviour on neonatal danger signs and identified associated factors among mothers in Tenta district, Northeast Ethiopia.

MATERIALS AND METHODS

Study area and period

The study was carried out in Tenta district, Northeast Ethiopia, from October 23 to November 17, 2015. Tenta district is located 608 km away from East of Bihar Dar and 528 km from North of Addis Ababa. This district has three urban and 25 rural kebeles (the *smallest administrative units).* Based on Tenta district health office report, there are nine health centres, 28 health post, three private lower clinics and two private drug stores. There were 3179 mothers who had infant age 28 to 364 days during study period ((unpublished Tenta District health office report, 2015).

Study design and population

A community-based cross sectional study design was employed. All mothers who had infant age of 28 to 364 days in the district were included in the study. Mentally and physically incapable women's to provide response during data collection period were excluded.

Operational definitions

Health care seeking behaviour

Seeking medical or non-medical care in response to neonatal danger signs to reduce severity and complication after recognizing the danger signs and perceived nature of illness. It was measured by calculating all individual answers to health care seeking questions and then categorized as having health care seeking behaviour (if participants initiate home care and necessitate seeking care at the health facility) or not having health care seeking behaviour (if participants do not initiate home care and care at the health facility).

Have newborn care practices

These are activities taken by the mothers to protect against new-born danger signs and perceived nature of illness. It is measured if participants practiced safe cord care, optimal thermal care and neonatal breast-feeding.

Have optimal thermal care practice

Mothers who bathed their new-born after 24 h of birth. It is measured if participants bathed their new-born after 24 h of birth.

Have decision-making ability

This is the way an individual put decision by him/herself or with somebody else. It is measured by calculating all individual answers of decision-making ability questions; and then categorize as having decision-making ability (if participants make decision by herself and with her husband to get medical care and to select treatment place for their ill infant) or not having decision-making ability (if participants do not make decision by herself and with her husband to get medical care and to select treatment place for their ill infant).

Sample size determination

The sample size was determined using single population proportion formula.

$$n = (Z\alpha/2)^2 \, p\,(1-p) / W^2$$

with considering the following assumptions where P=proportion of mothers who sought medical care for their newborn illness as 47.7% (p=0.477) (Ekwochi et al., 2015), W=margin error of 5%, design effect=1.5. Z α/2=critical value for normal distribution at 95% confidence level. With these assumptions, the formula yields 383. Since the number of mothers who had an infant age of 28 to 364 day in Tenta district were 3179 (which was less than 10,000), correction formula was used as follows:

$$cf = \frac{n}{1+\frac{n}{N}} = \frac{383}{1+\frac{383}{3179}} = 341.9{\sim}342$$

By adding 10% of non-response rate and design effect of 1.5, the total sample size was 564.

Sampling procedures

The study district was stratified into urban and rural kebeles. From each stratum, 1 out of 3 urban and 7 out of 25 rural kebeles were selected by simple random sampling technique. Family folder was used as sampling frame. These folders contained personal records of individual mothers: address, date of delivery, place of delivery, name of kebele, development group leader, and their house number. The calculated sample size was proportionally allocated to(one urban and seven rural) kebeles. The study participants were selected from the sampling frame through computer-generated method. Data collectors used name of kebeles, their house numbers, and health extension workers for guidance.

Data collection

Structured interviewer administered questionnaire was designed by researchers after reviewing literatures which had previously been done on this topic (Webair and Bin-Gouth, 2013; Mbagaya et al., 2005). The questionnaire was prepared in English language and then translated to Amharic (local language) and re-translated back to English to check for any inconsistencies.

The questionnaire was pre-tested on 5% of the sample in Mekidella district, which had similar socio-demographic characteristics with Tenta district and modification was done. Training was given for data collectors before the pre-test and the beginning of the actual interviews. The investigator checked data completeness. Double entry of data was carried out to prevent data entry errors.

Data processing and analysis

Data were entered in Epi-data version 3.1 and exported to SPSS version 20.0. The completeness and consistency of the data were checked and cleaned. Descriptive analysis was made and measures of central tendency were also determined. Logistic regression was applied to see the association between dependent and independent variables. Independent variables, which had association in bi-variable analysis with p-value <0.25 were included in multiple logistic regression model to handle potential confounding variables. Independent variables with p-value<0.05 in multiple logistic regression model were considered as significant predictors of health seeking behaviour of neonatal danger sign. The results were presented as odds ratios (OR) with 95% confidence intervals (CI).

Ethical consideration

Ethical approval was obtained from ethical review committee of Jimma University. Letter of permission was obtained from Tenta district administrative and health office. Informed verbal consent was also obtained from the study participants. To assure complete confidentiality, other identifying information including name were not recorded on the questionnaires.

RESULTS AND DISCUSSION

Socio demographic characteristics

A total of 527 mothers were interviewed which made the response rate of 93.4%. The mean age of respondents were 30.85 (± 6.16 SD). About fifteen present of respondents were urban and 84.4% were rural residents. Nearly two-third (59.1%) of mothers was Christians and 40.9% were Muslims. Larger proportions (82.9%) of respondents were married and 68.9% were farmers. Regarding educational levels, majority of respondents were illiterate (47.8%), while 5.1% of mothers had completed the grade. Concerning the number of children in the family, majority (87.5%) of mothers had less than five children in their houses (Table 1).

Mother's newborn care practice

From the total study participants, 67.7% of mothers did not apply any substance on their infant's umbilical cord. Of those mothers who applied substances to the infant's cord, nearly half (48.2%) of mothers applied animal muck. Sixty-five percent of mothers gave only breast milk and 68.5% of mothers initiated/started breast-feeding within the first hours. Two hundred two (38.3%) of mothers bathed their new-born before 24 h of birth, and 38.3% of mothers practiced optimal thermal care (Table 2).

Mother's experience on neonatal danger signs and their health seeking behavior

Four hundred four (76.7%) of mothers noticed one or more of their newborn danger signs. The most common neonatal danger signs recognized by mothers were unable to feed/poor sucking (43.5%) and fever (39.8%). Among 404 mothers who recognized neonatal danger signs, 41.3% of them sought medical care, while 55.2% of mothers sought non-medical care for neonatal danger signs. Among two hundred twenty-three mothers who sought non-medical care, 37.7% of them gave home remedies and 30.1% of mothers sought spiritual care. Long distance of the health facility (51.7%), perceived seriousness of neonatal danger signs (42.6%), and beliefs that some danger signs have been caused by evil spirits (34.8%) were the most common reasons cited by mothers who did not seek medical care (Table 3).

Factors associated with health seeking behavior on neonatal danger signs

Multivariable logistic regression model showed that four independent predictors of mother's health seeking behaviour towards neonatal danger signs. Mothers who completed their secondary education were 4.64 times more likely to seek medical care for their neonates compared to those who were illiterate (AOR=4.64; 95% CI=1.1, 19.81). Institutional delivery was found to be significantly associated with mother's health seeking behaviour towards neonatal danger signs. Mothers who delivered a child in health center were 3.35 times more likely to seek neonatal medical care compared to mothers who delivered at home (AOR=3.35, 95% CI=1.31-8.56). Likewise, mother's optimal thermal practice was another significant factor for health seeking behaviour. Mothers who practiced optimal thermal care were 2.52 times more likely to seek neonatal health care than mothers who did not practice optimal thermal care (AOR=2.52, 95%

Table 1. Sociodemographic characteristic of mothers in Tenta district, Northeast Ethiopia, 2015.

Variable	Categories	N	%
Age in year (n=527)	≤24	79	14.9
	25-30	154	29.2
	31-35	172	32.7
	≥36	122	23.2
Residence (n=527)	Urban	82	15.6
	Rural	445	84.4
Wealth quintiles (n=527)	Poorest	105	19.9
	Poor	106	20.1
	Middle	106	20.1
	Rich	106	20.1
	Richest	104	19.8
Number of children in the family (n=527)	<5	461	87.5
	≥5	66	12.5
Marital status (n=527)	Currently married	437	82.9
	Not currently married	90	17.1
Religion of respondent (n=527)	Christian	312	59.1
	Muslim	215	40.9
Educational status of respondent (n=527)	Illiterate	252	47.8
	Primary(1-8 grade)	168	31.9
	Secondary (9-12 grade)	80	15.2
	≥12	27	5.1
Husbands' educational status (n=527)	Illiterate	176	33.4
	Primary(1-8 grade)	224	42.5
	Secondary (9-12 grade)	81	15.4
	≥12	46	8.7
Occupation of the respondents (n=527)	Government employee	33	6.3
	Self-employee	94	17.8
	Farmer	363	68.9
	Daily Labour	37	7.0
Occupation of respondents husband (n=527)	Government employee	57	10.8
	Self-employee	100	19.0
	Farmer	370	70.2

CI=1.1, 5.85). In addition, mothers who had higher decision making abilities in seeking neonatal health care were 11.28 times more likely to seek medical care compared to mothers who had lower decision making ability (AOR=11.28, 95% CI=4.36, 29.22) (Table 4).

DISCUSSION

Seeking health care for neonatal danger signs have a great potential in reducing neonatal mortality (Workineh and Hailu, 2014). This study showed that, out of 404 mothers who experienced neonatal danger signs, about 41.3% of mothers sought medical care for their newborn danger signs. This finding was in agreement with study done in Dera district, Oromia (43.2%) (Assefa et al., 2012) and Enugu state, Nigeria (47.7%) (Ekwochi et al., 2015), but higher than study done in urban slum of India (18.1%) (Gupta et al., 2012) and Edo state, Nigeria (35.9%) (Aigbokhaode et al., 2015), and lower than

Table 2. New-born care practices of mothers in Tenta district, Northeast Ethiopia, 2015.

Variable	Categories	N	%
Applied substance to infant cord (n=527)	Yes	170	32.3
	No	357	67.7
Type of substance applied (n=170)	Oil or Shea butter	29	17.1
	Animal muck	82	48.2
	Shea butter with powder	36	21.2
	Ointment/body lotion	23	13.5
Pre-lacteal food given (n=527)	Yes	184	34.9
	No	343	65.1
Type of pre-lacteal food given (n=184)	Water or tea	78	42.4
	Spiritual water	5	2.7
	Butter/herbal concoction food	101	54.9
Initiated breast-feeding within 1 h (n=527)	Yes	361	68.5
	No	166	31.5
Feed colostrum (n=527)	Yes	445	84.4
	No	82	15.6
Bathed new born after 24 h (527)	Yes	202	38.3
	No	325	61.7
Practiced optimal thermal care (527)	Yes	206	39.1
	No	321	60.9

than studies in Bihar Dar (72.7%) (Awoke, 2013), Yemen (51.4%) (Webair and Bin-Gouth, 2013), peri-urban of India (92%) (Dongre et al., 2009), and Pakistan (81.1%) (Durrani et al., 2015). These discrepancies might be due to the difference in social environment that does not encourage health care seeking behaviour towards neonatal danger signs, differences in accessibility of health facilities. Educational levels also influence mother's health care seeking behaviour towards neonatal danger signs and health service utilization.

Educational status of parents and their work status had strong associations with child survival in developing countries (Ekwochi et al., 2015; Workineh and Hailu, 2014). In Yemen, mothers who attended secondary education were 5.8 times more likely to seek neonatal medical care for their sick neonate (Webair and Bin-Gouth, 2013). Similarly, in this study, mothers who attended secondary education were 4.6 times more likely to seek medical care for their sick neonate compared to illiterate mothers. The possible implications could be that formal education increases mother's knowledge about biological aspects of human beings, and health seeking habits. In addition, educated mothers are more likely to understand health education messages and seek neonatal medical care than illiterate ones.

In Rural Southern Tanzania (Mrisho et al., 2012), and Jabitenan district (Workineh and Hailu, 2014) revealed that mothers who delivered at health facilities were more likely to seek neonatal care than those who delivered at home. In this study, mothers who delivered in health facilities were 3.3 times more likely to seek neonatal medical care compared to those mothers who delivered at home. Thus, this finding further strengthens the argument that increasing institutional birth improves mother's health care seeking behaviour towards neonatal illnesses.

A study in Bihar Dar (Awoke, 2013) and Jabitanan district (Workineh and Hailu, 2014) showed that mother's decision-making level had significant effect on health seeking behaviour for child health services. Similarly, this study revealed that mothers who had higher decision-making levels were 11.28 times more likely to seek neonatal medical care compared with those mothers who had lower decision-making. The possible explanation could be that autonomous mothers have attended child health related conferences without any interference. It is also evident that autonomous mothers practiced behavioural change communications to increase medical care seeking for sick newborn, and needs scaling up with rising institutional deliveries.

Table 3. Mothers' health care seeking behaviour and experience of neonatal danger signs in Tenta District, Northeast Ethiopia, 2015.

Variable	Categories	N	%
Mothers who experienced neonatal danger signs (n=527)	Yes	404	76.7
	No	123	23.3
Type of experienced neonatal danger signs (n=404)	Unable to feed/ poor sucking	176	43.5
	Fever/ hot to touch	161	39.8
	Chest in drawing	103	25.5
	Cold to touch	97	24.0
	Umbilicus Infection	86	21.2
	Lethargic or unconscious	85	20.9
	Fast breathing	61	15.1
	Yellow sole	49	12.1
	Convulsion	33	8.2
	Others	11	2.7
Health seeking behaviour of mothers for neonatal danger signs (n=404)	Sought medical care	167	41.3
	Sought non-medical care	223	55.2
	Did not take action	14	3.5
Mothers who sought non-medical care (n=223)	Sought drug seller	19	8.5
	Sought traditional care	53	23.7
	Gave home remedies	84	37.7
	Sought spiritual care	67	30.1
Reasons for not seeking medical care (n=230)	Illness was not serious	98	42.6
	had no enough money	32	13.9
	Long distance to go health facility	119	51.7
	Occupied by different work	43	18.7
	Health workers are hostile	32	13.9
	Treatment expensive	8	3.1
	Herbs are more effective	73	31.7
	Illness was caused by evil sprit	80	34.8
Decision making levels of mothers in seeking neonatal health care (n=527)	Higher	334	63.4
	Lower	193	36.6

Mothers who practiced optimal thermal care were 2.52 times more likely to seek neonatal medical care compared to those mothers who were not practicing optimal thermal care. Mothers who practiced optimal thermal care could have better access to child health services, which influence mother's decisions in seeking health care towards neonatal danger signs.

Conclusion

Our study suggested that mothers' health seeking behaviour for neonatal medical care was low (41.3%) in the study area. This study also revealed that factors significantly associated with health-seeking behaviour of mothers towards neonatal danger sign including; educational status of mothers, health center delivery, optimal thermal care practice and mother's decision-making ability to seek neonatal health care.

As a recommendation, improving maternal education and their decision-making abilities, and promoting institutional delivery are the recommended interventions to improve mother's health care seeking for neonatal illness. Health facilities should integrate essential newborn care service during ANC and PNC follow up to improve the quality of health information about newborn danger signs. In addition, at the community level, health extension workers should educate mothers about newborn care practices and neonatal danger signs.

CONFLICT OF INTERESTS

The authors have not declared any conflict of interests.

Table 4. Multivariate analysis of health care seeking behaviour of mothers on neonatal danger signs in Tenta district, Northeast, Ethiopia, 2015.

Variable	Health seeking behaviour		Crude odds ratio (COR) (95% CI)	Adjusted odd ratio (AOR) (95%CI)
	Sought medical care (%)	Sought non-medical care (%)		
Mothers educational status				
Illiterate	54 (25.8)	155 (74.2)	1	1
Primary(1-8th)	63 (51.2)	60 (48.8)	3.01 (1.88-4.82)**	1.43 (0.59-3.43)
Secondary(9-12th)	43 (79.6)	11 (20.4)	11.22 (5.4-23.31)**	4.64 (1.1-19.81)*
≥12	15 (78.9)	4 (21.1)	10.74 (3.42-33.84)**	0.52 (0.11-2.40)
Place of delivery of last child				
Home	57 (24.5)	176 (75.5)	1	1
Health post	8 (44.4)	10 (55.6)	2.47 (0.93-6.56)	1.82 (0.38-8.77)
Health center	93 (73.8)	33 (26.2)	8.7 (5.29-14.30)**	3.35 (1.31-8.56)*
Hospital	17 (60.7)	11 (39.3)	4.77 (2.11-10.78)**	1.69 (0.36-7.92)
Optimal thermal care				
Yes	98 (67.1)	48 (32.9)	4.83 (3.12-7.47)**	2.52 (1.08-5.85)*
No	77 (29.7)	182 (70.3)	1	1
Decision making ability to seek neonatal health care				
Higher	155 (63.3)	90 (36.7)	12.06 (7.06-20.59)**	11.28 (4.36-29.21)**
Lower	20 (12.5)	140 (87.5)	1	1

1: Reference category; *P-Value <.05, **P-Value ≤.001.

ABBREVIATIONS

ANC, Antenatal care; **AOR,** adjusted odds ratio; **COR,** crude odds ratios; **OR,** odds ratios; **CI,** confidence interval; **HC,** health center; **SD,** standard deviation; **NMR,** neonatal mortality rate; **PNC,** post natal care; **WHO,** World Health Organization.

ACKNOWLEDGEMENTS

The authors are thankful for Jimma University for funding this study. They would like to thank Tenta district health office for their cooperation to give necessary information. They are also extremely grateful to mothers who participated in this study for their willingness to share their experiences on newborn care.

REFERENCES

Ababa A (2008). Maternal Health Care Seeking Behaviour in Ethiopia: Findings from EDHS 2005. pp. 1-35.

Aigbokhaode AQ, Isah EC, Isara AR (2015). Health seeking behaviour among caregivers of under-five children in Edo state, Nigeria. Southeastern Eur. J. Public Health 3(1):1-10.

Alex-Hart BA, Dotimi DA, Opara PI (2014). Mothers ' recognition of newborn danger signs and health seeking behaviour. Niger. J. Paediatr. 41(3):199-203.

Anyanwu FC, Okeke SR (2014). Health Care Provider and Client Satisfaction: Transforming Health Care Delivery System for Improved Health Care Seeking Behaviour. J. Mod. Educ. Rev. 4(10):846-53. Available at: https://www.researchgate.net/profile/Sylvester_Okeke/publication/285173552_Health_Care_Care_Provider_and_Client_Satisfaction_Transforming_Health_Care_Delivery_System_for_Improved_Health_Care_Seeking_Behaviour/links/579209d508aed51475ac1b7e.pdf

Assefa T, Belachew T, Tegegn A, Deribew A (2008). Mothers' health care seeking behavior for childhood illnesses in Derra district, Northshoa zone, Oromia regional state, Ethiopia. Ethiop. J. Health Sci. 18(3):87-94.

Awasthi S, Srivastava NM, Agarwal GG, Pant S, Ahluwalia TP (2009). Effect of behaviour change communication on qualified medical care-seeking for sick neonates among urban poor in Lucknow, northern India: a before and after intervention study. Trop. Med. Int. Health 14(10):1199-209.

Awoke W (2013). Prevalence of childhood illness and mothers'/caregivers' care seeking behavior in Bahir Dar, Ethiopia: A descriptive community based cross sectional study. Open J. Prev. Med. 3(2):155-9.

Beck D, Ganges F, Goldmaan S, Long P (2004). Care of the Newborn: A Reference Manual. Save the Children. Available at: http://www.chd.gov.np/downloads/Care_of_the_Newborn_Reference_Manual_2004.pdf

Chandwani H, Pandor J (2015). Healthcare-Seeking Behaviors of Mothers regarding their Children in a Tribal Community of Gujarat, India. Electronic Phys. 7(1):990.

Dongre AR, Deshmukh PR, Garg BS (2009). Awareness and health care seeking for newborn danger signs among mothers in peri-urban Wardha. Indian J. Pediatr. 76(7):691-3.

Durrani HM, Kumar R, Durrani SM (2015). Recognizing the Danger Signs and Health Seeking Behaviour of Mothers in Childhood Illness in Karachi, Pakistan. Univ. J. Public Health 3(2):49-54.

Ekwochi U, Ndu IK, Osuorah CD, Amadi OF, Okeke IB, Obuoha E,

Onah KS, Nwokoye I, Odetunde OI, Obumneme-Anyim NI (2015). Knowledge of danger signs in newborns and health seeking practices of mothers and care givers in Enugu state, South-East Nigeria. Ital. J. Pediatr. 41:18.

Ethiopia Demographic and Health Survey (EDHS) (2016). Central Statistical Agency (CSA) [Ethiopia] and ICF. Ethiopia Demographic and Health Survey 2016: Key Indicators Report. Addis Ababa, Ethiopia, and Rockville, Maryland, USA. CSA and ICF.

Gelaw YA, Biks GA, Alene KA (2014). Effect of residence on mothers' health care seeking behavior for common childhood illness in Northwest Ethiopia: a community based comparative cross-sectional study. BMC Res. Notes 7(705):1-8.

Gupta P, Srivastava VK, Kumar V, Jain S, Masood J, Ahmad N, Srivastava JP (2012). Care seeking behaviour of mothers during illness of newborn in urban slums of Lucknow City. Indian J. Commun. Health 24(3):179-183.

Herbert HK, Lee AC, Chandran A, Rudan I, Baqui AH (2012). Care seeking for neonatal illness in low-and middle-income countries: a systematic review. PLoS Med. 9(3):e1001183.

Marsh DR, Darmstadt GL, Moore J, Daly P, Oot D, Tinker A (2002). Advancing newborn health and survival in developing countries: a conceptual framework. J. Perinatol. 22(7):572-6.

Mbagaya GM, Odhiambo MO, Oniang RK (2005). Mothers health seeking behaviour during child illness in a rural western Kenya community. Afr. Health Sci. 5(4):322-327.

Mrisho M, Schellenberg D, Manzi F, Tanner M, Mshinda H, Shirima K, Msambichaka B, Abdulla S, Schellenberg JA (2012). Neonatal deaths in rural southern Tanzania: care-seeking and causes of death. Pediatrics 2012:1-8.

Sandberg J, Pettersson KO, Asp G, Kabakyenga J, Agardh A (2014). Inadequate knowledge of neonatal danger signs among recently delivered women in southwestern rural Uganda: a community survey. PLoS One 9(5):e97253.

Save the Children (2014). Ending newborn deaths ensuring every baby survives. 1 St John's Lane London EC1M 4AR UK. pp. 9-23.

Syed U, Asiruddin S, Helal MS, Mannan II, Murray J (2006). Immediate and early postnatal care for mothers and newborns in rural Bangladesh. J. Health Popul. Nutr. 24(4):508-518.

Webair HH, Bin-Gouth AS (2013). Factors affecting health seeking behavior for common childhood illnesses in Yemen. Patient Prefer. Adherence 7:1129-38.

Workineh YG, Hailu DA (2014). Factors affecting utilization of postnatal care service in Jabitena district, Amhara region, Ethiopia. Sci. J. Public Health 2(3):169-76.

Factors related with low back pain and pelvic pain at the early stage of pregnancy in Japanese women

Yuko Uemura[1,2]*, Toshiyuki Yasui[3], Kimiyo Horike[4], Kazuhisa Maeda[4], Hirokazu Uemura[5], Mari Haku[6], Reiko Sakae[1] and Keiko Matsumura[1]

[1]Department of Nursing, Kagawa Prefectural College of Health Sciences, Kagawa, Japan.
[2]Tokushima University Graduate School, Tokushima, Japan.
[3]Department of Reproductive and Menopausal Medicine, Institute of Biomedical Sciences, Tokushima University Graduate School, Tokushima, Japan.
[4]Shikoku Medical Center for Children and Adults, Kagawa, Japan.
[5]Department of Preventive Medicine, Institute of Biomedical Sciences, Tokushima University Graduate School, Tokushima, Japan.
[6]Department of Midwifery, Institute of Biomedical Sciences, Tokushima University Graduate School, Tokushima, Japan.

The aim of this study was to clarify the proportion of women with low back and/or pelvic pain (LBPP) and LBPP-related factors at the early stage of pregnancy and to clarify the differences between LBPP-related factors in primiparous women and multiparous women in Japan. 157 pregnant women were recruited. Information about the presence of LBPP, degree of pain by using a visual analog scale (VAS), location of pain, past history of LBPP and background characteristics were collected. Physical status was assessed by the pregnancy mobility index (PMI). The Ethics Committee of Tokushima University Hospital approved the study. The proportion of women who complained of LBPP was 65.6%. PMI score in women with LBPP was significantly higher than that in women without LBPP ($p<0.001$). The proportions of women with a past history of LBPP before pregnancy and with a past history of LBPP in the previous pregnancy were significantly higher in women with LBPP ($p<0.001$ and $p=0.002$, respectively). In women with LBPP, the score of VAS in multiparous women was significantly higher than that in primiparous women ($p=0.019$). Early management for women with a past history of LBPP before pregnancy and with a past history of LBPP in the previous pregnancy is important. Management for lumbar pain according to parity is needed for health guidance at the early stage of pregnancy.

Key words: Pregnancy, first trimester, low back pain, pelvic pain, parity.

INTRODUCTION

Low back and/or pelvic pain (LBPP) during and after pregnancy is a common complication of pregnancy and puerperium. Mogren and Pohjanen (2005) reported that the overall prevalence of LBPP was 71.7% and that the mean gestational age at the start of LBPP was 22.1 weeks. It has been reported that the proportions of pregnant women with LBPP were approximately 50% in the first trimester (Gutke et al., 2008), 40 to 70% in the second trimester (Olsson et al., 2012) and 70 to 80% in the third trimester (Kovacs et al., 2012). Also, 70% of postpartum women complained of LBPP immediately after delivery and 40% of women complained of LBPP

3 to 4 months after delivery (Ostgaard, 1992). Pain in the pelvic girdle and lumbar region that occurs at the early stage of pregnancy has been suggested to be a predictor for persistent pain after delivery (Gutke et al., 2008). For pregnant women, prevention of LBPP is an important issue since LBPP is not only the most frequent complaint during pregnancy but also persists for a long period of time.

Several factors related to LBPP have been demonstrated. The association of LBPP with age has been controversial. It has been reported that the age of women without lumbopelvic pain was significantly higher than that of women with lumbopelvic pain in the second trimester (Olsson et al., 2009). On the other hand, it has been reported that older pregnant women are more likely to have pain in the lower back, pelvis and buttock regions in the third trimester (Brown et al., 2013).

It has been reported that increase in parity was associated with increased risk for lumbar pain and that risk for lumbar pain in multiparous women was higher than that in primiparous women (Mota et al., 2015). A past history of lumbar and pelvic pain related or unrelated to previous pregnancy (Kovacs et al., 2012), low educational level (Chang et al., 2011), and high body mass index (BMI) and overweight (Mogren and Pohjanen, 2005) have been reported to be as factors related to LBPP. It has also been reported that a longer period of previous regular physical activity decreased the risk of LBPP during pregnancy and that a physically demanding occupation was associated with increased risk of LBPP during pregnancy (Mogren, 2005). Ostgaard et al. (1992) reported that persistent postpartum back pain was associated with the presence of back pain before pregnancy, the presence of back pain during pregnancy, physically heavy work and multipregnancy. Mogren (2006) reported that women with persistent LBPP at 6 months after delivery had significantly earlier onset of pain during pregnancy, higher maternal age and higher BMI, suggesting that the level and timing of onset of pain during pregnancy were strong predictors of persistent LBPP after delivery (Mogren, 2006). The aim of this study was to clarify the proportion of women with LBPP and LBPP-related factors at the early stage of pregnancy and to clarify the differences between LBPP-related factors in primiparous women and multiparous women in Japan.

MATERIALS AND METHODS

Study setting and date collection

This study was conducted from March in 2015 to January in 2016 in a birth center in Kagawa Prefecture in Japan. Number of delivery was approximately 500 per year in the hospital that was examined, and sample size was 184 by using permissible errors (5%), reliability (95%) and a ratio of a population (25%). The sample size was determined to be 215, considering the number of uncollected sample. 157 pregnant women were recruited at the first trimester in the birth center. Participants were informed of the purposes and procedure of the study.

The study protocol was reviewed and approved by the Ethics Review Board of Tokushima University Hospital (Approval No. 2201).

Questionnaire

A self-administered questionnaire was designed consisting of three parts that took about 20 min to complete. With respect to location of pain, the reference was cited (Al-Sayegh et al., 2012). VAS score was used, which was widely used as objective assessment for degree of pain. Ten women were tested using self-administered questionnaire for assessment of validity in advance and studied using revised self-administered questionnaire. The first part of the questionnaire consisted of questions regarding baseline characteristics such as age, marital status, education and week of pregnancy. The second part of the questionnaire consisted of questions regarding the presence of LBPP, location of pain and 10 cm visual analog scale (VAS) with the end-points of no pain (0 cm) and worst thinkable pain (10 cm). The third part consisted of questions on factors related to low back pain including employment, smoking, and menstruation before pregnancy and history of low back pain. Physical status was evaluated using the pregnancy mobility index (PMI) (Van et al., 2006). In the question for PMI, daily activities were categorized into three scales: (1) daily mobility in the house, (2) ability to perform normal household activities, and (3) mobility outdoors. Every item has a score option from 0 to 3 ('no problem in performing the task', 'some effort in performing the task' and 'not possible to perform the task or only possible with the aid of others'), which was transformed to a 0 to 72 scale. A higher score indicates limitation of the activity in daily life.

Data analyses

Differences in background characteristics, physical factors, LBPP-related factors, and PMI were evaluated by the χ^2 test or Mann-Whitney U test in all subjects and in women with LBPP. Odds rations (OR) and their corresponding to 95% confidence interval (CI) were calculated by using logistic regression analyses. All p values are two-tailed and those less than 0.05 were considered to be statistically significant. Statistical analyses for data evaluation were carried out using SPSS version 22 for Windows (IBM Crop., Aromonk, NY).

RESULTS

Baseline characteristics of the subjects are shown in Table 1. Mean age ± standard deviation (SD) of the subjects was 32.2 ± 5.1 years. The proportion of women whose age was more than 35 years was 31.8%. The mean week of pregnancy was 14.8 weeks, ranging from 9 to 20 weeks. The subjects included 38.9% primiparous

*Corresponding author. E-mail: uemura@chs.pref.kagawa.jp.

Table 1. Background characteristics of the subjects.

Age (year)	-	32.2 ± 5.1
Week of pregnancy (weeks)	-	14.8 ± 1.6
Height (cm)	-	157.0 ± 5.3
Weight (kg)	-	53.4 ± 9.8
Body mass index (kg/m^2)	-	21.6 ± 3.9
Marital status	Married	150 (95.5)
	Not married	7 (4.5)
Working	Yes	109 (69.4)
	No	48 (30.6)
Smoking	Current	2 (1.3)
	Previous	35 (22.3)
	Never	120 (76.4)
Parity	Primiparous	61 (38.9)
	Multiparous	96 (61.1)
Education level	High school	43 (27.4)
	Junior college or professional school	72 (45.9)
	College and/or graduate school	42 (26.7)
Presence of LBPP before pregnancy	Yes	81 (51.6)
	No	76 (48.4)
Past history of treatment for LBPP	Yes	37 (23.6)
	No	120 (76.4)
Past history of orthopedic diseases	Yes	32 (20.4)
	No	125 (79.6)
Past history of LBPP in the previous pregnancy (n=96)	Yes	67 (69.8)
	No	29 (30.2)

LBPP: Low back and/or pelvic pain. The values of age, duration of pregnancy, height, weight and BMI are presented as means ± standard deviation.

women and 61.1% multiparous women. The proportion of working women was 69.4% and the proportion of primiparous working women was significantly higher than that of multiparous working women (p=0.013). The proportion of women with a past history of LBPP before pregnancy was 51.6% and the proportion of women with a past history of LBPP in the previous pregnancy was 69.8%. As shown in Table 2, the proportion of women who complained of LBPP was 65.6%. The mean ± standard deviation (SD) of VAS score was 2.6 ± 2.4, ranging from 0 to 8.6. The proportion of women whose VAS scores were more than 7 was 6.4%. The proportion of women whose frequency of LBPP was once or twice per week was 45.7%. Only 40.8% of women coped with LBPP. The proportion of women who coped with pain in working women was lower than the proportion of women who did cope with pain in non-working women (p=0.019). The region in which women complained most frequently of pain was the lower back followed by the buttocks.

The subjects were classified into two groups: women with LBPP and women without LBPP as shown in Figure 1. As shown in Table 3, PMI score in women with LBPP was significantly higher than that in women without LBPP (p<0.001). The proportion of working women in women without LBPP was significantly higher than that in women with LBPP (p=0.032). The proportions of women with a past history of LBPP before pregnancy and with a past history of LBPP in the previous pregnancy were significantly higher in women with LBPP (p<0.001 and p=0.002, respectively). The presence of LBPP before

Table 2. Characteristics of LBPP in the subjects.

VAS score	-	2.6 ± 2.5
Frequency of LBPP	1-2 days/week	47 (45.7)
	3-6 days/week	26 (25.2)
	7 days/week	30 (29.1)
Coping with LBPP	Yes	42 (40.8)
	No	61 (59.2)
Location of LBPP (Multiple answers)	Back	71 (45.2)
	Left hip	27 (17.2)
	Right hip	26 (16.6)
	Around the pubis	17 (10.8)
PMI score	-	7.0 ± 7.6

LBPP: Low back and/or pelvic pain; PMI: pregnancy mobility index. The values of VAS score and PMI are presented as means ± standard deviation.

pregnancy was an increased risk for LBPP (OR 5.33, 95%CI 2.18-13.06).

There was no significant difference between the proportions of primiparous women with LBPP (62.2%) and multiparous women with LBPP (67.7%). In order to clarify the characteristics of women with LBPP according to parity, the women were classified into two groups: primiparous women with LBPP and multiparous women with LBPP (Figure 1). In women with LBPP, the proportions of primiparous women and multiparous women were 36.9 and 63.1%, respectively. As shown in Table 4, mean VAS scores were 3.3 in primiparous women and 4.2 in multiparous women and VAS score in multiparous women was significantly higher than that in primiparous women (p=0.019). In primiparous women with LBPP, the proportion of working women was higher than that of working multiparous women (p=0.013). In multiparous women with LBPP, the proportion of women who coped with LBPP was higher than that in primiparous women (p=0.047). The region of pain that primiparous women most frequently complained of was around the pubic bone (p=0.043), and the region of pain that multiparous women most frequently complained of was the lower back (p=0.04).

DISCUSSION

In the present study, we found that the prevalence of LBPP in women at the early stage of pregnancy was 65.6%, that pregnant women with LBPP had a past history of LBPP before pregnancy and a past history of LBPP in the previous pregnancy, and that LBPP-related factors were different in primiparous women with LBPP and multiparous women with LBPP.

Previous studies demonstrated that the prevalence of lumbar pain was approximately 50% at the first trimester (Gutke et al., 2008; Robinson et al., 2010) and that the prevalence of pelvic and low back pain was 59 to 66% in Japan (Shinkawa et al., 2009). The prevalence (65.6%) in the present study is consistent with those previous studies. The region of pain shown in the present study is also consistent with a previous study (Brown et al., 2013). On the other hand, it has been reported that 14.6% of pregnant women at the first trimester experienced pain in which the value of VAS was more than 7 (Brown et al., 2013). The proportion of such women in the present study (6.4%) was lower than that in the previous study. Also, the frequency of LBPP was shown to be once or twice per week. The relative low intensity and frequency of LBPP might have been the reason why 60% of the pregnant women did not have to cope with LBPP. However, it has been reported that pelvic girdle pain and lumbar pain at the early stage of pregnancy persist in the puerperium period (Gutke et al., 2008). Therefore, health guidance for LBPP at the early stage of pregnancy is important even if the intensity and frequency are low.

In the present study, high proportions of women with a past history of LBPP before pregnancy and with a past history of LBPP in the previous pregnancy were found in women with LBPP. These factors were shown in previous studies to be risk factors of lumbar pain during pregnancy (Ostgaard et al., 1992; Mogren and Pohjanen, 2005; Mohseni-Bandpei et al., 2009; Bjelland et al., 2011; Al-Sayegh et al., 2012). It has been reported that the proportion of women with chronic lower back pain increased from 20 to 30 years of age to 50 to 60 years of age (Meucci et al., 2015), suggesting that the occurrence of lumbar pain increases with advance of age. An increase in the number of women in Japan who have

Table 3. Comparison of characteristics of women with and without LBPP.

Parameter		Women with LBPP (n=103)	Women without LBPP (n=54)	*P*
Age (years)	-	31.8 ± 4.8	33.0 ± 5.4	0.143
Duration of pregnancy (weeks)	-	14.9 ± 1.5	14.6 ± 1.4	0.429
Height (cm)	-	156.7 ± 5.3	157.8 ± 5.1	0.206
Weight (kg)	-	53.5 ± 8.7	53.1 ± 11.7	0.357
Body mass index (kg/m^2)	-	21.8 ± 3.7	21.3 ± 4.1	0.218
Marital status	Married	98 (95.1)	52 (96.3)	0.546
	Not married	5 (4.9)	2 (3.7)	
Working	Yes	66 (64.1)	43 (79.6)	0.032
	No	37 (35.9)	11 (20.4)	
Smoking	Current	1 (1.0)	1 (1.8)	0.436
	Previous	26 (25.2)	9 (16.7)	
	Never	76 (73.8)	44 (81.5)	
Educational level	High school	30 (29.1)	13 (24.1)	0.719
	Junior college or professional school	45 (43.7)	27 (50.0)	
	College and/or graduate school	28 (27.2)	14 (25.9)	
Parity	Primiparous	38 (36.9)	23 (42.6)	0.299
	Multiparous	65 (63.1)	31 (57.4)	
Presence of LBPP before pregnancy	Yes	65 (63.1)	16 (29.6)	<0.001
	No	38 (36.9)	38 (70.4)	
Past history of treatment for LBPP	Yes	26 (25.2)	11 (20.4)	0.317
	No	77 (74.8)	43 (79.6)	
Past history of orthopedic diseases	Yes	24 (23.3)	8 (14.8)	0.148
	No	79 (76.7)	46 (85.2)	
Past history of LBPP in the previous pregnancy (n=96)	Yes	52 (80.0)	15 (48.4)	0.002
	No	13 (20.0)	16 (51.6)	
PMI	-	9.1 ± 8.1	3.2 ± 4.5	<0.001

LBPP: Low back and/or pelvic pain; PMI: pregnancy mobility index. The values of age, duration of pregnancy, height, weight, body mass index and PMI are presented as means ± standard deviation.

LBPP before pregnancy is expected since the age of birth has recently been increasing in Japan (Ministry of Health, Labour and Welfare, 2015). Health guidance for prevention of lumbar pain at the early stage of pregnancy is important since lumbar pain in women with a past history of LBPP before pregnancy may become worse throughout pregnancy.

Previous studies showed that the proportion of women who were working was not significantly different between women with lumbar pain and women without lumbar pain (Gutke et al., 2008; Olsson et al., 2009; Mohseni-Bandpei et al., 2009). It has been reported that women without LBPP were more likely to work than women with LBPP in the late stage of pregnancy (Kovac et al., 2012). In the early stage of pregnancy, the proportion of working women in women without LBPP was we shown to be higher than that in women with LBPP. However, a causal relationship between LBPP and working was not found. Given that physical and psychological factors related to jobs have also been reported to be predictors for lumbar

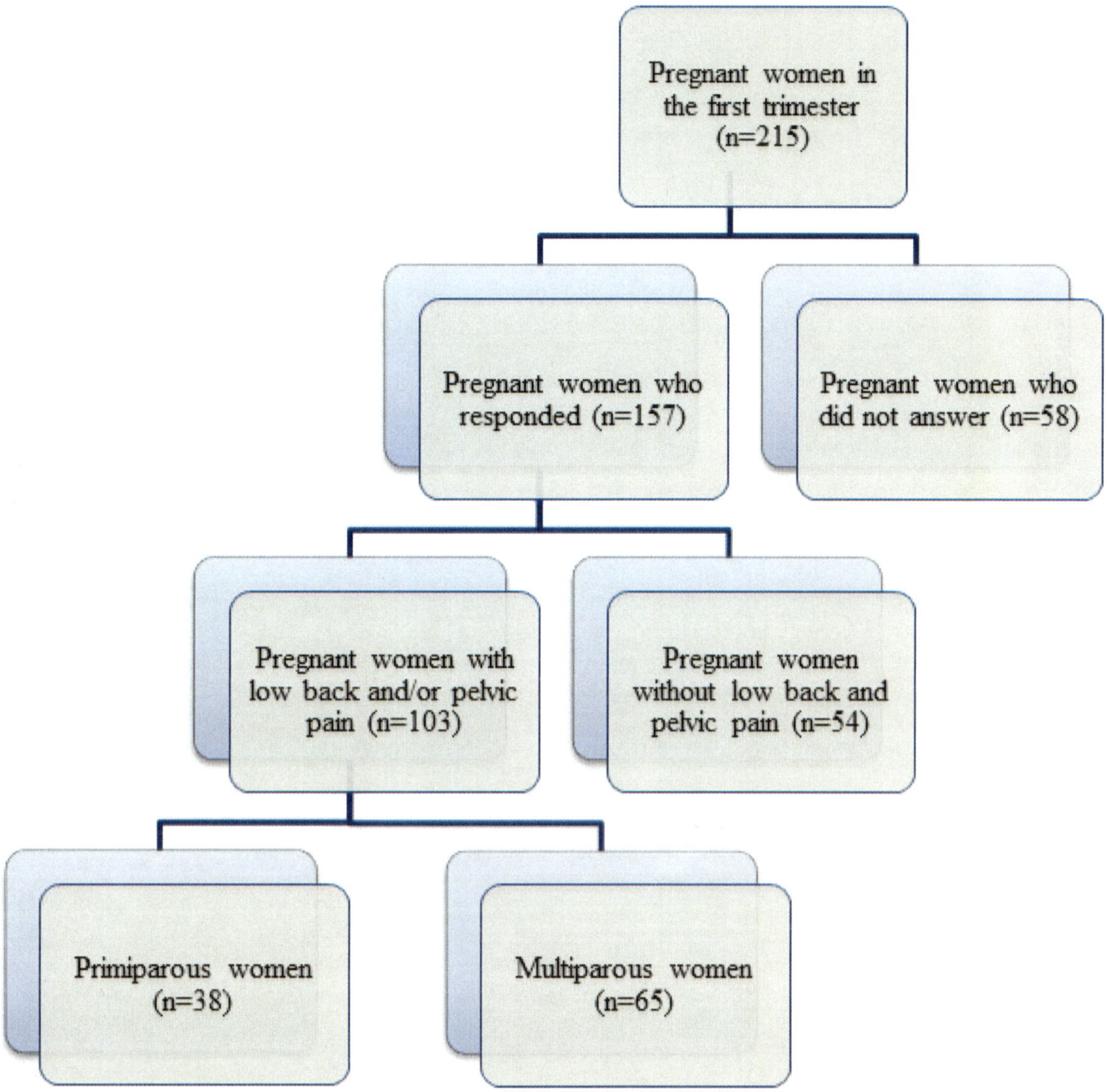

Figure 1. Classification of subjects.

pain (Wáng et al., 2016), a prospective longitudinal study is needed to determine the relationship between LBPP and working.

The mean PMI score (7.0) in the present study was higher than that (3.5 at 12 weeks of age) in a previous study (Bakker et al., 2013). Bakker et al. (2013) suggested that PMI score at the first trimester can predict PMI score at the third trimester since PMI score increases with advance of gestational weeks. Therefore, PMI at the early stage of pregnancy is important. Since PMI score in women with LBPP was high, activity in daily life was limited due to pain in women with LBPP. In addition, Bakker et al. (2013) reported that PMI score caused by lumbopelvic pain was significantly associated with psychological determinants during all stages of pregnancy (Bakker et al., 2013). Management for LBPP at the early stage of pregnancy may also be involved in prevention of the development of a poor psychological condition.

The characteristics of primiparous and multiparous pregnant women with LBPP might be different. A previous study showed that multiparty was a risk factor for LBPP during pregnancy (Mogren and Pohjanen, 2005). Since a past history of lower back pain in the previous pregnancy has been suggested to be a risk factor for LBPP (Mogren and Pohjanen, 2005; Mohseni-Bandpei et al., 2009), the risk of LBPP in multiparous women may be higher than that in primiparous women. The fact that 80% of multiparous women with LBPP in the present study had a past history of LBPP in their previous pregnancy suggests

Table 4. Comparison of primiparous and multiparous women with LBPP.

Parameter		Primiparous (n=38)	Multiparous (n=65)	*P*
Age (year)		30.5 ± 5.0)	32.6 ± 4.5	0.028
pregnancy duration (weeks)		14.7 ± 1.2	14.9 ± 1.8	0.428
Height (cm)		155.6 ± 5.0	157.3 ± 5.4	0.110
Weight (kg)		52.5 ± 10.4	54.1 ± 7.7	0.140
Body mass index (kg/m^2)		21.7 ± 4.2	21.9 ± 3.4	0.335
Marital status	Married	34 (89.5)	64 (98.5)	0.061
	Not married	4 (10.5)	1 (1.5)	
Working	Yes	30 (78.9)	36 (55.4)	0.013
	No	8 (21.1)	29 (44.6)	
Smoking	Current	0 (0.0)	1 (1.5)	0.543
	Previous	8 (21.1)	18 (27.7)	
	Never	30 (78.9)	46 (70.8)	
Educational level	High school	8 (21.1)	22 (33.8)	0.291
	Junior college or professional school	20 (52.6)	25 (38.5)	
	College or Graduate school	10 (26.3)	18 (27.7)	
Presence of LBPP before pregnancy	Yes	28 (73.7)	37 (56.9)	0.067
	No	10 (26.3)	28 (43.1)	
Past history of treatment for LBPP	Yes	12 (31.6)	14 (21.5)	0.184
	No	26 (68.4)	51 (78.5)	
Past history of orthopedic diseases	Yes	11 (28.9)	13 (20.0)	0.212
	No	27 (71.1)	52 (80.0)	
Past history of LBPP in the previous pregnancy	Yes	-	52 (80.0)	
	No	-	13 (20.0)	
Coping with LBPP	Yes	11 (28.9)	31 (47.7)	0.047
	No	27 (71.1)	34 (52.3)	
Location of LBPP				
Back	Yes	22 (57.9)	49 (75.4)	0.040
	No	16 (42.1)	16 (24.6)	
Left hip	Yes	12 (31.6)	15 (23.1)	0.250
	No	26 (68.4)	50 (76.9)	
Right hip	Yes	11 (28.9)	15 (23.1)	0.348
	No	27 (71.1)	50 (76.9)	
Around the pubis	Yes	10 (26.3)	7 (10.8)	0.043
	No	28 (73.7)	58 (89.2)	
VAS score	-	3.3 ± 1.6	4.2 ± 2.1	0.019
PMI score	-	6.8 ± 5.5	10.3 ± 9.2	0.100

LBPP: Low back and/or pelvic pain; VAS: visual analog scale; PMI: pregnancy mobility index. The values of age, duration of pregnancy, height, weight, body mass index, VAS and PMI are presented as means ± standard deviation.

that multiparous women generally have LBPP. However, the proportion of multiparous women with LBPP was not significantly different from the proportion of primiparous women with LBPP being in line with the results of previous studies (Mohseni-Bandpei et al., 2009; Mota et al., 2015). Mogren and Pohjanen (2005) reported that mean gestational age at the onset of LBPP was 22.1 weeks. The reason for no significant difference between proportions of multiparous and primiparous women with LBPP in the present study might be that the subjects were in the early stage of pregnancy.

The proportion of working women was shown to be high in primiparous women with LBPP. Previous studies showed that occurrence of lumbar pain were not associated with working status (Olsson et al., 2009; Mohseni-Bandpei et al., 2009). To the best of our knowledge, there has been no report regarding the association of LBPP with working status according to parity. It was found that VAS level in multiparous women with LBPP was higher than that in primiparous women with LBPP. Since subjective and personal experiences in the past contribute to the feeling of pain, a high VAS level may be associated with a past history of LBPP in the previous pregnancy in multiparous women. It is important to obtain information regarding a past history of LBPP in the previous pregnancy.

Multiparous women with LBPP were likely to cope with pain, while primiparous women with LBPP did not cope with pain sufficiently. Given that a past history of LBPP in the previous pregnancy is a risk factor for LBPP, coping with LBPP is important for primiparous women, and active management for LBPP is needed. Primiparous women with LBPP were likely to have pain around the pubic bone, while multiparous women with LBPP were likely to have pain at the lower back. It has been reported that the areas of pain for which the VAS score was more than 7 were the lower back (12.4%) and pelvis (9.8%) in the first trimester. However, to the best of our knowledge, a difference in location of pain according to parity has not been demonstrated.

A significant relationship between LBPP and age was also not found in our study. In previous studies, both younger age (Olsson et al., 2009; Mohseni-Bandpei et al., 2009; Bjelland et al., 2011; Kovacs et al., 2012) and older age (Gutke et al., 2008) were shown to be risk factors for LBPP. Wu et al. (2004) reported that both youngest age and oldest age were higher risks for lower back pain. Increase in abdominal girth and change in posture do not occur at the early stage of pregnancy. This might be the reason for no significant association of LBPP with age being found in the present study.

This study has several limitations. First, the proportions of primiparous women and multiparous women were not similar, though the difference was not significant. Further study with a large sample size may be needed. Second, this study is of a cross-sectional nature. Prospective studies including subjects in middle and late gestational stages and puerperium may be required to clarify the characteristics of LBPP in each stage.

In conclusion, 65% of women complained of LBPP at the early stage of pregnancy and daily life of women with LBPP was limited. Early management for women with a past history of LBPP before pregnancy and with a past history of LBPP in the previous pregnancy is important. Management for lumbar pain according to parity is needed for health guidance at the early stage of pregnancy.

Conflict of Interests

The authors have not declared any conflict of interests.

ACKNOWLEDGEMENTS

The authors are grateful to doctors, midwives and medical assistants in Shikoku Medical Center for Children and Adults for supporting this research. They also thank the women who participated in this study. This work was supported by JSPS KAKENHI Grant Numbers JP16K12104.

REFERENCES

Al-Sayegh NA, Salem M, Dashti LF, Al-Sharrah S, Kalakh S, Al-Rashidi R (2012). Pregnancy-related lumbopelvic pain: prevalence, risk factors, and profile in Kuwait. Pain Med. 13(8):1081-1087.

Bakker EC, van Nimwegen-Matzinger CW, Ekkel-van der Voorden W, Nijkamp MD, Völlink T (2013). Psychological determinants of pregnancy-related lumbopelvic pain: a prospective cohort study. Acta Obstet. Gynecol. Scand. 92(7):797-803.

Bjelland EK, Eberhard-Gran M, Nielsen CS, Eskild A (2011). Age at menarche and pelvic girdle syndrome in pregnancy: a population study of 74973 women. BJOG 118(13):1646-52.

Brown A, Johnston R (2013). Maternal experience of musculoskeletal pain during pregnancy and birth outcomes: significance of lower back and pelvic pain. Midwifery 29(12):1346-1351.

Chang HY, Jensen MP, Yang YL, Lee CN, Lai YH (2011). Risk factor of pregnancy-related lumbopelvic pain: a biopsychosocial approach. J. Clin. Nurs. 21(9-10):1274-1283.

Gutke A, Ostgaard HC, Oberg B (2008). Predicting persistent pregnancy-related low back pain. Spine 33(12):E386-393.

Kovacs FM, Garcia E, Royuela A, González L, Abraira V (2012). Prevalence and factors associated with low back pain and pelvic girdle pain during pregnancy: a multicenter study conducted in the Spanish National Health Service. Spine 37(17):1516-1533.

Meucci RD, Fassa AG, Faria NM (2015). Prevalence of chronic low back pain: systematic review. Rev. Saude. Pub. 49(1):3-22.

Ministry of Health, Labour and Welfare (2015). Vital Statistics. (In Japanese). Available at : http://www.mhlw.go.jp/english/database/db-hw/vs01.html

Mogren IM (2005). Previous physical activity decreases the risk of low back pain and pelvic pain during pregnancy. Scand. J. Public Health 33(4):300-6.

Mogren IM (2006). BMI, pain and hyper-mobility are determinants of long-term outcome for woman with low back pain and pelvic pain during pregnancy. Eur. Spine. J. 15(7):1093-1102.

Mogren IM, Pohjanen AI (2005). Low back pain and pelvic pain during pregnancy: prevalence and risk factors. Spine 30(8):983-991.

Mohseni-Bandpei MA, Fakhri M, Ahmad-Shirvani M, Bagheri-Nessami

M, Khalilian AR, Shayesteh-Azar M, Mohseni-Bandpei H (2009). Low back pain in 1,100 Iranian pregnant women: prevalence and risk factors. Spine J. 9(10):795-801.

Mota MJ, Cardoso M, Carvalho A, Marques A, Sá-Couto P, Demain S (2015). Women's experiences of low back pain during pregnancy. J. Back Musculoskelet. Rehabil. 28(2):351-357.

Olsson C, Buer N, Holm K, Nilsson-Wikmar L (2009). Lumbopelvic pain associated with catastrophizing and fear-avoidance beliefs in early pregnancy. Acta Obstet. Gynecol. Scand. 88(4):378-385.

Olsson CB, Nilsson-Wikmar L, Grooten WJ (2012). Determinants for lumbopelvic pain 6 months postpartum. Disabil. Rehabil. 34(5):416-422.

Ostgaard HC, Andersson GB (1992). Postpartum Low-Back Pain. Spine 17(1):53-55.

Robinson HS, Veierød MB, Mengshoel AM, Vøllestad NK (2010). Pelvic girdle pain-associations between risk factors in early pregnancy and disability or pain intensity in late pregnancy: a prospective cohort study. BMC Musculoskeletal Disorders 11(1):91.

Shinkawa H, Shimada M, Hayase M, Inui T (2009). A survey of the variety, incidence rate, and frequency of minor symptoms currently experienced by expectant mothers. J. Jpn. Acad. Midwif. 23(1):48-58. (In Japanese).

Van de Pol G, de Leeuw JR, van Brummen HJ, Bruinse HW, Heintz AP, van der Vaart CH (2006). The Pregnancy Mobility Index: a mobility scale during and after pregnancy. Acta Obstet. Gynecol. Scand. 85(7):786-791.

Wáng YX, Wáng JQ, Káplár Z (2016). Increased low back pain prevalence in females than in males after menopause age: evidences based on synthetic literature review. Quant. Imaging. Med. Surg. 6(2):199-206.

Wu WH, Meijer OG, Uegaki K, Mens JM, van Dieën JH, Wuisman PI, Ostgaard HC (2004). Pregnancy-related pelvic girdle pain (PPP), I: Terminology, clinical presentation, and prevalence. Eur. Spine. J. 13(7):575-589.

7

Breastfeeding skills in Arba Minch Zuria: The positioning and attachment initiatives

Dessalegn Tamiru[1] and Hunduma Jisha[2*]

[1]College of Public Health and Medical Science, Arba Minch University, Ethiopia.
[2]College of Health Science, Jimma University, Ethiopia.

Proper child positioning and attachment initiates the production of optimal amounts of breast milk and contribute to the comfort of a child during suckling. Poor breastfeeding practices like early cessation and poor breastfeeding skills, introduction of unclean artificial feeding have been widely documented in the world. This cross-sectional community based study was carried out between October 7 and 25, 2013 in Arba Minch Zuria. Structured questionnaires and observational-checklist were used to collect data. The missing values and outliers, data, were checked and entered in double. Multivariable logistic regression was done to identify the predictors of poor and good positioning and attachment to breast. More than one-fifth of 384 (20.1%) infants was poorly positioned and attached to breast. Poor attachment of children to the breast were negatively associated with infant's age below 6 (AOR=0.03 (0.01, 0.11)), attending breast feeding education (AOR=0.42(0.19, 0.93)) and positively associated with having an uneducated husband (AOR=0.07(0.01, 0.51)). Poor child positioning were also negatively associated with infant's age below 6 (AOR=0.03(0.01, 0.10)), lack of information on breastfeeding (AOR=0.42(0.19, 0.94)), and early introduction of additional food (AOR=0.44(0.20, 0.97). Overall, in more than one-fifth of mothers (20.1%), the breastfeeding attachment and positioning were found to be lower than the national and global recommendations. It is highly related to infant's age, paternal educational and an exposure to breastfeeding education. Thus, continuous community based nutritional health education were needed to promote optimal breastfeeding skills using health workers, religious leader and local community resource people as key actors.

Key words: Positioning, attachment, breastfeeding, Arba Minch.

INTRODUCTION

There is a universal consensus on the dietary benefit of optimal breastfeeding practices for children's optimal growth and mental health benefits. Currently, breastfeeding is the focus of multi-professional interest because of its nutritional value and psychological benefits for both mother and her child. Breastfeeding benefits are short-term and long-term protection of children against malnutrition and infectious disease (WHO, 2002, 2003).

Effective breastfeeding is achieved when the mother and baby are properly positioned and child is attached to the mother's breast. Breastfeeding is an art that could be learned. It has been documented that very few women

*Corresponding author. E-mail: hunjisha@gmail.com.

breastfeed without difficulty from the first day, but majority encounter problems somewhere along the way (FMOH, 2004; WHO and UNICEF, 2008). These difficulties are due to limited feeding time, lack of sureness or poor attachment of the baby at the breast. Study showed an unsettled, hungry and angry baby, breast engorgement, and maybe obstructed milk ducts and reduced milk production are the most common cause of ineffective breastfeeding (FMOH, 2004; WHO and UNICEF, 2008; Belachew, 2003). Mothers and babies should be comfortable during breastfeeding. Proper child positioning and attachment initiate the production of adequate amounts of breast milk and give comfort to a child during sucking and it helps in preventing sore nipples, engorgement and mastitis. For good attachment and successful breastfeeding, it is important to properly position the baby's body (ThaKre et al., 2012; Goyal et al., 2011; CSA, 2012; FMOH, 2005).

Right positioning and attachment of the baby at the breast are critical in establishing and effective breastfeeding. Early initiation of breastfeeding, skin to skin contact between mothers and babies, breastfeeding on demand, and help with positioning and attaching the baby increase the opportunity of successful breastfeeding. Successful breastfeeding is a result of the appropriate positioning and attachment of the child to the breast (ThaKre et al., 2012; Goyal et al., 2011; CSA, 2012; FMOH, 2005, 2008; Kimani-Murage et al., 2011).

Poor breastfeeding practices have been well documented both in emerging and developed countries. Suboptimal breastfeeding practices like discarding colostrum, overdue initiation of breastfeeding, introduction of dirty and unreliable artificial feeding and poor breastfeeding skills are common constraints to tackling an infant and child mortality in developing countries like Ethiopia (CSA, 2012; FMOH, 2005, 2008; Kimani-Murage et al., 2011).

The baby's head, neck and trunk should be positioned in neutral alignment to optimize breastfeeding performance. Otherwise it compromises an infant's ability to feed effectively, as it disturbs respiratory mechanisms, oral motor control and swallowing. If the baby is not properly attached to the breast, it might cause nipple pain and even damage. Limited feeding can result in engorgement of breast, which in turn can lead to poor attachment (WHO, 2002; FMOH, 2008; Kimani-Murage et al., 2011; WHO and UNICEF, 2009; Heck et al., 2006). Although, many scholars recommend that a proper positioning and attachment technique reduces breastfeeding related problems and increases long-term breastfeeding, no studies have been done in the area of Arba Minch Zuria.

METHODS

Study setting and sample

A cross-sectional community based study was conducted from October 7 to 25, 2013 in Arba Minch Zuria in GamoGofa zone, in the southern part of Ethiopia. The district has an estimated total population of 165,680 of which 82,751 were males and 82,929 were females as it was shown by 2007 published Central Statistical Agency (2008). Nine administrative units (kebeles) were randomly selected from 31 kebeles of the district.

A total of 384 breastfeeding women were included in the study through a single population proportion formula. Since there has been no study done in this area, an estimated 50% prevalence of proper breastfeeding skill and practice was considered with a 5% margin of error, 95% confidence interval. The study included mothers who had children in the last two years and were permanent resident of selected kebeles. Breastfeeding women were randomly selected using a simple random sampling technique.

Data collection procedure

Structured questionnaires and observational-checklist were used to collect socio-demographics characteristics, child feeding practices and environmental health characteristics. Moreover, women's knowledge on breast milk and breastfeeding skills was also included in the questions. Questionnaires were prepared in English and translated to Amharic, then retranslated back to English by language experts who can speak both languages to check its reliability. The questionnaires were pre-tested for simplicity and clarity. Based on pre-test, additional adjustment was made in terminologies and formatting questionnaires.

Statistical analysis

The data were checked for missing values and outliers and entered in double and analysed using SPSS version 16.0. Descriptive statistics like frequencies and proportion were used to describe the study population in relation to relevant variables. Bivariate associations between predictors and breastfeeding skills were described to see the strength of association using odds ratios and 95% of confidence intervals. Then, to identify the predictors of positioning and attachment grade, only variables that were significantly associated with bivariate analyses were entered into the multivariable logistic regression model with good positioning and attachment as a dependent variable. Multicollinearity among independent variables was checked and no multicollinearity was detected (Egata et al., 2013). All tests were two-sided and $P<0.05$ was considered as statistically significant.

The observation was evaluated in accordance with criteria set by national breastfeeding recommendations. If infant body and head is straight; head and body is facing breast and well supported with skin-to-skin contact and if the infant's whole body is supported and all of these four signs are present, breastfeeding skills were graded as well positioned. Missing one or two criteria was graded as average and achieving one criteria or missing all was considered as poor positioning. A child is well attached, if the chin touches the breast and lip is opened widely; lower lip turned downward and areola is more visible above than below. If one of the criteria was not fulfilled, it was considered as an average attachment and achieving one criteria or missing all was considered as poor attachment.

Ethical considerations

Ethical clearance and official permission was obtained from an ethical clearance committee of Arba Minch University and Arba Minch Zuria Woreda administration before the study commenced. And an informed verbal consent was obtained from each study participant for their willingness of participation.

Table 1. Breastfeeding skills in Arbaminch Zuria, 2013.

Breastfeeding skills	Categories	Number (n)	Percent (%)
Positioning grade	Poor positioning	77	20.1
	Average positioning	196	51.2
	Good positioning	110	28.7
Attachment grade	Poor attachment	77	20.1
	Average attachment	197	51.4
	Good attachment	109	28.5

RESULTS

From 384 breastfeeding women, 98.2% gave complete response. The mean (±SD) age of the mothers was 25.08 years (±6.65) with the range of 15 to 40 years. More than one-fourth of infants were well positioned and attached to breast. Inversely, more than one fifth of mothers poorly positioned and attached their infants to breast (Table 1).

Women who had infants below 6 months and 6 to 12 months were 99.92 (AOR=0.03(0.01, 0.11)) and 99.77% (AOR=0.08(0.02, 0.27)) that poorly attached their infants to breast than who had one year and above, respectively. Women who had infants below 6 months were 8 times more well attached (AOR=8.54(8.44, 84.39) than those that had 12 months and above infants (Table 2).

Women who have been informed about the dietary importance of breastfeeding and poorly attached their children to breast were 58% less (AOR=0.42(0.19, 0.93)) than who had no information. Similarly, women who had uneducated husband and poorly attached their children to breast were 99.93% (AOR=0.07(0.01, 0.51)) more than those that had educated husband (Table 3).

Similar to breastfeeding attachment, women who had infants below 6 and 6-12 months were 14% times (AOR=8.14(3.04, 1.87)) more well positioned and 99.02% (AOR=0.08(0.02, 0.26)) less poorly positioned than those that had 12 months and above. Women who had information on breastfeeding and attached their children (AOR=0.42(0.19, 0.94)) poorly to breast were 58% less than those that had no information. Women who gave additional food before 6 months and poorly positioned (AOR=0.44(0.20, 0.97) their children to breast were 56% more than those that did not give additional food (Table 4).

DISCUSSION

The promotion of optimal breastfeeding has been recognized as a global public health concern. Effective breastfeeding is crucial in getting all the benefits of breastfeeding. Breastfeeding has a unique combination of nutritional and immunological benefits for infants and their mothers. Only 28.5% of women appropriately attached their children to breast during breastfeeding, which was relatively low as compared to the study done in Arjo, were 35.97% mothers well attached their children to breast (Tamiru et al., 2012). Similarly, small number of women (28.8%) appropriately positioned their children during breastfeeding which is less than the findings from Jimma Arjo were 33.79% of women appropriately positioned their children during breastfeeding (Rea et al., 1999). As compared to the study done in india, child positioning and attachment during breastfeeding were also relatively low which might be due to lack of knowledge on optimal child feeding practices (ThaKre et al., 2012).

Breastfeeding skills were significantly associated with infant's age, breastfeeding education and paternal educational levels. Women who had infants aged less than 6 months were more appropriately attached and positioned their infants during breastfeeding as compared to those who had one year and above. This might be due to the size of a child, easy to hold and poor breastfeeding skills. This study also showed that an exposure to breastfeeding education had a significant input for proper child attachment to breast. Women who had information on breastfeeding practised relatively less child attachment to breast. This might be due breastfeeding education given along with other health issues for women. Studies from india and other countries also showed that pre-education is a determinant factor of appropriate child feeding practices (WHO, 2002, 2003; Tamiru et al., 2012).

Paternal education level was significantly associated with good attachment of child to breast. This might be due to the influences of husband involvement and psychological support to optimal breastfeeding practices. Fathers with more education are better informed and aware of the benefits of breastfeeding and encourage their wife on optimal breastfeeding. Women need full support of their families and government to feed their children and family appropriately. Studies also found the positive trends of optimal child feeding improvement with paternal education status (Tamiru et al., 2012; Rea et al., 1999; Tamiru et al., 2012; Law et al., 2007; Kristiansen et al., 2010).

Women who attended breastfeeding education and

Table 2. Maternal characteristics and breastfeeding skills in Arba Minch Zuria, 2013.

Characteristics	Categories	Positioning grade			Attachment grade		
		Poor	Average	Good	Poor	Average	Good
		No. (%)	No. (%)	No. (%)	No. (%)	No. (%)	No. (%)
Marital status	Married	75(97.4)	193(98.5)	108(98.2)	75(97.4)	194(98.5)	107(98.2)
	Unmarried	2(2.6)	3(1.5)	2(1.8)	2(2.6)	3(1.5)	2(1.8)
Family size	< 5	39(50.6)	104(53.1)	60(54.5)	39(50.6)	109(55.3)	55(50.5)
	>5	38(49.4)	92(46.9)	50(45.5)	38(49.4)	88(44.7)	54(49.5)
Maternal age (in years)	>20	10(13)	13(6.6)	5(4.5)	10(13.0)	13(6.6)	5(4.6)
	20-24	44(57.1)	117 (59.7)	69 (62.7)	44(57.1)	120(60.9)	66(60.6)
	> 25	23(29.9)	66(33.6)	36(32.8)	23(29.9)	64(32.5)	38(34.9)
Attended Antenatal Care	Yes	66(85.7)	162(82.7)	91(82.7)	66(85.7)	162(82.2)	91(83.5)
	No	11(14.3)	34(17.3)	19(17.3)	11(14.3)	35 (17.8)	18(16.5)
	TBA	35(45.5)	98(50.0)	64(58.2)	35(45.5)	99(50.3)	63(57.8)
Delivery Assistant	Health Workers	12(15.6)	14(7.1)	15(13.6)	12(15.6)	16(8.1)	13(11.9)
	Relatives	30(39.0)	84(42.9)	31(28.2)	30(39.0)	82(41.6)	33(30.3)
Child Age (in months)	0-6	14(18.2)	108(55.1)	46(41.8)	14(18.2)	109(55.3)	45(41.3)
	7-12	41(53.2)	84(42.9)	60(54.5)	41(53.2)	84(42.6)	60(55.0)
	13-24	22(28.6)	4(2.0)	4(3.6)	22(28.6)	4(2.0)	4(3.7)
Delivery Type	Caesarean section	1(1.3)	3(1.5)	2(1.8)	1(1.3)	3(1.5)	2(1.8)
	Vaginal delivery	76(98.7)	193(98.5)	108(98.2)	76(98.7)	194(98.5)	107(98.2)
Place of delivery	Home	71(92.2)	191(97.6)	108(98.2)	71(92.2)	192(97.5)	107(98.2)
	Health institution	6(7.8)	5(2.5)	2(1.8)	6(7.8)	5(2.5)	2(1.8)
Maternal education	No education	48(62.3)	122(62.2)	65(59.1)	48(62.3)	122(61.9)	65(59.6)
	Read and write	14(18.2)	38(19.4)	27(24.5)	14(18.2)	39(19.8)	26(23.9)
	Elementary & above	15(19.5)	36(18.4)	18(16.4)	15(19.5)	36(18.3)	18(16.5)
Ethnicity	Gamo	57(74.0)	149(76.0)	93()84.5	57(74.0)	154(78.2)	88(80.7)
	Wolaita	5(6.5)	12(6.1)	2(1.8)	5(6.5)	12(6.1)	2(1.8)
	Others *	15(19.5)	35(17.9)	15(13.6)	15(19.5)	31(15.7)	19(17.4)
Farm land owners	No	54(70.1)	154(78.6)	81(73.6)	54(70.1)	153(77.7)	82(75.2)
	Yes	23(29.9)	42(21.4)	29(26.4)	23(29.9)	44(22.3)	27(24.8)
Religion	Protestant	51(66.2)	119(60.7)	64(58.2)	51(66.2)	119(60.4)	64(58.7)
	Orthodox Christian	24(31.2)	71(36.2)	43(39.1)	24(31.2)	72(36.5)	42(38.5)
	Others**	2(2.6)	6(3.1)	3(2.7)	2(2.6)	6(3.0)	3(2.8)

*Zeyse, Amhara, Ganta, Gofa; ** Muslim, Traditional.

poorly positioned their children to breast were less than those that did not attend, this could be due to health extension support. This shows that basic education in the promotion of optimal breast-feeding should be heartened. Studies also showed health education given at different juncture regarding breastfeeding practices is the predetermining factors to promote optimal breastfeeding practices (WHO, 2002, 2003; Rea et al., 1999).

Women who introduced complementary food early and poorly positioned their children to breast were 56% more than those that did not introduce complementary food early. This might be due to complementing of breastfeeding with food and maternal gap of knowledge on the breastfeeding skills. Studies from Arjo and national report also demonstrated that maternal knowledge and their educational status has significant input on optimal child feeding practices (FMOH, 2005; Rea et al., 1999).

Conclusions

More than one-fifth of women poorly positioned and attached their children to breast as compared to national and international recommendations. Poor breastfeeding skills were significantly associated with infant's age, pre-education on the benefits of breastfeeding and educational status of husband. Hence, sustained community based nutritional education were recommended for pregnant and lactating mothers to encourage optimal breastfeeding skills during the period of attending health care and community meeting through education on breastfeeding using health extension

Table 3. Factors associated with breastfeeding attachment during breastfeeding in Arba Minch Zuria, 2013.

Variables	Categories	Attachment grade during breastfeeding					
		Poor attachment		Average attachment		Good attachment	
		COR	AOR (95%CI)	COR	AOR	COR	AOR (95%CI)
Maternal education	No education	0.74	0.40(0.07, 2.27)	1.51	1.44(0.36, 5.78)	1.11	2.01(0.25, 16.06)
	Read and write	0.54	0.39(0.07, 2.25)	1.23	1.24(0.30, 5.09)	0.81	1.77(0.21, 14.88)
	Elementary	0.83	0.65(0.11, 3.73)	1.67	1.43(0.34, 6.05)	2.00	2.23(0.29, 16.94)
	High school	1	1	1	1	1	1
ANC Follow up	Yes	1.21	1.32(0.48, 3.64)	0.83	0.80(0.37, 1.74)	1.42	2.44(0.71, 8.40)
	No	1	1	1	1	1	1
Child age	Below 6	0.05**	0.03(0.01, 0.11)**	1.96	1.59(0.36, 7.01)	1.99	1.05(1.01, 2.42)
	6 to 12	0.12**	0.08(0.02, 0.27)**	1.07	0.80(0.18, 0.49)	1.42	8.54(8.44, 84.39)
	Above 12	1	1	1	1	1	1
Maternal age	>20	3.00	4.23(0.68,26.35)	1.20	1.52(0.32, 7.16)	0.90	1.05(0.12,9.10)
	20-24	1.02	0.99(0.24, 4.19)	0.89	1.07(0.35, 3.31)	0.50	0.45(0.10, 2.12)
	25-29	0.89	0.69(0.15, 3.15)	0.71	0.77(0.24, 2.47)	0.56	0.48(0.10,2.42)
	≥30	1	1	1	1	1	1
Having a radio	Yes	0.86	0.77(0.37, 1.62)	1.14	1.16(0.66, 2.04)	0.68	0.65(0.26, 1.62)
	No	1	1	1	1	1	1
Breastfeeding refusal	Yes	0.87	1.10(0.29, 1.10)	1.34	0.96(0.37, 2.51)	2.16	2.71(0.75, 9.74)
	No	1	1	1	1	1	1
EBF knowledge	Yes	1.68	1.41(0.42, 4.76)	1.93*	1.93(0.69, 5.42)	3.53**	1.61(0.39, 6.70)
	No	1	1	1	1	1	1
EBF to 6 months	Yes	0.56	0.58(0.12, 2.90)	0.71	0.46(0.11, 1.90)	0.19(*	0.25(0.05, 1.19)
	No	1		1	1	1	1
Breastfeeding information	Yes	0.61	0.42(0.19, 0.93)*	1.18	1.16(0.59, 2.26)	0.44*	0.41(0.16, 1.07)
	No	1		1	1	1	1
Breastfeeding initiation	Within 1 hour	0.60	0.65(0.32, 1.33)	0.57	0.62(0.36, 1.07)	0.73	1.15(0.50, 2.68)
	After one hour	1	1	1	1	1	1
Giving additional food	Yes	0.92	0.69(0.25, 1.91)	0.47	0.59(0.28, 1.25)	0.48	0.47(0.16, 1.34)
	No	1	1	1	1	1	1
Twins	Yes	2.84	2.45(0.19,32.16)	2.12	2.34(0.21,25.60)	5.54	6.77(0.48, 96.53)
	No	1		1	1	1	1
Breastfeeding frequency	Below 8	2.25	2.73(0.19, 6.30)	1.01	0.90(0.50, 1.61)	1.12	1.37(0.56, 3.35)
	8 and above	1	1	1	1	1	1
Paternal education	No education	0.41	0.77(0.11, 5.43)	0.61	0.44(0.09, 2.23)	0.20*	0.07(0.01, 0.51)**
	Reading and writing	0.20	0.46(0.06, 3.39)	0.57	0.60(0.12, 3.11)	0.14*	0.08(0.01, 0.59)**
	Elementary	0.30	0.38(0.06, 2.36)	0.63	0.50(0.11, 2.37)	0.26	0.23(0.04, 1.35)
	High school &above	1	1	1	1	1	1
Deliver assistant	TBA	0.63	0.48(0.22, 1.02)	0.50*	0.49(0.27, 0.86)*	1.57	1.48(0.60, 3.66)
	Health Workers	1.02	0.58(0.19, 1:81)	0.53	0.54(0.22, 1.35)	0.25	0.23(0.03, 2.20)
	Relatives	1	1	1	1	1	1

*Significant at <0.05; **significant at <0.01; COR: crude odd ratio; AOR: adjusted odd ratio.

Table 4. Factors associated with child positioning during breastfeeding in Arba Minch Zuria, 2013.

Variables	Categories	Child positioning Grade during breastfeeding					
		Poor positioning		Average positioning		Good positioning	
		COR	AOR (95%CI)	COR	AOR (95%CI)	COR	AOR (95%CI)
Maternal education	No education	0.74	0.44(0.08, 2.53)	1.46	1.54(0.37, 6.34)	1.25	3.55(0.45, 27.66)
	Reading and writing	0.52	0.37(0.06, 2.17)	1.00	0.94(0.22, 3.96)	1.22	2.97(0.37, 23.41)
	Elementary	0.83	0.69(0.12, 3.99)	1.75	1.61(0.37, 6.87)	1.75	2.39(0.31, 18.30)
	High school	1	1	1	1	1	1
ANC Follow up	Yes	1.27	1.33(0.46, 3.65)	0.90	0.82(0.37, 1.82)	1.43	2.04(0.64, 6.42)
	No	1	1	1	1	1	1
Child age	Below 6	0.05*	0.03(0.01, 0.10)*	1.89	1.48(0.33, 6.57)	1.71*	8.14(3.04, 1.87)*
	6 to 12	0.12*	0.08(0.02, 0.26)*	0.97	0.69(0.15, 3.04)	1.63*	7.81(6.81, 8.81)**
	Above 12	1	1	1	1	1	1
Maternal age	>20	3.0	4.14(0.66,26.05)	1.20	1.47(0.30, 7.11)	0.90	1.29(0.15, 11.11)
	20-24	0.98	0.94(0.22, 3.99)	0.82	0.94(0.29, 2.97)	0.50	0.48(0.10, 2.26)
	25-29	0.95	0.75(0.16, 3.44	0.70	0.72(0.21, 2.40)	0.85	0.89(0.18, 4.38)
	≥30	1	1	1	1	1	1
Having a radio	Yes	0.81	0.68(0.32, 1.43)	1.07	1.00(0.55, 1.78)	0.62	0.44(0.18, 1.06)
	No	1	1	1	1	1	1
BF refusal	Yes	0.87	1.11(0.29, 4.26)	1.32	0.90(0.33, 2.44)	2.23	3.17(0.92, 10.84)
	No		1	1	1		1
EBF knowledge	Yes	1.21	1.62(0.48, 5.41)	2.46*	2.68(0.91, 7.89)	1.08	2.11(0.53, 8.33)
	No	1	1	1	1	1	1
EBF to 6 months	Yes	0.70	0.71(0.15, 3.37)	0.97	0.58(0.14, 2.41)	0.27*	0.39(0.08, 1.79)
	No	1	1	1	1	1	1
Breastfeeding information	Yes	0.66	0.42(0.19, 0.94)	1.34	1.24(0.62, 2.46)	0.55	0.47(0.18, 1.19)
	No	1	1	1	1	1	1
Breastfeeding initiation	Within 1 hour	0.57	0.61(0.29, 1.24)	0.53	0.57(0.32, 0.99)	0.60	0.86(0.38, 1.92)
	After one hour	1	1	1	1	1	1
Giving additional food	Yes	0.76	0.56(0.19, 1.58)	0.36	0.44(0.20, 0.97)	0.36	0.32(0.11, 1.90)
	No	1	1	1	1	1	1
Twins	Yes	1.42	1.27(0.14,11.11)	0.74	0.78(0.09, 6.68)	2.40	2.96(0.31, 28.61)
	No	1	1	1	1	1	1
Breastfeeding frequency	Below 8	2.13	2.55(0.10, 5.90)	0.97	0.85(0.46, 1.55)	0.89	0.99(0.43, 2.297)
	8 and above	1	1	1	1	1	1
Paternal education	No education	0.39	0.67(0.09, 4.73)	0.55	0.36(0.07, 1.85)	0.19*	0.04(0.01, 1.35)**
	Reading and writing	0.25	0.49(0.06, 3.66)	0.55	0.68(0.13, 3.63)	0.23	0.09(0.01, 1.66)
	Elementary school	0.31	0.38(0.06, 2.39)	0.62	0.49(0.10, 2.33)	0.33	0.27(0.04, 1.61)
	High school and above	1	1	1	1	1	1
Deliver assistant	TBA	0.58	0.46(0.21, 1.00)	0.45*	0.45(0.25,0.83)**	1.14	1.31(0.56, 3.04)
	Health Workers	0.83	0.50(0.16, 1.53)	0.41*	0.43(0.17, 1.09)	1.37*	0.74(0.07, 4.23)
	Relatives	1	1	1	1	1	1

*Significant at <0.05; **significant at <0.01; COR: crude odd ratio; AOR: adjusted odd ratio.

workers, religious personel and development army as key actors.

CONFLICT OF INTERESTS

The authors have not declared any conflict of interest.

ACKNOWLEDGEMENTS

The authors sincerely thank the Arba Minch University, that financially supported this study. They also thank the data collectors. Last but not the least, the authors also thank the mothers who gave their valuable time during data collection.

REFERENCES

Belachew T (2003). Human Nutrition for Health Science Students Jimma, 2003. Published by: Jimma University, Faculty of Public Health.

Central Statistical Agency (CSA) (2008). Summary of statistical report of 2007; Population and housing census. Addis Ababa: CSA; 2008 Available at: www.csa.gov.et/newcsaweb/images/ documents/pdf

Central Statistical Authority (CSA) (2012). Ethiopia Demographic and HealthSurvey 2011. Addis Ababa and Calverton: CSA; 2012 Available at: www.unicef.org/ethiopia/ET_2011_EDHS.pdf

Egata G, Berhane Y, Worku A (2013). Predictors of non-exclusive breastfeeding at 6 months among rural mothers in east Ethiopia: A community-based analytical cross-sectional study. Int. Breastfeed. J. 8:8.

Federal Ministry of Health (FMOH) (2005). National strategy for child survival in Ethiopia. Addis Ababa: FMOH; 2005. Available at: http://can-mnch.ca/wp-content/uploads/2012/09/National-Strategy-for-Child-Survival-in-Ethiopia.pdf

Federal Ministry of Health (FMOH) (2008). Program Implementation Manual of National Nutrition Program. Addis Ababa: FMOH; 2008. Available at: www.pronutrition.org/files/Ethiopia_NutHIV_ Manual_ 2008.pdf

Federal Ministry of Health: National strategy for infant and young child feeding. Addis Ababa: (FMOH) (2004). Available at: http://www.aedlinkagesethiopia.org/My_Homepage_Files/IYCFStrategy.pdf

Goyal RC, Banginwar AS, Ziyo F, Toweir AA (2011). Breastfeeding practices: Positioning, attachment (latch-on) and effective suckling-A hospital-based study in Libya. J. Fam. Commun. Med. 18(2):74.

Heck K, Braveman P, Cubbin C, Chavez, G, Kiely J (2006). Socioeconomic Status and Breastfeeding Initiation among California Mothers. Public Health Rep. 121(1):51-59.

Kimani-Murage E, Madise N, Fotso J, Kyobutungi C, Mutua M, Gitau T, Yatich N (2011). Patterns and determinants of breastfeeding and complementary feeding practices in urban informal settlements, Nairobi Kenya. BMC Public Health 11:396.

Kristiansen AL, Lande B, Øverby NC, Andersen LF (2010). Factors associated with exclusive breast-feeding and breast-feeding in Norway. Public Health Nutr. 13(12):2087-2096.

Law SM, Dunn OM, Wallace LM, Inch SA (2007). Breastfeeding Best Start study: training midwives in a 'hands off'positioning and attachment intervention. Maternal Child Nutr. 3(3):194-205.

Rea MF, Venancio SI, Martines JC, Savage F (1999). Counselling on breastfeeding: assessing knowledge and skills. Bull. World Health Organ. 77:492-498.

Tamiru D, Belachew T, Loha E, Mohammed S (2012). Sub-optimal breastfeeding of infants during the first six months and associated factors in rural communities of Jimma Arjo Woreda, Southwest Ethiopia. BMC Public Health 12(1):363.

Thakre SB, Thakre SS, Ughade SM, Golawar S, Thakre AD, Kale P (2012). The breastfeeding practices: the positioning and attachment initiative among the mothers of rural Nagpur. J. Clin. Diagn. Res. 6(7):1215-1218.

WHO and UNICEF (2008). Strengthening action to improve the feeding of infants and young children 6-23 months of age in nutrition and child health programmes. Geneva: WHO; 2OO8 Available at: www.unicef.org/nutrition/files/BFHI_2009_s3.1and2

WHO and UNICEF (2009). Breastfeeding promotion and support in a baby-friendly hospital. Geneva: WHO; 2OO9. Available at: www.unicef.org/nutrition/files/BFHI_2009_s3.1and2

World Health Organization (WHO) (2002). The optimal duration of exclusive breastfeeding: A systematic review. Geneva: WHO; 2002. Available at: http://www.who.int/nutrition/publications/infantfeeding/WHO_NHD_01.08 /en/

World Health Organization (WHO) (2003). Global Strategy for Infant and Young Child Feeding. A joint WHO/UNICEF statement. Geneva: WHO; 2003. Available at: www.who.int/nutrition/publications/gs_infantfeeding.

Pain as 5th vital sign: impact of pain assessment training program on Nigerian nurses' knowledge of pain management

Patricia Obiajulu Onianwa[1], Temitope O. Alonge[2], Jesse A. Otegbayo[2], Elizabeth U. Ike[2], Felicia O. Chukura[2], Olufunke O. Are[2], Folashade O. M. Akanbi[2], Mary O. Ayorinde[2*], Iyanuoluwa O. Adubi[2] and Olaoluwa S. Yaya[3]

[1]Department of Clinical Nursing, University College Hospital Ibadan, Ibadan, Nigeria.
[2]Department of Medicine, University College Hospital Ibadan, Ibadan, Nigeria.
[3]Department of Statistics, University of Ibadan, Ibadan, Nigeria.

Pain is subjective and it can only be described by the individual experiencing it. It is the main reason why people seek medical help. Nurses play a major role in the management of pain; hence they must be highly knowledgeable to ensure their practices are of high quality. The aim of this study was to evaluate the impact of Nurses' Pain Educational Program (NPEP) on nurses' knowledge of pain management. The quantitative design was employed in the study; five lectures on the Nurses Pain Educational Program (NPEP) were conducted for 500 nurses. All participants were given 15 items questionnaires in a pre and post test design. The study location was the University College Hospital Ibadan and the duration of the study was between March to December, 2015. The pre and post-test on nurses' knowledge were analyzed using descriptive and inferential statistics and the overall improvement in knowledge and management of pain was analyzed using the student t-test. The participants were divided into groups; each group was trained for two days in a week using the Nurses Pain Educational Program Package (NPEP). Findings revealed an improvement in knowledge which was found to be statistically significant (*P* < 0.000). This was evident by the results of the pre-test and post-test values; pre-test mean score was 2.6 ± 0.05 while that of the post test score was 4.0 ± 0.04. This indicated that knowledge was impacted. The Nurses Pain Educational Program had a positive effect on nurses' knowledge of pain assessment and pain management.

Key words: Nurses' Pain Education Program (NPEP), nursing, pain management.

INTRODUCTION

Pain is a universal experience, and it is the most frequent reason why people seek health care. It is described as the way the brain interprets information about a particular sensation that the body is experiencing (Ojong et al.,

*Corresponding author. E-mail: niksem@yahoo.com.

2014).

Mansour et al. (2016), stated that quality of life and performance of patients is worsened if pain is under diagnosed by health care providers. There is a growing recognition that pain is a complex experience, yet it is among the most neglected and under-treated amidst patient's complaints (Ali and Thompson, 2009). According to Zhang et al. (2008), inadequate treatment of pain is a pervasive clinical problem in hospitalized patients, resulting in significant physiological, psychological, and financial consequences which include poor recovery, a higher rate of complications, anxiety, sleep disturbance, and lowered quality of life.

In a study conducted by Nahin (2015), it was estimated that within a previous three-month period, 25 million U.S. adults had daily chronic pain, and 23 million more reported severe pain. Those with serious pain need and use more health care services and suffer a greater disability than persons with less severe pain (America Society of Pain, 2015).

The International Association of the Study of Pain (IASP) (2011) defines pain as an unpleasant, sensory, emotional and subjective experience associated with tissue damage. Also, Puntillo et al. (2008), stated in their article, that pain is what the patient experiencing it says it is. Patients can experience pain from preexisting diseases, invasive procedures and trauma. If ineffectively managed, acute pain can lead to negative physiological and psychological ramifications, including the development of chronic pain syndromes (Kehlet et al., 2006; Bower and Reuter, 2009). Despite substantial advances in pain research and management, people continue to suffer because of inadequate pain assessment and pain control, thereby leaving gaps in the quality and safety of pain management provided to patients (International Association for the Study of Pain, 2011). Pain that is not well controlled can lead to discomfort and suffering which can include unwanted consequences such as delayed healing, an increased risk of morbidity, a prolonged hospital stay, and the risk of developing chronic persistent pain (Wells et al., 2008; Morton and Fontaine, 2013).

Nurses play a pivotal role in the assessment, relief, and evaluation of pain. Maintaining an optimal level of comfort for patients is a universal goal for physicians and nurses because pain is one of the major experiences that can minimize patient comfort (Kizza et al., 2016). The consequences of unrelieved pain can be devastating as opined in a survey by the National Health Service (NHS) trusts in England (2007) that reported 67% of patients experienced pain whilst in hospital; despite relief efforts, this experience can be reduced if nurses have adequate knowledge of pain assessment and management.

In achieving the goal of pain management, nurses have numerous responsibilities and shouls have adequate knowledge required (Craige, 2014; Coulling, 2005; Courtenay and Carey, 2008). Zhang et al. (2008) stated that many nurses lack pain management knowledge and a varying number of studies indicated knowledge deficits and inadequate pain assessment as the most important barriers for health care professionals in implementing pain management. Bakshi et al. (2014), posit that pain education for health professionals at all levels has been repeatedly identified as an important step to changing ineffective pain management practices.

According to Khomerian et al. (2006), nurses' theoretical knowledge influences their ability to meet practice expectation in order to improve quality care. Nursing education has evolved to meet the changing demand in health care, of which continuing educational program is one such effective method of educating nurses in pain management, since there is a major poor performance in pain assessment and management (Latchman, 2014).

In Nigeria, no study has been done to evaluate the nurses' knowledge of pain assessment and management, compared to other developing countries such as Uganda and Zimbabwe, where nurses' knowledge and practice related to pain assessment and management were studied. In Zimbabwe registered nurses had low knowledge levels and poor attitude regarding pain management of adult medical patients (Manwere et al., 2015). Also, in a study conducted in Uganda by Kizza et al. (2016), nurses generally had adequate knowledge about pain assessment principle, but there was a lack of knowledge about some key concepts such as value for patients' autonomy in pain assessment and pre-emptive analgesia concepts. This knowledge gap may affect their ability to provide quality pain assessment and management.

However, it was observed in University College Hospital Ibadan that most patients who were present in the hospital have mild, moderate to severe pain which is not measured to know the quality and intensity. Pain is managed in this institution using multidisciplinary approach which had little effect on patients' recovery. This is due to inadequate knowledge on pain management and assessment of the health care provider. It was also observed that nurses have a poor attitude towards pain assessment and management, for example by fostering patient addiction to opiates. In pain control nurses play an essential role, however, in order to meet with practice expectation nurses need to have adequate effective training in pain assessment/management which brought about the need for NPEP.

Therefore, evaluating the impact of Nurses' Pain Educational Program (NPEP) on nurses' knowledge of pain management is a paramount step in constructing a foundation for better strategies in effective management of pain, ensuring patients' comfort and ultimate improvement of nursing practice in giving quality care to patients. Findings from this study will add important information to the literature regarding nurses' knowledge on pain management/assessment in Nigeria and also assist in designing continuing professional development programs for nurses in clinical settings to further scale up their pain assessment skills of clients towards ensuring total quality /holistic care. The objectives of the study includes: 1, general objective which is to evaluate the impact of Nurses' Pain Educational Program (NPEP) on nurses' knowledge of pain management and 2 the specific objective which includes to assess the knowledge of clinical nurses on pain management and to evaluate the impact of the training on clinical Nurses' knowledge.

METHODS

A pre and post-test intervention study was used to evaluate the impact of Nurses' Pain Educational Program (NPEP) on nurses' knowledge of pain management in the University College Hospital Ibadan. Samples of 500 nurses were selected using systematic random sampling. Data was collected using a self administered structured questionnaire which was developed after an extensive literature review. The questionnaire consists of two sections; section A assessed the demographic data of nurses and section B assessed the knowledge of nurses on pain assessment and management. The content validity of the research instrument was examined by expert in pain management in the University College Hospital Ibadan. Approval for the study was obtained from the management board of University College Hospital. The questionnaires were anonymous and the nurses consented to participate in the study. Data analysis was performed using statistical package for social sciences version (SPSS) 22.0.

Descriptive and inferential statistics were employed in analyzing the significance level of $p < 0.05$ data.

Sampling technique

A systemic random sampling method was used to select 500 nurses that participated in the training out of 1195 nurses in the setting. The nurses were divided into 28 groups and each group contained 17-18 nurses. The selected nurses participated in pain assessment training for a period of 28 weeks. The group's nucleus members included all cadres of nurses. This same set of nurses had two days training in a week lasting 4-5 h daily: Day 1 all participants were given a set of questions with a participant specific code and were allotted 30 min to answer 15 questions prior to the beginning of the training to access their basic knowledge on pain management. This was followed by training and a practicum section using hypothetical cases. This same set of questions was answered at the end of the training to ascertain if knowledge was impacted; Day 2 included training and practicum demonstration on patients on the use of pain assessment tools. Consent was taken and patient who volunteered was used for the demonstration and the nurses pain assessment skills were assessed. After which they were requested to answer the same set of questions as a post test at the end of teaching activities. The practicum demonstrated assessment of the patient's level pain by using various pain rating scales. The training also instructed the group members in the correct way to document the pain ratings, pain quality, pain location and impact of pain on a Pain Assessment Record Booklet (PARB). The participant code was used to identify each participant's pre and post tests.

The educational package for the training

The Nurses' Pain Educational Program (NPEP) aimed to promote nurses' knowledge regarding pain measurement and management and build nurses' skills to perform better pain management behaviors (such as use a pain assessment tool in clinical practice). The NPEP consist of two components: an education program and clinical demonstration to implement pain assessment and management. To ensure administrative support of NPEP, a pain assessment group was led by the principal investigator and the nursing staff of the Continuing Education/ Research Unit. The NPEP intervention included, focused education, group activity, and individual instruction. Teaching materials included handbook, standardized pain assessment materials and a pocket numeric pain rating / Wong baker pain scale tool. The standardized procedure for assessing pain using the numeric pain rating / Wong baker pain scale tool were provided to nurses in every unit.

The Nurses' Pain Educational Program Package included five lectures on: introduction to pain; concept of pain and pain assessment; common myths about pain; pain assessment tools; newly Modified Vital signs Chart to include pain as the 5th vital signs.

Instruments for data collection

The instrument for data collection is a self-administered questionnaire for the pre and post assessment. The questionnaire items were structured to collect information about: Section A, the socio-demographic characteristics of nurses which addresses participant age, sex, years of experience level of education and nurses' professional cadres; Section B: addressed questions on nurses' knowledge of pain assessment tools and pain management.

RESULTS

As shown in Table 1, the sex distribution of the participants' shows that majority 467(96.9%) were females. The participant mean age was 40±7.1years, majority of the participants had above 10yrs of experience 179 (37.1). The professional qualification of the nurses shows that 82.0% were registered nurses/ midwife (RN/RM), 17.4% had a degree in nursing while 0.6% had Master degree in nursing. Professional cadres of nurses revealed that 34.6% of the nurses were Nursing Officer I&II (NOI& NOII), 7.9% were Senior Nursing Officer (SNO), 36.5% were Assistant Chief Nursing Officer (ACNO), 20.3% were Chief Nursing Officer (CNO) and 0.6% were Assistant Director of Nursing(ADN).

As reflected in Table 2, the mean score of the pre and post-test of the participant revealed significant difference with t value = -22.039 and p = 0.000.

In Table 3, the mean score of the pre and post-test of the participant demonstration skills revealed significant difference with t value = -7.249 and p = 0.000.

DISCUSSION

A total of 482 questionnaires was retrieved which gives

Table 1. Socio-demographic characteristics of nurses.

Variables	Level	Frequency	Percentage
Sex	Male	15	3.1
	Female	467	96.9
Total		482	100.0
Age in years(M=40.1,SD=7.1)	25-30	17	3.5
	31-35	125	25.9
	36-40	126	26.1
	41-45	101	21.0
	46-50	69	14.3
	51-55	34	7.1
	56-60	10	2.1
Total		482	100.0
Year of experience	1-5 years	136	28.2
	6-10 years	167	34.6
	Above 10 years	179	37.1
Total		482	100.0
Level of Education	RN/RM	395	82.0
	BNSc	84	17.4
	MSc	3	0.6
Total		482	100.0
Professional Cadre	NO I/NO II	167	34.6
	SNO	38	7.9
	ACNO	176	36.5
	CNO	98	20.3
	AND	3	0.6
Total		482	100.0

Table 2. Pretest and Posttest mean scores of nurses' level of knowledge on pain management.

Parameter	Mean ± SE	SD	T	P-value
Pre-test	2.6307±0.04551	0.99924	-22.039	0.000***
Post-test	4.0228±0.04380	0.96158		

96.4% participation rate, the majority of the nurses were within the age bracket of 36 to 40 years which gives 26.1%; this could be due to the fact that this age range lies within the productive age in the workforce in the hospital. Female nurses constitute 96.9% of the target sampled. The high percentage of female nurses in this study revealed nursing as a female dominated profession in Nigeria. The majority of the nurses had above ten years of professional experience (37.1%) and had attained diploma level (82.0%) of education in nursing. Also, majority of the nurses that participated in the study happens to be an Assistant Chief Nursing Officer (ACNO) (36.5%), who are wards managers in various wards thereby enabling them to become trainers.

The results of the pre-test showed a deficiency in the baseline pain knowledge amongst the participants (2.6 ± 0.05) while that of the post test score was 4.0± 0.04; this show an improvement in knowledge which was found to be statistically significant ($p < 0.000$). A similar finding was found by Ellis et al. (2007) in a study, to examine the

Table 3. Pretest and Posttest mean scores of the nurses' skill demonstration on pain management.

Parameter	Mean ±SE	SD	T	P-value
Pretest	1.4667 ± 0.18404	1.00801	-7.249	0.000***
Posttest	3.1± 0.12999	0.71197	-	-

implementation of a comprehensive program to improve the practices of pain management in a pediatric hospital. They reported a statistically significant improvement in their pain assessment and management practice after the implementation of the program with the p=0.004, 0.17 respectively as opposed to a study by Kaur (2017), on knowledge and attitude regarding pain management among staff nurses at Kular Hospital, Bija (Punjab), where nurse were reported to have average knowledge and attitudes towards pain management.

Furthermore, in a related study by Odutayo et al. (2013), on impact of an educational program on the use of standardized nursing languages for nursing documentation among public health nurses in Nigeria, a significant difference with the t value = -27.61, d.f. 99, p = 0.0001 in the mean score of pretest and posttest of their experimental group was reported which also revealed that knowledge was impacted. However, Ho et al. (2013), in their study reported that respondents possessed good knowledge (99.12±14.810) and attitude (66.00±10.415) towards pain management after an educational program.

This shows that, health practitioners, including nurses, would embrace and implement new ideas and practices, such as the use of pain assessment tools, if they are informed, educated, and have a congruent understanding of the relevant concepts. This is in line with the American Nurses Association (2006) which states that nurses would acquire adequate knowledge when trained consistently through seminars/workshops, in-service training, and higher education.

Regarding the evaluation on the impact of the training on clinical Nurses' knowledge, result revealed that nurses had good demonstration of the use of pain rating tools with a mean score 3.1±0.1 post test. The result also showed a significant difference in the pretest and posttest with t= -7.249, p= 0.000. This result is similar to a study in Uganda by Kizza (2012), that almost all the nurses knew the pain assessment tool (90%), assessment and documentation of pain are very important (93%) and averagely, the nurses scored 71.8% with a median score of 71.43% on theoretical knowledge. This as well also indicates that nurses have reasonable knowledge about pain assessment tools. The findings from this study support the opinion of Williams (2007), that when nurses have a good knowledge of pain their patients receive a higher standard of pain assessment and management. This is because knowledge is an important factor that brings about change.

On the contrary, in a study by Rampanjoto et al. (2007), more than three quarters of nurses could not assess pain using the provided Visual Analogue Scale. This may imply that provision of tools and presence of a protocol on how to use them are not enough to ensure the use of the tools. There is increasing evidence on the effect of continuing education programs on pain assessment practices (Bedard et al., 2006; Abdalrahim, 2009). For example, in Jordan a well planned and implemented education program conducted for nurses coupled with supervision of the application of knowledge shows that nurses developed a habit of assessing post-operative pain intensity using numerical rating scales and improved documentation practices (Abdalrahim, 2009).

Limitation

Undoubtedly, the study was confronted with some limitations that need to be addressed in further studies that have a similar focus. One of the major limitations of the study was the use of a questionnaire as a self-report assessment tool designed to tap information on variables in the study. We report this as a limitation because respondents can fake their responses in order to present themselves in a desired manner, which could affect the general opinion of the subject matter in the population sampled. The study was also limited to the clinical nurses only.

CONCLUSION AND RECOMMENDATION

The questionnaire study found that the current knowledge about pain assessment and management is deficient and with the introduction of the nurses' pain educational program, there was a positive effect on nurses' knowledge, practice, and demonstration related to pain assessment and pain management.

Based on the findings from this study, there is need to design and implement a continuous professional education program on pain and its assessment with special focus on the methods of assessment, guidelines, protocols and documentation of pain in patients. In addition, we recommend that the management of the hospitals should continually supply tools, charts and protocols for pain management and assessment. Implementation of these recommendations will require a multifaceted approach which will combine input from the hospital management, nurse leaders in conjunction with clinical nurse-educators of the continuing education unit.

To ensure the proper and continued use of tools, protocols and charts, there is a need for a supportive environment which can be attained through improving staffing, provision of monitoring and support supervision by experienced and skilled nurses.

A study employing mixed methods involving more than one hospital is recommended to gain more insight on the knowledge and practices of nurses related to pain assessment so that the study could be more generalized. The study was also limited to the clinical nurses only. It was also observed that, some of the nurses did not return the questionnaires which led to the reduction in sample size. There is a need for more research in Nigeria on how pain assessment tools can be adapted to client care and the impact of pain management on client care.

CONFLICT OF INTERESTS

The authors declare that they have no financial or personal relationships that may have inappropriately influenced them in writing this article.

ACKNOWLEDGEMENTS

We thank the management of the University College Hospital, Ibadan-Nigeria, the Department of Medicine and staff of the clinical Nursing Department. Their support and motivation has helped us to achieve this level of excellence in our project.

REFERENCES

Abdalrahim MS (2009). Postoperative pain assessment and management; the effects of educational program of Jordanian nurses' practices, knowledge and attitudes. Available at: https://gupea.ub.gu.se/handle/2077/20316

Ali N, Thompson DA (2009). Comparison of the knowledge of chronic pain and its management between final year physiotherapy and medical student. Eur. J. Pain 13:38-50.

America Society of Pain (2015). NIH study shows the prevalence of chronic or severe pain in US adults. Available at: http://americanpainsociety.org/about-us/press-room/nih-study-shows-prevalence-of-chronic-or-severe-pain-in-u-s-adults

American Nurses Association (2006). ANA recognized terminologies and data element sets. Available at: https://www.scribd.com/document/54800799/ANA-Recognized-Terminologies-and-Data-Element-Sets

Bakshi SE, Jain PN, Kannan S (2014). An assessment of basic pain knowledge and impact of pain education on Indian anesthesiologists-a pre and post questionnaire study. Indian J. Anesth. 58(2):127-131.

Bedard D, Purden M, Certosini C (2006). The pain experience of post-surgical patients following implementation of evidence based approach pain management. Nursing 7(3):80-92.

Bower TC, Reuter JP (2009). Analgesia sedation and neuromuscular blockade in the trauma patient. Quillam, KA, Makic MBF, Whalen E, eds. Trauma nursing from resuscitation through rehabilitation. 4th edition. Philadelphia: Saunders, Elsevier, pp. 372-421. Available at: https://musculoskeletalkey.com/analgesia-sedation-and neuromuscular-blockade-in-the-trauma-patient/

Coulling S (2005). Nurses' and doctors' knowledge of pain after surgery. Nurs. Standard 19(34):41-49.

Courtenay M, Carey N (2008). The impact and effectiveness of nurse-led care in the management of acute and chronic pain: a review of the literature. J. Clin. Nurs. 17(15):2001-2013.

Craig JA (2014). Nursing Knowledge and Attitudes toward Pain Management. Gardner-Webb University. Available at: http://digitalcommons.gardner-webb.edu/nursing_etd/8/

Ellis JA, McCleary L, Blouin R, Dube K, Rowley B, MacNeil M, Cooke C (2007). Implementing best practice pain management in a pediatric hospital. J. Spec. Pediatr. Nurs. 12(4):264-277.

Ho SE, Ho CC, Pang Yuen H, Lexshimi R, Choy YC, Jaafar MZ, Cardosa M, Das S (2013). A study of knowledge and attitudes of registered nurses towards pain management in an urban hospital. Clin. Ter. 164(3):215-219.

International Association for the Study of Pain (IASP) (2011). Pain terminology: A list with definitions and notes on usage. Changes in 2011. Pain, pp. 209-214. https://www.iasp-pain.org/Education/Content.aspx?ItemNumber=1698

Kehlet H, Jensen TS, Woolf CJ (2006). Persistent postsurgical pain: risk factors and prevention. Lancet 367(9522):1618-1625.

Khomeiran RT, Yekta ZP, Kiger AM, Ahmadi F (2006). Professional competence: factors described by nurses as influencing their development. Int. Nurs. Rev. 53(1):66-72.

Kizza IB (2012). Nurses' knowledge of the principles of acute pain assessment in critically ill adult patients who are able to self report. 20-27. MSN (Critical Care and Trauma) Dissertation Muhimbili University of Health and Allied Sciences November 2012.

Kizza IB, Muliira JB, Kohi TW, Nabirye RS (2016). Nurses' knowledge of the principles of acute pain assessment in critically ill adult patients who are able to self report. Int. J. Africa Nurs. Sci. 4:20-27.

Kaur K (2017). Knowledge and Attitude Regarding Pain Management among Staff Nurses. Nurs. Care Open Access J. 2(1):00024.

Latchman J (2014). Improving pain management at the nursing education level: Evaluating knowledge and attitude. J. Adv. Pract. Oncol. 5(1):10-16.

Manwere A, Chipfuwa T, Mukwamba M.M, Chironda G (2015). Knowledge and Attitude of Registered Nurses towards pain management of adult medical patients: A case of Bindura Hospital. Health Sci. J. 9(4):3.

Mansour A, Fatemeh S, Sakineh S, Yones J, Maryam R, Mohammad E, Nezar G, Abbas B (2016). Effects of training programs on knowledge and attitudes of nurses about postoperative pain. Der Pharm. littre 8(4):108-111.

Morton P, Fontaine D (2013). Essentials of critical care nursing: a holistic approach. Lippincott Williamson Wilkins ISBN/ISSN 978160913693 Published on October 15, 2013. https://www.amazon.com/Essentials-Critical-Care-Nursing-Holistic/dp/1609136934

Nahin RL (2015). Estimates of pain prevalence and severity in adults: United States, 2012. J. Pain 16(8):769-780. Available online at: http://www.sciencedirect.com/science/article/pii/S1526590015006793

National Health Service (NHS) (2007). Adult Inpatient Survey Results. Available at: http://www.nhssurveys.org/survey/613

Odutayo PO, Olaogun AA, Oluwatosin AO, Ogunfowokan AA (2013). Impact of an Educational Program on the Use of Standardized Nursing Languages for Nursing Documentation Among Public Health Nurses in Nigeria. Int. J. Nurs. knowl. 24(2):108-112.

Ojong IN, Ojong-Alasia MM, Nlumanze FF (2014). Nurses' assessment and management of pain among surgical patients in secondary health facility in Calabar metropolis, Cross River State, Nigeria European. J. Exp. Biol. 4(1):315-320.

Puntillo K, Li D, Miaskowski C (2008). A review of objective pain measures for use with critical care patients unable to self-report. J. Pain 9(1):2-10.

Rampanjoto RM, Mukarugiwa F, Ndimubanzi CP, Finucane BF (2007). Factors influencing pain management by nurses in emergency departments in central Africa. J. Emerg. Med. 24(47):475-476.

Wells N, Pasero C, Mc Caffery M (2008). Improving the quality of care through pain assessment and management. An evidence based Handbook for Nurses. Rockville; Agency for healthcare research and quality. Available at: https://www.ncbi.nlm.nih.gov/books/NBK2658/?report=reader

Williams B (2007). Nurses' knowledge of pain. J. Clin. Nurs. 16(6):1012-1020.

Zhang CH, Hsu L, Zou BR, Li JF, Wang HY, Huang, J. (2008). Effect of a pain education program on Nurses' pain knowledge, attitudes and assessment practice in china. J. Pain Symptom Manag. 36(6):616-627.

9

Nutrition education during pregnancy: Are final year midwifery trainees ready to offer this service?

Christiana Nsiah- Asamoah[1]* and Evelyn Asamoah Ampofo[2]

[1]Department of Health Sciences Education, University of Cape Coast, Cape Coast, Ghana.
[2]School of Nursing and Midwifery, University of Cape Coast, Cape Coast, Ghana.

Midwives provide most of the maternity services, including nutritional counseling and education services. In Ghana, there is scarce evidence regarding the competency of midwives in providing sound nutritional advice to pregnant women. Therefore, the aim of this research was to assess the nutritional knowledge levels of final year midwifery students. A descriptive cross-sectional study was conducted, in which 562 final year midwifery students from six Midwifery Training Institutions answered 20 multiple-choice questions on nutritional-related issues during pregnancy. An average score of 9.8 (approximately 49%) was obtained by the respondents. Most (>70%) of the respondents were knowledgeable of the ideal time to start taking folic acid when planning to be pregnant and the effects of high alcohol intake during pregnancy. Key areas that require attention included recommended weight gain during pregnancy, sources and functions of micronutrients, such as folic acid, iron, vitamin C, calcium and iodine during pregnancy, and nutritional management of pregnancy-related conditions like pregnancy-induced hypertension, nausea and heartburn. The findings of this study support other reports that midwives need more training in human nutrition; and it has important implications for professional planning of curricula for midwifery education.

Key words: Midwifery students, nutrition education, diet during pregnancy.

INTRODUCTION

Healthy eating is very critical before, during and after pregnancy. The nutritional status of a woman during the child-bearing stages of life has significant long-term consequences on the health and well-being of the mother, the growing foetus and newborn child (Marangoni et al., 2016; Darnton-Hill and Mkparu, 2015). It is therefore important that reliable nutrition information is given to pregnant women, and that midwives, the major health service providers of maternity care, have the requisite knowledge to execute their roles as nutrition counselors and educators (Elias and Green, 2007). Indeed, studies have established that nutrition education during pregnancy is associated with positive pregnancy outcomes (Streuling et al., 2010). Specifically in Ghana, previous studies have also highlighted the importance of nutritional counseling by health workers (Yawson et al., 2017; SPING/Ghana, 2013).

A systematic review to assess whether health

*Corresponding author. E-mail: cbuxton@ucc.edu.gh.

professionals had the capacity to provide nutritional advice during pregnancy and if pregnant women were receiving such nutritional counselling services revealed that, generally, women in their reproductive age were not receiving adequate nutrition education during pregnancy. Although healthcare practitioners perceived nutrition education to be important, barriers to providing education to clients included lack of time, lack of resources and lack of relevant training (Lucas et al., 2014).

However, a literature review to explore the extent to which the role of midwives in nutrition education during pregnancy has been reported led to a conclusion that there is limited research available on the role of midwives in nutrition education during pregnancy. The authors therefore recommended that more research is required to explore the educational needs of midwives to enhance nutritional care of pregnant women (Arrish et al., 2014).

It has been asserted that midwives often lack the essential knowledge and skills to provide adequate and reliable nutrition advice to pregnant and lactating women on how to meet increased nutrient requirements during these critical and nutrient-demanding stages of their lives (Morton et al., 2014). Improving the quality of nutrition training of midwifery trainees is vital for building the necessary human resource capacity to provide effective nutrition education and counselling services in order to tackle the public health issue of malnutrition among vulnerable groups in Ghana (Yawson et al, 2017; Sodjinou et al., 2014).

In a review paper, Arrish et al. (2014) asserted that few studies have explored the nutrition knowledge of midwives. This study was therefore undertaken to assess the current status of nutritional knowledge of final year midwifery students who were in their last semester of training in six diploma awarding midwifery training tertiary institutions in Ghana.

METHODS

This was a descriptive cross-sectional study designed to assess the nutritional knowledge of midwifery students at six diploma awarding midwifery training institutions in Ghana. The study was carried out to identify 'gaps' in the nutritional knowledge of these midwifery trainees who were in the last semester of their 3-year training programme.

Study participants

The inclusion criterion for participation was for a study participant to be in the final year of the three- year training programme. Hence only third (3rd) year midwifery students qualified to participate in the study since they had completed more than 75% of their course load required for their training and were more likely to have completed nutrition-related courses in the curriculum. Students in the first (1st) and second (2nd) years were excluded because they had not completed at least 75% of their course work.

Regarding sampling of the respondents after obtaining permission from the principals in the school, all final year students were approached and those who gave their consent to participate in the study signed an informed consent form and were given the questionnaire to complete. Therefore, participation was voluntary. Out of a total number of 571 questionnaires that were administered to students who consented to participate in the study in the six selected Midwifery training schools, 562 completed the questionnaire representing approximately 98.4% of the population. Participants were individually approached to seek for their consent to voluntarily participate in the study. The consenting process entailed thoroughly explaining the purpose of the study, confidentiality and the freedom to opt out of the study without any penalty. After the study had been thoroughly explained to the participants, they were only recruited to participate in the study after they gave their consent by signing an informed consent form. Confidentiality was maintained and anonymity of responses was ensured by avoiding the use of any form of identity of participants.

Data collection

The data was collected between November and December, 2016. A self-administered questionnaire was distributed to students who voluntarily gave their consent to participate in the study after the purpose for the study had been explained to them. The questionnaire used in this study is a modified version of nutritional knowledge questionnaires employed in similar studies among midwives in Australia (Arrish et al., 2016), New Zealand (Elias and Green, 2007) and Sudan (Elkhalifa and Kuppuswamy, 2014).

Information sought from the study participants included demographic data, educational background, knowledge about nutrition during pregnancy and respondents' views regarding the relevance of nutrition as part of their school's curriculum and their ability to thus apply nutritional knowledge in their career as professional midwives.

Quality assurance

Standard procedures were used to ensure accurate and consistent collection of data in each of the six schools. The data was collected by final year health science education university students who were undergoing their teaching practice in these six schools. They were trained on how to explain the purpose of the study to the students and issues on voluntary participation, informed consent, ensuring anonymity and confidentiality of responses given by the study participants.

The questionnaire was also pre-tested among 30 final year students to assess for reliability, clarity and simplicity of the test items at one midwifery training institution not selected for the final study. To ensure that responses given by the students were a true reflection of their knowledge levels, the students were not allowed to send the questionnaire out of their lecture rooms, but had to sit and answer the questions on their own without consulting any textbook or fellow student. Therefore it was ensured that students completed the questionnaire independently in a quiet lecture room setting.

Data analysis

The data was analysed using the Statistical Package for the Social Sciences (SPSS) programme, (version 21.0). Each correct multiple choice question was assigned a score of 1 mark (with a maximum possible score of 20 marks). In addition, the proportion of students who provided correct answers to each question was assessed and presented in tables. Descriptive statistics were run to summarize the data collected; and the results were displayed in frequencies, percentages and means.

Table 1. Information on nutritional education and application of knowledge acquired by midwifery students.

Variable/statement	N	Percentage
Completion of a nutrition –related course at the Midwifery Training College		
Yes	562	100.0
No	0	0.0
Number of nutrition courses studied		
One(1)	530	94.3
Two(2)	32	5.7
Ability to apply nutrition knowledge acquired later as a professional midwife		
Yes	538	95.7
No	24	4.3
If No, reason for inability to apply the knowledge acquired in nutrition		
Knowledge acquired is inadequate	10	41.7
Knowledge acquired sounds abstract	8	33.3
No practical application of the theoretical knowledge was included in nutrition course	6	25.0
Main source of nutritional information		
Nutrition Lessons taught by tutor	472	84.0
Magazines, newspapers	18	3.2
Internet	50	8.9
Television/Radio	8	1.4
Journals	4	0.7
Nutrition Books	8	1.4
Not applicable	2	0.4
Did you ever had an interaction with a nutritionist or dietician when you studied the nutrition course(s)		
Yes	0	0.0
No	562	100.0
Opinion with regard to adequacy of/time allocated for nutrition instruction in their institutions		
Adequate	94	16.7
Not adequate	406	72.3
Do not know	62	11.0
Opinion with regard to the importance of teaching and learning of nutrition courses in NMTC		
Not important	4	0.7
Important	68	12.1
Very Important	490	87.2

RESULTS

All the study participants were females as the profession of midwifery is dominated by females with so few men in this profession. Most of the respondents, 514 (91.5%), were between the ages of 18 and 24 years.

Nutrition education and application of knowledge acquired by study participants

Information on nutrition education and application of knowledge acquired by the surveyed midwifery students are presented in Table 1.

The study revealed that all the study participants, 562 (100.0%) had completed and passed a nutrition course as required in their training. Majority 530 (94.3%) indicated that they had studied one nutrition course. A higher proportion of the respondents, 538 (95.7%), indicated that they had the ability to apply the nutrition knowledge acquired during their training later when they start working as professional midwives. Out of the 24, who indicated that they did not have the ability to apply the knowledge acquired later as professional midwives, most of them 10 (41.7%) pointed out that the knowledge acquired was not adequate, 8 (33.3%) indicated that the knowledge acquired sounds abstract, whereas for 6 (25%), they were not in a better position to apply the knowledge acquired in nutrition because no practical application of the theoretical knowledge was included in nutrition course. Most of the respondents (84.0%) indicated that their main source of nutritional information was from their nutrition course tutor rather than nutrition books or the internet. With regard to their opinion on the

Table 2. Percentage of midwifery students that correctly answered nutrition knowledge questions.

S/N	Abbreviated form of question	Correct answer	N (%)
1	Nutrient strongly associated with the prevention of neural tube defects	B. Folate	280 (49.8)
2	Recommended average weight gain range during pregnancy for a women with BMI of 18.5 to 24.9 kg/m^2	B. 11.3 to 15.8 kg	70 (12.5)
3	Recommended time to start taking a folic acid supplement when planning to become pregnant	A. at least 1 month before pregnancy	420 (74.7)
4	Recommended folic acid intake level for pregnant women	A. 400 mcg per day.	262 (46.6)
5	Not a good source of folic acid	B. Milk	250 (44.5)
6	No need for an increased intake during pregnancy	A. Vitamin A	324 (57.7)
7	Not a reason why a pregnant woman should take adequate levels of vitamin C	C. Needed to prevent microcephaly (small head)	254 (45.2)
8	Not a rich or good food source of iron	C. banana	222 (39.5)
9	Not an importance or role of calcium during pregnancy	C. needed for normal vision/ eye sight	278 (49.5)
10	Nutrient helps to increase absorption of iron from plant food sources	B. Vitamin C	304 (54.1)
11	Advice not recommended to a pregnant woman who complains of nausea morning sickness	B. Drink some liquids at mealtime	312 (55.5)
12	Advice not recommended to a pregnant woman who complains of constipation	C. Reducing one's daily exercise or physical activity level	480 (85.4)
13	Advice not recommended to a pregnant woman who complains of heartburn	A.drinking liquids with meals to relieve burning feeling	322 (57.3)
14	Not a dietary management of Pregnancy-induced hypertension (PIH)	C. Reducing intake of magnesium rich foods in daily diet	302 (53.7)
15	Deficiency can result in megaloblastic anaemia during pregnancy	B.folate deficiency	98 (17.4)
16	Ideal gestation period to screen for gestational diabetes mellitus	B. 24 and 28 weeks	222 (39.5)
17	Nutrient works with calcium to help in the development of a baby's bones during pregnancy	C. vitamin D	218 (38.8)
18	Average amount of iron required by a pregnant woman each day to meet her iron needs	B. 27 mg/day	54 (9.6)
19	Result of Heavy alcohol intake during pregnancy	C. Fetal Alcohol Syndrome(FAS)	488 (86.8)
20	Inadequate intake increases risk of mental impairment and cretinism in newborn baby	C. Iodine	320 (56.9)

relevance of studying nutrition as part of their midwifery curriculum, majority 486 (86.5%) indicated that it is very important to study nutrition as midwifery students.

The percentage distribution of students who gave correct answers to the nutrition knowledge questions is presented in Table 2. The mean score for correctly answered questions for all the study participants was 9.8 (49%) out of the total 20 questions (approximately 49%). Some of these questions assessed respondents' knowledge of the importance of taking folic acid supplements during pregnancy, recommendations on weight gain during pregnancy, importance of micronutrients such as vitamin C, B, calcium, iron, iodine, dietary management of pregnancy-related minor disorders and complications such as heartburn, constipation, pregnancy induced hypertension and effect of alcohol intake during pregnancy.

Three questions were answered correctly by less than 20% of the respondents. One of questions assessed respondents' knowledge of the recommended average weight gain during pregnancy for women with normal/healthy BMI of 18.5 to 24.9 kg/m^2 of which only 70 (12.5%) had it correct. The other question tested respondents' knowledge of the nutrient whose deficiency can result in megaloblastic anaemia during pregnancy, of which only 98 (17.4%) were able to provide the right answer. Again, the third question which evaluated respondents' knowledge on the approximate average iron intake per day during pregnancy was answered correctly by 9.6% of the respondents. Three questions were answered correctly by more than 30% but less than 40% of the respondents. One of the questions required that respondents should identify one out of five food sources given which was not a rich or good food source of iron, of which 222 (39.5%) provided the right answer. The other question assessed respondents' knowledge on the gestation period in weeks which is ideal to screen pregnant women for gestational diabetes, of which 222 (39.5%) provided the correct answer. The third questionnaire assessed respondents' knowledge on the nutrient that works with calcium to help in the development of a baby's bones during pregnancy, of which 38.8% had it correct.

Five questions were answered correctly by more than 40%, but less than 50% of the respondents. These five (5) questions assessed respondents' knowledge on the nutrient associated with the prevention of neural tube defects, the recommended folic acid intake level for pregnant women, food sources of folic acid, reasons why a pregnant woman should take adequate levels of vitamin C and the importance of calcium during pregnancy. Six (6) questions were answered correctly by more than 50% but less than 60% of the respondents. Some of these six (6) questions assessed respondents' knowledge on the nutrient that helps to increase absorption of iron from plant sources, nutritional advices that must be given to manage pregnancy induced hypertension (PIH), nausea, morning sickness and heartburns. Two (2) questions were answered correctly by more than 80% of the respondents. One of these questions sought to evaluate the knowledge levels of respondents on the dietary advice that must be given to pregnant women who complains of constipation. The other question sought to assess respondents' knowledge on the result of heavy alcohol intake during pregnancy, of which 488 (86.8%) of the respondents provided the correct answer.

DISCUSSION

The results of the present study indicated that the mean score for correctly answered questions for all the study participants was approximately 49%, suggesting that the nutritional knowledge of midwifery students was poor as has been reported in similar studies previously conducted among midwives in Sudan (Elkhalifa and Kuppuswamy, 2014); Australia (Schmied et al., 2011) and the United Kingdom (Lee et al., 2010). The poor performance of the final year students in general in the present study can perhaps be attributed to the little emphasis or priority given to nutrition education during the training of midwives (Arish et al., 2016; Sodjinou et al., 2014). Other factors include the level of nutritional competences exhibited by tutors (Sethuraman et al., 2015) and issues related to the lack of essential aspects of human nutrition in courses taught (Shrimpton et al., 2016). In this study, majority (94.3%) of the final year students indicated that they studied only one nutrition course throughout the entire three year duration of the training programme.

Out of the 20 questions that were asked on maternal nutritional issues during pregnancy, 11 questions were answered correctly by less than 50% of the respondents. With regard to folic acid intake during pregnancy, only 46.6% knew the recommended folic acid intake level for pregnant women. It has been reported based on studies conducted in developing countries that majority of health professionals have insufficient knowledge on benefits, correct dose, particular time when folic acid should be administered to prevent Neural Tube Defects (NTDs) (Abedi et al., 2011) and food sources of folic acid (Demilew and Nigussie, 2017).

With respect to the importance of vitamin C during pregnancy, only 45.2% of the respondents knew the benefits of meeting the recommended intakes of vitamin C during pregnancy. The study also shows that 54.1% knew that vitamin C helps to increase absorption of iron from plant food sources. The fact that only 45.2% of the respondents knew the importance of vitamin C during pregnancy in a country like Ghana where about 42% of Ghanaian women aged between 15 and 49 are anaemic and 66% of children aged between 6 and 59 months are anaemic (Ghana Statistical Service (GSS), Ghana Health Service (GHS), 2015) warrants much attention. This is because of the important role that vitamin C plays in facilitating the absorption of non-heam iron.

With regard to calcium intake during pregnancy, only 49.5% knew about its role during pregnancy. In addition only 38.8% of the respondents knew the nutrient (vitamin D) which works with calcium to help in the development of a baby's bones during pregnancy. Regarding, the importance of iodine during pregnancy, a little over half (56.9%) of the participants knew that inadequate intake of iodine increases risk of mental impairment and cretinism in a newborn baby. Pregnant women have much higher iodine requirements as compared to all other population groups. The fact that midwives lack adequate knowledge about the importance of iodine during pregnancy has implications on the awareness of pregnant women and even their dietary intakes of good iodine food sources.

On the issue of gestational weight gain (GWG), only 12.5% knew the recommended average weight gain during pregnancy for women with healthy BMI of 18.5 to 24.9 kg/m^2. Generally, it has been reported in some studies that generally, midwives give low priority to GWG, lack adequate knowledge in GWG and its management and in most cases fail to educate clients on weight gain management issues (Fieldwick et al., 2014; Willcox et al., 2012).

With respect to knowledge on gestational diabetes mellitus (GDM), only 39.5% knew that pregnant women should be screened for the condition between 24 and 28 weeks of pregnancy. The findings of this study suggest that midwifery trainees might not have been introduced to the need for screening pregnant women to early detect cases of women affected with gestational diabetes. Similarly, it has been reported that midwives knowledge about screening, management practices especially with diet and sensitization of women about gestational diabetes is low (Utz et al., 2016; Antos et al., 2013).

With regard to Pregnancy Induced Hypertension (PIH), only 53.7% could indicate out of five options given that reducing intake of magnesium rich foods is not a recommended dietary management of PIH. Generally, it has been indicated based on the findings of studies that the knowledge of midwives is deficient regarding management of PIH (Stellenberg and Ngwekazi, 2016; Munirathnamma and Lakshmamma, 2013). Munirathnamma and Lakshmamma (2013) reported that generally midwives are more knowledgeable in the area of nursing management than in the area of dietary management of PIH.

Findings from this study also revealed that majority (91.4%) of the final year midwifery trainees did not know the approximate average iron intake per day during pregnancy. Again, only 39.5% could indicate out of five food sources given (Meat, Spinach, Fish, Banana and Eggs) that banana is not a good food source of iron. This finding supports reports made in a similar study where most of the midwives failed to recognize rich food sources of iron (Elkhalifa and Kuppuswamy, 2014). This finding is worrying and warrants great attention particularly considering WHO reports that more than 40% of pregnant women worldwide are anaemic and that at least half of this anaemia burden is assumed to be due to iron deficiency (WHO, 2017).

Findings from this study demonstrate and reiterate the need for continued education to improve midwifery trainees' nutrition knowledge which will boost their confidence as they carry out their duties. Recommendations include the need to update and strengthen the content of the nutrition curriculum in collaboration with experts in nutrition such as dieticians and public health nutritionists. In addition, developing a maternal nutrition resource toolkit which can be approved and adopted for use by all midwifery training institutions and conducting regular refresher workshops for midwifery tutors who teach nutrition-related courses are also worth considering. It is also worthwhile considering giving midwifery students the opportunity to apply their theoretical knowledge on the field while being mentored by a dietician or a public health nutritionist as part of the curriculum for their training.

Conclusion

Generally, majority of midwifery students who are in their final semester of their three-year training lacked basic knowledge of nutrition requirements during pregnancy. Their poor nutritional knowledge was evident in the fact that less than 50% of them could provide the right answers to most of the questions asked (11 out of 20 questions). Lack of knowledge in areas in maternal nutrition which were evident among the final-year midwifery diploma students include weight gain during pregnancy, role and food sources of critical micronutrients in pregnancy such as iron, folic acid, calcium, vitamin D and vitamin C. Other areas which were deficient in the knowledge levels of the study participants include screening for gestational diabetes, and dietary management of problems such as nausea, heartburn and pregnancy-induced hypertension (PIH) during pregnancy.

CONFLICT OF INTERESTS

The authors have not declared any conflict of interests.

REFERENCES

Abedi G, Abdollahi F, Etemadinejad S (2011). Health behaviors of health practitioners about folic acid in Mazandaran province, Sari, Iran. World Appl. Sci. J. 12:944-50.

Antos E, Nowak B, Olszewski J (2013). The analysis of midwives' knowledge on the education of women with gestational diabetes and preparation for it. J. Public Health, Nurs. Med. Rescue 19(4):29-36.

Arrish J, Yeatman H, Williamson M (2014). Midwives and nutrition education during pregnancy: A literature review. Women Birth 27(1):2-8.

Arrish J, Yeatman H, Williamson M (2016). Australian midwives and provision of nutrition education during pregnancy: A cross sectional survey of nutrition knowledge, attitudes, and confidence. Women Birth 29(5):455-464.

Darnton-Hill I, Mkparu UC (2015). Micronutrients in pregnancy in low- and middle-income countries. Nutrients 7(3):1744-1768.

Demilew YM, Nigussie AA (2017). Knowledge of Health Professionals on Folic Acid Use and Their Prescribing Practice in Bahir Dar City Administration, Northwest Ethiopia: Cross-Sectional Study. PloS One 12(1):e0170116.

Elias S, Green T (2007). Nutrition knowledge and attitudes of New Zealand registered midwives. Nutr. Diet. 64(4):290-294.

Elkhalifa AEO, Kuppuswamy SB (2014). Evaluation of Midwifery Knowledge on Antenatal Care in Omdurman Maternity Hospital Sudan. Int. J. Health Sci. Educ. 2(2):127-142.

Fieldwick D, Paterson H, Stephen M, Cameron A, Egan R, McFadden S, Pienaar J, Sinclair C, Struthers T, Taplin K, Watson C (2014). Management of excess weight in pregnancy in Otago, New Zealand: a qualitative study with lead maternity carers. NZ Med. J. 127(1392):27-37.

Ghana Statistical Service (GSS) (2014). Ghana Health Service (GHS), ICF International (2015). Ghana Demographic and Health Survey 2014. Rockville, Maryland, USA: GSS, GHS, and ICF International.

Lee D, Haynes C, Garrod D (2010). Exploring health promotion practice within maternity services. National Health Service Foundation Trust. Stockport, UK: National Health Service.

Lucas C, Charlton KE, Yeatman H (2014). Nutrition advice during pregnancy: do women receive it and can health professionals provide it? Matern Child Health J. 18(10):2465-2478.

Marangoni F, Cetin I, Verduci E, Canzone G, Giovannini M, Scollo P, Corsello G, Poli A (2016). Maternal Diet and Nutrient Requirements in Pregnancy and Breastfeeding. An Italian Consensus Document. Nutrients 8(10):629.

Morton SM, Grant CC, Wall CR, Carr PEA, Bandara DK, Schmidt JM, Ivory V, Inskip HM, Camargo CA (2014). Adherence to nutritional guidelines in pregnancy: evidence from the Growing Up in New Zealand birth cohort study. Public Health Nutr. 17(9):1919-1929.

Munirathnamma M, Lakshmamma T (2013) Knowledge of Staff Nurses Regarding Management of Pregnancy Induced Hypertension (PIH). Int. J. Soc. Sci. Humanit. Invent. 2(11):8-12.

Schmied VA, Duff M, Dahlen HG, Mills AE, Kolt GS (2011). 'Not waving but drowning': a study of the experiences and concerns of midwives and other health professionals caring for obese childbearing women. Midwifery 27(4):424-430.

Sethuraman K (2015). Development of a public health nutrition workforce: Nurses and midwives in Ghana. In 2015 APHA Annual Meeting and Expo (Oct. 31-Nov. 4, 2015). APHA.

Shrimpton R, du Plessis LM, Delisle H, Blaney S, Atwood SJ, Sanders D, Margetts B, Hughes R (2016). Public health nutrition capacity: assuring the quality of workforce preparation for scaling up nutrition programmes. Public Health Nutr. 19(11):2090-2100.

Sodjinou R, Bosu WK, Fanou N, Déart L, Kupka R, Tchibindat F, Baker S (2014). Nutrition training in medical and other health professional schools in West Africa: the need to improve current approaches and enhance training effectiveness. Glob. Health Action 2014:7.

Stellenberg EL, Ngwekazi NL (2016). Knowledge of midwives about hypertensive disorders during pregnancy in primary healthcare. Afr. J. Prim. Health Care Fam. Med. 8(1):1- 6.

SPING/Ghana (Strengthening Partnerships, Results and Innovations in Nutrition Globally) (2013). Breastfeeding Basics Mean Better Nutrition: The Important Role of Nutrition Counseling in Ghana. United States Agency for International Development (USAID) and JSI Research and Training Institute, Inc.

Streuling I, Beyerlein A, von Kries R (2010). Can gestational weight gain be modified by increasing physical activity and diet counseling? A meta-analysis of interventional trials. Am. J. Clin. Nutr. 2010:29363.

Utz B, Assarag B, Essolbi A, Barkat A, Benkaddour YA, De Brouwere V (2016). Diagnosis a posteriori? Assessing gestational diabetes screening and management in Morocco. Glob. Health Action 2016:9.

Willcox JC, Campbell KJ, van der Pligt P, Hoban E, Pidd D, Wilkinson S (2012). Excess gestational weight gain: an exploration of midwives' views and practice. BMC Pregnancy Childbirth 12(1):102.

Yawson AE, Amoaful EO, Senaya LK, Yawson AO, Aboagye PK, Mahama AB, Selenje L, Ngongalah V (2017). The lancet series nutritional interventions in Ghana: a determinants analysis approach to inform nutrition strategic planning. BMC Nutr. 3(1):27.

Focused antenatal care: Re-appraisal of current practices

T. Ebunoluwa Oshinyemi[1], J. Ojo Aluko[2] and O. Abimbola Oluwatosin[2]

[1]Department of Nursing Science, College of Medicine, University of Lagos, Nigeria.
[2]Department of Nursing, College of Medicine, University of Ibadan, Oyo State, Nigeria.

Focused antenatal care has been viewed to be a better option to the previously existing orthodox model of antenatal care. The orthodox antenatal care otherwise known as traditional model of antenatal care requires a number of routine and frequent visits by pregnant women to the healthcare facility. This traditional model of antenatal care has been observed to require numerous materials such as financial and human resources for its continuous implementation. The observable cumbersome nature of the traditional model necessitates the recent exploration of alternative model of antenatal care referred to as focused antenatal care (FANC) model. The FANC model emanated during the era of evidenced based practice and evidence based approach to care. Evidence-based ensures that the care rendered are based on previous outcomes of care and are focused on what can be achieved during the less regular but specific visit, which is characterized by being client friendly with reduced cost of implementation. Despite this importance of FANC, antenatal care continues to be centered around clinical assessment, and regular attendance at the clinic. Thus, the objective of this paper is to review the traditional care model and the focused antenatal care model because antenatal care remains a mixture of both art and science, and to re-appraise current antenatal practices.

Key words: Focused antenatal care, pregnancy, clinical assessment.

INTRODUCTION

Recently, focused antenatal care (FANC) has proven to be a better option to the traditional model of antenatal care (ANC). The traditional model of ANC otherwise known as orthodox model of ANC requires regular clinical assessment and frequent visits to the antenatal clinic, thus it consumes more time and larger resources. The traditional model of ANC is also centered on quantity of care rather than quality of care (World Health Organization, 2015).

Antenatal care (Prenatal care) is the care provided to a pregnant woman before delivery. The care includes the clinical assessment of the pregnant woman and her fetus during the pregnancy period in order to achieve a favorable outcome for both the mother and child. ANC services require detailed history taking, physical examination, laboratory and diagnostic investigations.

While rendering these services activities are directed at sustaining the maternal physical and psychological health and improving the fetal wellbeing to ensure the delivery of a live healthy neonate, and also prepare the family for

*Corresponding author. E-mail: iseoluwatope@yahoo.com.

parenthood (Women's Healthcare, 2014; Lincetto et al., 2006).

World Health Organization (WHO) (2006), defined antenatal care as "activities directed at screening for health and socio-economic conditions that are likely to increase the possibility of specific adverse pregnancy outcomes, and providing therapeutic interventions known to be effective; educating pregnant women about planning for safe birth or how to deal with emergencies during pregnancy". Focused antenatal care is a goal oriented antenatal care with activities directed at clinical assessment and specific decision making processes when rendering care to the pregnant woman while also maintaining targeted and individualized care.

Traditional approach to antenatal care (ANC)

Traditional approach to antenatal care dates back to the 1900, it was introduced by social reformers in the United States, and in 1978 the World health Organization integrated the risk based approach to antenatal care still with the aim of improving the quality and outcome of care. During the risk based approach, pregnant women are expected to make frequent visits to the health care facility, they are then classified into low and high risk with the aim of early identification of those at risk of developing complications from their previous history such as medical, obstetrics and gynecology and social history (Kearns et al., 2014).

WHO's Maternal Health and Safe Motherhood Program in 1994 initiated the "Mother-Baby Package: implementing safe motherhood in countries" and under it identified the four pillars of Safe Motherhood Initiative as family planning, antenatal care (ANC), clean/safe delivery, and essential obstetric care. This package was not expected to operate on its own but was to be integrated into the existing health systems, and the existing model of antenatal care was the risk based approach under the traditional model of ANC. The weakness of the high risk approach include its uncertainty at predicting pregnant women at risk because all women can be regarded as being at risk of different complications which may not be identified during the frequent antenatal visits thus improved quality of care is essential to all women in order to achieve better outcomes in maternal and child health (WHO, 1994).

The traditional model of antenatal care visits were: once a month till 32 weeks gestation, twice a month till 36 weeks gestation, and weekly till delivery, a pregnant woman is therefore expected to make up to 14 antenatal visits to the hospital before delivery. Emphasis is placed on the number/quantity of visit rather than the quality of visit, routine risk indicators such as maternal height and weight were used to identify those at risk of developing complications during delivery and there seems to be little difference in outcome of care between the frequent antenatal visit and the focused antenatal visit. Currently, the trend is shifting towards reducing the number of antenatal visit, while at the same time establishing clearly defined objectives to be achieved at each visit and improving quality of care rendered at each visit (Women's Health care, 2014).

In the traditional model of ANC, pregnant women were classified as being at low risk or high risk based on predetermined criteria, this was difficult to implement effectively since women usually had at least one risk factor, even the low risk women develop complications particularly during childbirth while in the focused model of ANC, specific evidence-based interventions are provided for all women, carried out at certain critical times in the pregnancy (Lincetto et al., 2006).

The traditional model assumes that the more the number of visits, the more favorable the outcome, therefore pregnant women were expected to make up to 16 antenatal visit regardless of their risk status to the healthcare facility and only pregnancy related issues are addressed during this visit, the model relies on routine risk indicators, such as a maternal height that is lesser than 150 cm, weight lesser than 50 kg presence of edema of the legs, and mal-presentations before 36 weeks gestation (Assegid et al., 2017).

Focused antenatal care (FANC)

The focused antenatal care was instituted in 2002 by the WHO in an attempt to overcome the challenges posed by the traditional antenatal model of care such as classifying pregnant women into high risk or low risk group based on pre-identified criteria, and the possibility of the low risk group developing complications at delivery (Kearns et al., 2014; Assegid et al., 2017).

For the adoption of the FANC model to be evidenced based, a multi-country randomised trial was conducted in 2001 to assess the effectiveness of the focused antenatal care, compared to the traditional antenatal care model, findings revealed that healthcare providers tolerated the focused antenatal care model, women in both models of care were generally satisfied with services, and FANC financial implications were the same or lesser than the traditional antenatal care (Kearns et al., 2014; Villar et al., 2001).

Another review of randomised controlled trials by WHO in 2001 compared interventions with a lower number of antenatal visits to the traditional ANC model, findings revealed similar results (Carroli et al., 2001; Kearns et al., 2014). Together, these studies led to the WHO's conclusion that care models with reduced antenatal visits could be implemented in both developed and developing countries without negatively affecting health outcomes of pregnant women or their infants.

The FANC focuses on quality of antenatal care than the frequency of visits, emphasis are laid on providing individualized care accordingly rather than categorizing groups of women into high risk or low risk, the FANC assumes that all pregnant women are at risk of developing complications therefore care is focused on early identification of complication as they arise, targeted and individualized care and the use of evidenced based practice in developing care (USAID, 2007; Assegid et al., 2017). This model of care makes pregnancy a family responsibility, the husband and the woman are fully informed of the potential complications, birth preparedness, postnatal care and planning for future child spacing/childbirth.

Women who present with pre-existing risk factors or medical conditions as well as women who are identified as having complications throughout their care are enrolled in a specialized care model that includes additional assessments, visits, and evaluation. The focused antenatal care model separates pregnant women into two groups: those likely to need only routine antenatal care (some 75% of the total population of pregnant women), and those with specific health conditions or risk factors that necessitate special care (25% of pregnant women). For the first group, a standard program of four antenatal visits is recommended (with additional visits should conditions emerge which require special care). The WHO guidelines are also specific as regards the timing and content of antenatal care visits according to gestational age. The guidelines stipulate that "only examinations and tests that serve an immediate purpose and that have been proven to be beneficial should be performed" (Abou-Zahr et al., 2003).

A study conducted in Zaire in 1984 on 3614 pregnant women showed that majority (71%) of the women who developed obstructed labor were previously categorized as 'not at risk', while 90% of women who were identified as 'at risk' did not develop obstructed labor, this shows evidence that most pregnancy problems are unpredictable (Assegid et al., 2017).

Benefits of focused antenatal care

Antenatal care aims at achieving positive pregnancy outcome in pregnancy; this outcome is to ensure improved maternal and neonatal health. The reduced visits by pregnant women to the healthcare settings provides reduction in the financial implication thus the saved money can be channeled to other use such as for specialized investigations. Also less visit to the healthcare personnel enable them to be available for other purposes especially in resource constrained environments. Specifically, adopting the FANC model is expected to produce the following outcomes (USAID, 2007, Assegid et al., 2017):

(1) Targeted assessments of pregnant women.
(2) Prompt identification and treatment of diseases.
(3) Early detection of complications and other potential problems that can affect the outcomes of pregnancy.
(4) Providing prophylaxis and treatment for anemia, malaria, and sexually transmitted infections (STIs) including HIV, urinary tract infections and tetanus.
(5) Providing individualized approach to care of pregnant women.
(6) Health promotion activities focused on birth preparedness, complication readiness, adequate nutrition, benefits of immunization to both the mother and the child, personal hygiene and postnatal care.
(7) Counseling on warning signs necessitating urgent attention.

Principles of focused antenatal care

Focused antenatal care model operates under the following principles (WHO, 2002; USAID, 2007; Assegid et al., 2017):

(1) Principle of woman friendliness: Antenatal care should be rendered in a cordial environment, healthcare providers should be accommodating, clinic hours should be friendly and convenient enough to accommodate the need of clients and their schedule of work. Health care providers should make all pregnant women feel welcomed at the clinic, it has been shown that the number of women seeking antenatal care increases proportionally with increases in hours of operation (USAID, 2007). Antenatal interventions or investigations should be carefully planned with the woman to increase their satisfaction with care while at the same time making room for improved outcome of care.
(2) Individualization of care: All information known about the woman from the detailed health history (medical, surgical, obstetrics and social history) should be used to individualize care and plan care with the woman.
(3) Targeted assessment and management : Targeted assessment of pregnant women under the FANC model assist in early identification and treatment of already established disease and early detection of complications and other potential complications, it is also used in categorizing pregnant women into groups of those that require routine care of the four visit only and those that require specialized care. Early management of these conditions that are identified can lead to improved maternal and fetal outcome.
(4) Family participation: The health care provider respect the opinion of the spouse in decision- making process, the entire family watches out for signs of complications and participates in birth preparedness, complication readiness and emergency planning. Family participation ensures compliance on the part of the woman and a fuller and safer reproductive health experience for the woman, her newborn and her family.

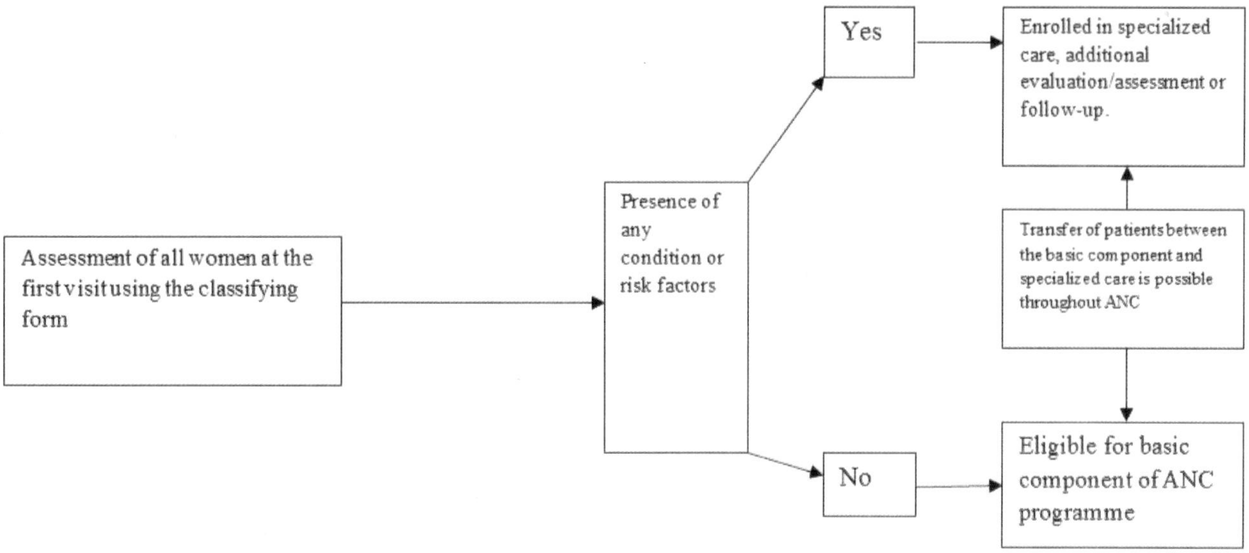

Figure 1. The focused antenatal care model.

(5) Culturally acceptable and appropriate: All activities in the focused antenatal care model must be culturally acceptable and appropriate as every culture has specific myths and beliefs, taboos and practices surrounding pregnancy and childbirth thus information should be centered around the necessity of certain healthcare interventions.

(6) Health promotion: Focused antenatal care should include health promotion activities by disseminating information, health education and counseling on balanced diet, personal and environmental hygiene, birth preparedness, emergency readiness and delivery. The steps in newborn care, importance of breastfeeding and immunization should be emphasized.

(7) Community commitment: Many of the components of FANC can be provided at the community level; therefore, linkage with the formal health care system is imperative to ensure adequate training and supervision of community health workers and implement functional referral systems.

(8) Integration of care: FANC should include other activities such as sexually transmitted infection and HIV testing/ counseling, malaria detection and prevention, micronutrient provision, birth planning, emergency planning and family counseling.

(9) Referral: The focused antenatal care model should adequately plan for referral and transportation to the appropriate health facility, a simple referral form should be created, this can be used to easily identify women with special health conditions or those at risk of developing complications and utilized to refer women to a higher level of care.

(10) Appropriate examinations/ tests: Only examinations and tests that serve an immediate purpose and that have been proven to be beneficial should be performed (WHO, 2002; USAID, 2007).

The WHO focused antenatal care model

The model segregates pregnant women into two groups: those eligible to receive routine ANC called the basic component and those who need special care based on their specific health conditions or risk factors (figure 1). Pre – set criteria are used to determine the eligibility of the women for basic component. The women who need special care will represent, on average, approximately 25% of all pregnant women attending antenatal care (WHO, 2002; USAID, 2007).

The classifying form for FANC

The classifying form as designed by the WHO is used at the first antenatal visit to the clinic to decide which women will follow the basic component or the specialized care (figure 1). The format of the form can be adapted to the format to be used in each clinic setting (WHO, 2002). The form contains 18 checklists, composed of closed ended questions that require a 'yes or no' response. They cover the patient's obstetric history, current pregnancy and general medical conditions.

Obstetric history

(1) Previous still birth or neonatal loss.
(2) History of three or more consecutive spontaneous abortions.

(3) Birth weight of last baby < 2500 g.
(4) Birth weight of last baby > 4500 g.
(5) Last pregnancy: hospital admission for hypertension or pre-eclampsia.
(6) Previous surgery on reproductive tract.

Current pregnancy

(1) Diagnosed or suspected multiple pregnancies.
(2) Age less than 18 years.
(3) Age more than 40 years.
(4) Iso-immunization: Rhesus negative in current or previous pregnancy.
(6) Vaginal bleeding.
(7) Pelvic mass.
(8) Diastolic blood pressure 90 mmHg or more at booking.

Medical

(1) Insulin-dependent diabetes mellitus.
(2) Renal disease.
(3) Cardiac disease.
(4) Known substance abuse (including heavy alcohol drinking).
(6) Any other severe medical disease or condition.

The basic component of the focused antenatal care is composed of four visits, the World Health Organization clinical guideline for each of the visit are as follows (WHO, 2002):

The first FANC visit should occur before 16 weeks gestation but some pregnant women may present later than that, activities are directed at using the pre-set criteria to categorize women into those eligible for the basic component of the antenatal care and those who require specialized care (WHO, 2002; Lincetto et al., 2006). The objectives of the first FANC visit are to:

(1) Obtain a detailed medical and obstetrics history and carry out physical examination and observation of vital signs.
(2) Assess hemoglobin level to determine the presence of anemia, perform urinalysis to identify abnormalities.
(3) Perform abdominal examination, and correlate the last menstrual period date with the fundal height measurement to determine the gestational age of the fetus.
(4) Initiate the individualized birth plan.
(5) Health educate on balanced diet, routine antenatal medications such as iron and folic acid supplementation and the use of insecticide treated bed nets (ITNs) and intermittent preventive treatment of malaria in pregnancy using sulfadoxine-pyrimethamine.
(6) Provide HIV counseling and prevention of mother to child transmission of HIV (PMTCT) services. Offer immunization services such administration of tetanus toxiod.
(7) Provide information on birth preparedness, complication readiness, blood transfusion and transportation.

The second FANC visit should occur between 24 to 28 weeks gestation. The objective of the second visit is to follow-up on the first visit, monitor the progress of pregnancy and address any complaints of the woman, the individualized care plan is reviewed and modified appropriately. The third FANC visit should occur between 30 to 32 weeks of gestation. In addition to what is expected of the second visit the objectives of the third visit are:

(1) To identify presence of multiple pregnancy necessitating referral
(2) Detect for the presence of protein in urine
(3) Determine the need for referral based on risk assessment
(4) Health educate on exclusive breastfeeding, birth preparedness, signs of labor, postnatal care and family planning.

The fourth FANC visit should occur between 36 to 40 weeks gestation, in addition to the objectives of the third visit the activities in the fourth visit are to:

(1) Confirm fetal position and fetal presentation during the abdominal examination
(2) Review the individualized birth plan

DISCUSSION

The introduction of FANC is associated with questions such as the appropriateness or adequacy of the four antenatal visits, the adequacy of the contact time required to get to know patients and care providers, social aspects of ANC and identifying if the clients actually desire a reduction in the number of their antenatal visits. Several studies identify the number and spacing of antenatal visits as potential areas of concern in FANC (Villar and Bergsjo, 2002).

According to Umeora et al. (2008), the recommended WHO focused antenatal care is yet to be implemented in many communities in rural Nigeria. In their study on the attitude of antenatal clients in a rural mission hospital to the new antenatal model, focused group discussions were carried out for 12 weeks; findings revealed that out of the 144 clients interviewed, none had heard of the new antenatal care model. More than half of them will prefer the traditional model with multiple visits than the new model. The traditional visit was said to be more reassuring and provides the clients time away from their routine chores/occupations and afford them the opportunity to interact with other expectant mothers and get acquainted with the health care providers (Umeora et al., 2008). The study concluded that to realize the goals of the new antenatal model in Nigeria, mass enlightenment and education must precede its gradual and cautious introduction.

Aluko and Oluwatosin (2008) conducted a research on the pattern and outcome of antenatal care among women attending a Catholic mission hospital in Ibadan, Nigeria using the records of 581 women who attended antenatal clinic, findings of the research showed that women had low rate of booking at first trimester and irregular visits to antenatal clinics, their finding also showed that antenatal visits were initiated by the presence of symptoms of illness, thus they recommended that antenatal care settings should adopt the modified antenatal care model (focused antenatal care), to improve compliance and also stress the importance of early booking at antenatal settings.

Aniebue and Aniebue (2011) evaluated the attitude of pregnant women to the new antenatal care model with four antenatal visits (focused antenatal care) using a cross-sectional survey in Enugu, Nigeria. Only 20.3% of the women desired a change to the new model, respondents who defaulted from antenatal care three or more times, those dissatisfied with their current antenatal care, senior civil servants and those who received secondary school education or less most commonly desired a change to the new model. Default from antenatal care and dissatisfaction with current antenatal care were factors associated with the desire for change. The most common reasons for desiring the change were convenience and cost considerations. Reasons given for the rejection of the new model were: fear of inadequate learning during antenatal care, the suspicion that four visits were inadequate for familiarization with healthcare providers, the need for early detection of disease and social satisfaction from antenatal visits, however the researches stated that these factors can be changed by health education and social mobilization (Aniebue and Aniebue, 2011).

Ajayi et al. (2013) conducted a study on quality assessment of the practice of focused antenatal care (FANC) in rural and urban primary health centres in Ekiti State, Nigeria, their study made an attempt at analysis of the practice of FANC according to the recommendation of WHO at the most basic level, and to determine the facilitating factors and challenges to the practice of FANC in urban and rural areas, that is comparing the primary Health centers in both urban and rural areas. Their study utilized two hundred (200) respondents each from urban and rural areas, simple random sampling was used to select 18 primary health centres for the study, in-depth interviews were conducted with the heads of selected facilities. Their findings showed that, 58 (29.3%) respondents from the urban areas had the minimum contents of the FANC compared to 41 (20.7%) of the rural respondents and 178 (90.8%) of the urban were taught a range of health education topics compared to 177 (88.5%).

Furthermore their study revealed that urban respondents were more likely to receive the minimum contents than rural respondents. In-depth interview results showed that the facilitating factor was free health service scheme in place in the state and the major challenge to focused antenatal care was inadequate number of skilled health workers especially in the rural areas studied. They concluded that, basic contents of focused antenatal care in Ekiti state were received by a small proportion of the respondents, suggesting that focused antenatal care had not fully translated into quality service.

In another study by Oluwatosin and Aluko (2014), on the compliance with intermittent preventive treatment of malaria during pregnancy among postpartum women in selected Hospitals in Ibadan, the descriptive survey study collected data from 346 women attending postnatal and child welfare clinics of the selected Hospitals using questionnaires, part of the findings from their study revealed that the settings still operate the traditional model of antenatal care and not the focused antenatal care model, and respondents in their study were not regular at antenatal visits, thus they recommended that focused antenatal care which is characterized by fewer visits be adopted by antenatal care settings to improve compliance.

The acceptability of focused antenatal care by pregnant Nigerian women in Lagos University Teaching Hospital and factors influencing the acceptability was examined by Olamijulo et al. (2015), their findings revealed that a greater proportion of women (56.1%) indicated their acceptance for FANC model. Their study went further to identify that a greater percentage of those with secondary and tertiary level of education accepted FANC when compared with those with primary level of education. In their study majority of their respondents' related acceptability of the FANC model by the WHO to convenience of the new model while others who still indicated preference for the traditional model of antenatal care preferred it because of fear of complications arising in the course of pregnancy if antenatal visits are reduced.

The study on "Determinants of Focused Antenatal Care Uptake among Women in Tharaka Nithi County, Kenya," using a descriptive cross-sectional survey design revealed that the level of uptake of focused antenatal care among respondents was slightly more than half (52%) and the determinants of uptake of focused antenatal care are level of education, type of employment, household income, parity, and marital status of the pregnant women. The study therefore concluded that irrespective of the high attendance of at least one antenatal visit in Kenya, the uptake of focused antenatal care is proportionally low (Gitonga, 2017).

Ekott et al. (2017) in their study on acceptability of focused antenatal care by antenatal clinic attendees in Obio Cottage Hospital, Port Harcourt, Nigeria found out that 75.7% of pregnant women were willing to accept making fewer visits that still met their health needs, while 24.3% would not accept making fewer visits. The main reason for accepting reduced visits by these women was to save time 40.6%, and the main reasons given for rejecting reduced visits were for better monitoring of pregnancy (35.1%) and early detection of problems (21.6%) in pregnancy.

The world health organization new guidelines for ANC

In 2016, the WHO designed new recommendations/ guideline for ANC for pregnant women and adolescent, these recommendations are expected to complement existing WHO guidelines on the management of specific pregnancy- related complications in order to achieve a positive pregnancy experience from ANC because recent evidence in 2015 suggests that a higher frequency of antenatal contacts by pregnant women and adolescent girls to the healthcare facility creates an opportunity to know the women better and detect potential complications therefore likely leading to reduction in the number of still births. Eight or more contacts for antenatal care can reduce perinatal deaths by up to 8 per 1000 births when compared to 4 visits (WHO, 2016), thus producing a positive pregnancy experience for both mother and child. 'A positive pregnancy experience is defined as maintaining physical and socio-cultural normality, maintaining a healthy pregnancy for mother and baby (including preventing or treating risks, illness and death), having an effective transition to positive labour and birth, and achieving positive motherhood (including maternal self-esteem, competence and autonomy)' (WHO, 2016). The new WHO recommendations are related to five types of interventions:

A. Nutritional interventions,
B. Maternal and fetal assessment,
C. Preventive measures,
D. Interventions for common physiological symptoms, and
E. Health system interventions to improve utilization and quality of ANC.
E7: Antenatal care models with a minimum of eight contacts are recommended to reduce perinatal mortality and improve women's experience of care

The 2016 WHO ANC model recommended an increase in the number of ANC visit from 4 visit to 8 contacts. This was necessary because the evidence from review of literature suggests that there has been lesser satisfaction of women with the four-visit model (also known as focused or basic ANC), thus the recommended number of contacts between the mother and the health-care providers may facilitate assessment of well-being and provision of interventions to improve outcomes if problems are identified. Globally, during the period from 2007–2014, only 64% of pregnant women attended the WHO recommended minimum four contacts for ANC, suggesting that much more work needs to be done to address ANC utilization and quality. Furthermore, evidence suggests that more ANC visits, irrespective of the resource setting, are probably associated with greater maternal satisfaction than less ANC visits (WHO, 2016).

Recommendation E.7 in the 2016 WHO ANC model under antenatal care schedule states that antenatal care models with a minimum of eight contacts are recommended to reduce perinatal mortality and improve women's experience of care (WHO, 2016). Thus, the Guideline Development Group (GDG) emphasized that the focused ANC (FANC) model does not offer women adequate contact with health-care practitioners and is no longer recommended. The GDG uses the word "contact" to "visit", as it implies an active connection between a pregnant woman and a health-care provider. The first contact is scheduled to take place in the first trimester (up to 12 weeks gestation), two contacts should be scheduled in the second trimester (at 20 and 26 weeks gestation) and five contacts scheduled in the third trimester (at 30, 34, 36, 38 and 40 weeks gestation) (WHO, 2016).

The list of interventions at each contact are to be adapted to the individual woman and not just prescriptive, it is also expected to be flexible as seen in the FANC Model. If the quality of ANC is poor and women's experience of it is negative, evidence shows that women will not attend ANC, irrespective of the number of recommended contacts in the ANC model. Thus, the aim of the 2016 WHO ANC model is to provide pregnant women with respectful individualized, person-centered care at every contact with the healthcare facility (WHO, 2016) (Table 1).

Challenges of focused antenatal care

The implementation of focused antenatal care is not yet attainable in developing countries like Nigeria for the following identified reasons:

(1) Political factor: Lack of political will on policy change and implementation of favorable policies on the issue of maternal and neonatal morbidity/mortality and the diversion of state funds needed for infrastructural development to personal usage negatively affected the outcome of maternal and child health services (Ekabua et al., 2011).

(2) Resistance to change: Difficulty in changing from the present traditional model of antenatal care of frequent visit to the practice of focused ANC of reduced antenatal visit by health care workers and clients (Ekott et al., 2017).

Table 1. The WHO FANC model and the 2016 WHO ANC model.

WHO FANC model	2016 WHO ANC model
First trimester	**First trimester**
Visit 1: 8-12 weeks	Contact 1: up to 12weeks
Second trimester	**Second trimester**
Visit 2: 24-26 weeks	Contact 2 : 20 weeks
-	Contact 3: 24 weeks
Third trimester	**Third trimester**
Visit 3: 32 weeks	Contact 4: 30 weeks
-	Contact 5: 34 weeks
Visit 4: 36-38 weeks	Contact 6: 36 weeks
-	Contact 7: 38 weeks
-	Contact 8: 40 weeks

Return at 41 weeks for delivery, if birth has not occurred

(3) Paucity of human and material resources: Inadequacy of both human and material resources adversely affects the implementation of focused antenatal care services. Health care providers such as doctors, nurses and others are inadequate in number to man the various antenatal centers and some are unwilling to live in rural areas of low infrastructural facilities, also, the migration of trained healthcare workers to industrialized nations negatively affects the implementation of focused antenatal care (Kearns et al., 2014).
(4) Economic factor: The current economic climate and commercialization of health services (antenatal care services) may impede the effective implementation of focused antenatal care in certain settings.
(5) Cultural factors: Prevailing cultural norms, illiteracy and myths about pregnancy and child birth make some women consult unskilled birth attendant/traditional healers instead of the professional health workers as pregnancy is perceived as a natural health process.

In line with the aforementioned stated barriers to ANC, Lincetto et al. (2006), opined that general health system weakness, social, economic, and cultural barriers and presence of weak health referral systems to support case management of complications of pregnancy inevitably reduces the overall impact of ANC.

(1) Poor communication among formal health care providers, traditional birth attendants (TBA) and other community health workers may be the cause of low utilization of ANC services in certain communities.

(2) The attitudes and behaviors of health care providers in ANC clinics, of lack of respect for privacy, confidentiality, and traditional beliefs of the women, may negatively influence the use of ANC as well as maternal and child health services at large (USAID, 2007).

Steps for strengthening antenatal care

Steps for strengthening focused antenatal care as identified by Lincetto et al. (2006) are as follows:

(1) Formulation of favorable health policies: Establishing favorable health policies will positively impact maternal and child health outcomes, and reduce the rate of maternal and infant mortality and morbidity.
(2) Setting attainable benchmarks for focused antenatal care: Focusing on attainable standards makes the objective of the new antenatal care model to be achievable in a stepwise way, thereby leading to the implementation of the objective of each antenatal care visit.
(3) Improving supply of human and material resources: Effective implementation of quality antenatal care service require the presence of adequate and qualified healthcare personnel, this will reduce the number of hours women spend waiting to be attended to while at the same time provides for quality service. Subsidizing and providing resources and infrastructure would encourage both pregnant women utilizing care and the provider of care.
(4) Increasing awareness: Dissemination of information on the importance of utilization of antenatal care services increases compliance to treatment regimen.
(5) Quality improvement: Quality improvement allows for the identification of constraints to providing client-orientated, antenatal care and ensures that care is based on evidenced based practice (Lincetto et al., 2006).

CONCLUSION

Antenatal care remains an essential tool in reducing the maternal and neonatal mortality ratio, and improving maternal and neonatal health. However, the traditional model of antenatal care requires frequent visits to the antenatal care center and in resource-constrained environment this model was observed to be encumbered with numerous challenges. This became a justification for the focused antenatal care model which was instituted about a decade ago. The focused antenatal care model is centered on quality of visits rather than quantity of visits. It operates under the principle of individualization of care and views all pregnant women as being potentially at risk of developing complications thus, it aims at early identification and treatment using evidenced based practice. Practice and satisfaction with focused antenatal care has not being adequate and it has produced lesser positive pregnancy outcome thus the WHO instituted the 2016 WHO ANC model that recommends that contacts during pregnancy should be increased from 4 visits to eight contacts.

CONFLICT OF INTERESTS

The authors have not declared any conflict of interests.

REFERENCES

Abou-Zahr I, Lidia C, Wardlaw TM (2003). Antenatal care in developing countries: promises, achievements and missed opportunities: an analysis of trends, levels and differentials, 1990-2001. World Health Organisation. Available at: http://whqlibdoc.who.int/publications /2003/9241590947.

Ajayi IO, Osakinle DC, Osakinle EO (2013). Quality assessment of the practice of focused antenatal care (FANC) in rural and urban primary health centres in Ekiti State. Open Journal of Obstetrics and Gynecology 3(3):319-326.

Aluko JO, Oluwatosin OA (2008). Pattern and outcome of antenatal care among women attending a Catholic mission hospital in Ibadan, Nigeria. Africa Journal of Medicine and Medical Sciences 37(3):231-238.

Aniebue UU, Aniebue PN (2011). Women's perception as a barrier to focused antenatal care in Nigeria: the issue of fewer antenatal visits. Health Policy and Planning, Oxford Journals 26(5):423-428.

Assegid M, Balew AG, Berhan Y, Davey B, Fesseha N, Gebrehiwot Y, Hailemariam M, Tadesse E (2017). Providing focused antenatal care, Antenatal Care module 13, Part 2, The HEAT Team, HEAT Programme, The Open University. Available at http://www.open.edu/openlearncreate/mod/oucontent/view.php ?id=44&printable=1

Carroli G, Villar J, Piaggio G, Khan-Neelofur D, Gülmezoglu M, Mugford M, Lumbiganon P, Farnot U, Bersgjø P (2001). WHO systematic review of randomised controlled trials of routine antenatal care. Lancet 357(9268):1565-1570. Available at: https://www.ncbi.nlm.nih.gov/pubmed /11377643

Ekabua J, Ekabua K, Njoku C (2011). Proposed framework for making focused antenatal care services accessible: a review of the Nigerian setting. Obstetrics and Gynecology, International Scholarly Research Notices. Volume 2011, Article ID 253964. Available at: http://www.hindawi.com/journals/isrn/2011/253964/

Ekott MI, Edet E, Ovwigho U, Ameh S, Udo A, Akinwunmi F, Babatunde F (2017). Acceptability of focused antenatal care by antenatal clinic attendees in Obio Cottage Hospital, Port Harcourt, Nigeria. Research Journal of Women's Health 4(1):1-6.

Gitonga E (2017). Determinants of focused antenatal care uptake among women in Tharaka Nithi County, Kenya. Advances in Public Health. Article ID 3685401, Available at: https://www.hindawi.com/journals/aph/2017/3685401/

Kearns A, Hurst T, Caglia J, Langer A (2014). Focused antenatal care in Tanzania: Delivering individualized, targeted, high-quality care. Country level Programme. Women and Health Initiative, Maternal Health Task Force. Available at: http://www.mhtf.org/wp-content/uploads/sites/32/2014/09/HSPH-Tanzania5.pdf

Lincetto O, Mothebesoane-Anoh S, Gomez P, Munjanja S (2006). Antenatal Care, Opportunities for Africa's Newborn: Practical data, policy and programmatic support for newborn care in Africa. Available at: http://www.who.int/pmnch/media/publications/aonsectionIII_2.pdf

Olamijulo JA, Oluwole AA, Babah OA, Aderolu MB, Okunola HA, Sanusi MM (2015). Acceptability of Focused Antenatal care by pregnant Nigerian Women and Factors Influencing it. Tropical Journal of Obstetrics and Gynaecology 32(2):90-96.

Oluwatosin OA, Aluko JO (2014). Compliance with intermittent preventive treatment during pregnancy among postpartum women in Ibadan, Nigeria. Africa Journal of Medicine and Medical Sciences 43(1):67-74

Umeora OUJ, Ejikeme BN, Sunday-Adeoye I, Ogu RN (2008). Implementing the new WHO antenatal care model: Voices from end users in a rural Nigerian community. Nigerian Journal of Clinical Practice 11(3):260-264.

United States Agency for International Development (USAID) (2007). Focused antenatal care: Providing integrated, individualized care during pregnancy. Access Program. Available at: https://cdn2.sph.harvard.edu/wp-content/uploads/sites/32/.../ HSPH-Tanzania5.pdf

Villar J, Ba-aqeel H, Piaggio G, Lumbiganon P, Miguel Belizán J, Farnot U, Al-Mazrou Y, Carroli G, Pinol A, Donner A, Langer A, Nigenda G, Mugford M, Fox-Rushby J, Hutton G, Bergsjø P, Bakketeig L, Berendes H, Garcia J (2001). WHO antenatal care randomised trial for the evaluation of a new model of routine antenatal care. The Lancet 357(9268):1551-1564. Available at: https://www.researchgate.net/publication/11960357_WHO_antenatal _care_randomised_trial_for_the_evaluation_of_a_new_model_of_rou tine_antenatal_care

Villar J, Bergsjo P (2002). WHO antenatal care randomized trial: manual for the implementation of the new model. World Health Organization. Geneva. Available at: http://apps.who.int/iris/handle/10665/42513

Women's Health care (2014). Antenatal care. Available at: http://www.wellbeingforwomen. com /pregnancy_topics/antenatal-care/

World Health Organization (1994). Mother-Baby Package: Implementing safe motherhood in countries. Practical Guide. Maternal Health and Safe Motherhood Programme. Available at: http://www.who.int/maternal_child_adolescent/documents/who_dhe_ msm_9411/en/

World Health Organization (2002). Antenatal Care Randomized Trial: Manual for the Implementation of the New Model. Geneva. http://apps.who.int/iris/handle/10665/42513

World Health Organization (2006). Antenatal care coverage. http://www.who.int/whosis/whostat2006AntenatalCareCoverage.pdf

World Health Organization (2015). Global Health Observatory (GHO) data. http://www.who.int/gho/en/

World Health Organization (2016). WHO recommendations on antenatal care for a positive pregnancy experience. http://www.who.int/reproductivehealth/publications/maternal_perinatal _health/anc-positive-pregnancy-experience/en/

11

Nutritional knowledge, attitude and practices among pregnant women who attend antenatal care at public hospitals of Addis Ababa, Ethiopia

Zelalem Tenaw[1], Mikyas Arega[2*] and Erdaw Tachbele[3]

[1]School of Nursing and Midwifery, College of Medicine and Health sciences, Hawassa University, Ethiopia.
[2]School of Nursing and Midwifery, College of Medicine and Health sciences, Debre Berhan University, Ethiopia.
[3]School of Nursing and Midwifery, College of Medicine and Health sciences, Addis Ababa University, Ethiopia.

During pregnancy, maternal nutrition requires considerable attention; however, pregnant women's nutritional knowledge, attitudes, and practices are less understood. The objective of this study was to assess nutritional knowledge, attitude, and practices among pregnant women who attend antenatal care at public hospitals of Addis Ababa, Ethiopia. An institution based cross-sectional study was conducted to collect relevant data of 322 pregnant women, who attended antenatal care service in selected public hospitals in Addis Ababa, Ethiopia from April to May, 2015. Simple random sampling procedure was used to select the public hospitals and systematic sampling techniques were used to select pregnant mothers by using hospitals' registration lists. Data were coded and entered to computer using Epi data version 3.1 and exported to statistical package for social sciences (SPSS) program version 21.0 for further analysis. Multivariable logistic regression analyses were used to identify independent predictors of knowledge, attitude, and practices of pregnant women regarding nutrition. The study revealed that of the 322 pregnant women surveyed, 87(27%), 156(48.4%), and 111(34.5%) of them had knowledge, favorable attitude, and good practices of nutrition during pregnancy, respectively. There was a positive significant association between educational status of women (AOR=3.047, 95%CI (1.046 to 8.873)), family income (AOR=3.093, 95%CI (1.076 to 8.890)), attitude (AOR=4.4, 95%CI (2.315 to 8.299)), number of pregnancies (AOR=2.175, 95%CI (1.034 to 4.573)) and nutrition knowledge during pregnancy. Whereas knowledge, family income, husband education and occupation had a positive association with good practices of nutrition during pregnancy. Knowledge, attitude and practices of pregnant mothers regarding nutrition during pregnancy were low in the study area.

Key words: Knowledge, attitude, practice, nutrition; malnutrition, pregnancy, Ethiopia.

INTRODUCTION

All human beings need a balanced amount of nutrients for proper functioning of the body system. Nutrition is a fundamental pillar of human life, health and development throughout the entire lifespan (Daba et al., 2013). There are approximately 40 different nutrients that are essential for health. If any one of these is deficient in the diet, the person will not be fully healthy and able to resist the agents of disease (Collins, 2007).

Malnutrition is an umbrella term for poor nutrition, whether that is excess consumption of nutrients (overnutrition) or inadequate consumption or absorption of one or more nutrients undernutrition) while undernutrition includes being underweight for one's age, too short for one's age (stunted), dangerously thin (wasted) and deficient in vitamins and minerals (micronutrient malnutrition). Malnutrition is now a problem in both poor and rich countries. In developing countries, while widespread under nutrition and micronutrient deficiencies persist, obesity is also fast emerging as a problem (Shekar et al., 2006).

In Ethiopia, nutritional disorders are among the main causes of morbidity and mortality. The major problems are protein-energy malnutrition and micronutrient deficiencies such as vitamin A, iron, and iodine (Federal Democratic Republic of Ethiopia MoH. Health Sector Development Programme, 2010). 27% of women in Ethiopia are undernourished with a body mass index (BMI) of less than the 18.5 cutoff points; only 4% are obese with a BMI of more than 25.0. These figures put Ethiopia among sub-Saharan countries with the highest proportion of malnourished women (IYCN, 2011).

Pregnancy is a time of increased energy and nutrient needs for a woman in order to meet the needs of the growing fetus and of maternal tissues associated with pregnancy, proper dietary balance is necessary to ensure sufficient energy intake for adequate growth of fetus without drawing on mother's own tissues to maintain her pregnancy (Subarnalata and Panda, 2006).

The poor health and nutrition of women and the lack of care that contributes to their death in pregnancy and child birth also compromises the health and survival of the infants and children (Abdella, 2010). Undernutrition has the most damaging effect on the fetus during pregnancy and in the first two years of life, and the effects of this early damage on health, brain development, intelligence, educability, and productivity are largely irreversible (Shekare et al., 2006).

The pregnant and lactating woman's diet should include a substantial increase in calories, protein, calcium, folic acid, iodine and iron. Pregnant women at particular risk for nutritional deficiencies are adolescents, underweight women, obese women, women with chronic nutritional problems, women who smoke or ingest alcohol or drugs, low income women, and women with chronic illnesses such as diabetes or anemia (Edris et al., 2005). Knowledgeable about nutrition during pregnancy was low in previous studies conducted in 2013 in East Wollega, Ethiopia (64.4%) and in 2012 in Malaysia (70%) (Daba et al., 2013; Mitra et al., 2012).

Practices of eating fresh vegetables and daily milk consumption, is low in the previous studies conducted in America (58.9 and 42.7%) respectively (Federal Democratic Republic of Ethiopia, 2013). While many studies and projects focus on maternal health in Addis Ababa, less attention is given to maternal nutrition in this study area (Berg et al., 2011). It is clear that maternal nutrition is crucial in reducing maternal and infant morbidity and mortality, but no study has been conducted to assess nutritional knowledge, attitude and practices of pregnant mothers in the study area. Therefore, the aim of this study was to assess nutritional knowledge, attitude, and practices among pregnant women who attend antenatal care at public hospitals of Addis Ababa, Ethiopia.

MATERIALS AND METHODS

The study was conducted in Addis Ababa, the capital city of Ethiopia. Established in 1887, by Emperor Menilik II, the city is divided into ten sub-cities. In 2014, Addis Ababa had a projected population of 3,194,999 million of whom 1,679,998 (53%) were females and 1,515,001 (47%) were males (Marías and Glasauer, 2014). According to the information from Ministry of Health, in Addis Ababa there are eight hospitals that provide antenatal services to the public. Based on the information provided from each of these hospitals, the average number of pregnant mothers attending antenatal clinics antenatal care (ANC) is estimated at 2527 per month. The study was conducted from April to May, 2015.

The study population included randomly selected pregnant women who had visited public hospitals in Addis Ababa during the month of April 2015 for antenatal care. The sample size was determined using single population proportion formula at 95% of confidence interval with assumption of prevalence of knowledge of pregnant mothers towards nutrition 64.4% (Daba et al., 2013) with (α=0.05) 5% marginal error (d=0.05). Since the total study population in the study area is below 10,000, reduction formulas were employed. By factoring in a 10% non-response rate, the final sample size was 340.

The calculated sample size was proportionally allocated to randomly select four public hospitals in Addis Ababa based on the number of clients attending antenatal care (ANC). To select study subjects from each antenatal care unit systematic random sampling technique was applied by using client's registration order to get ANC care during the data collection period. Then every 7th person, as they registered, was included in the study at each antenatal care unit until the desired sample size was attained.

An unstructured, semi-structured and structured questionnaire was prepared in English. The questionnaire was translated to Amharic and after data collection it was translated back to English to check for consistency by experts. Data were coded and entered to computer using Epi data version 3.1 and exported to SPSS program version 21.0 for further analysis. The result was presented using frequency tables and percentage. Bivariate analysis was done to determine association between factors and knowledge, attitude and practice among pregnant mothers. Multivariate logistic regressions were performed to identify the independent predictors of knowledge, attitude and practice among pregnant mothers.

*Corresponding author. E-mail: miky24real@gmail.com.

Data were supervised by BSc midwives who were trained on the objective of the study, methods of data collection, and content of questionnaire in order to avoid any ambiguity raised during data collection. Data was checked for completeness, accuracy, and consistency by supervisors and principal investigator after the data collection on daily base. The prepared questionnaire was pre-tested on 5 % of pregnant mothers who were not being included in the study to identify the clarity and sequence of question.

Operational definitions

Knowledge

This refers to an individual's knowledge of nutrition, including the ability to remember and recall food and nutrition related terminology.

Knowledgeable

If respondents score ≥ 70% (out of 100%) on the knowledge questions.

Not knowledgeable

If respondents score < 70% (out of 100%) on the knowledge questions.

Attitudes

Pregnant women's feeding or eating behavior which is influenced by her emotions, motivations, perceptions and thoughts.

Favorable attitude

The respondents attitude score > median

Unfavorable attitude

The respondents 'attitude score less than or equal to the median.

Practice

This is the observable action of the mothers that could affect her nutrition such as eating, feeding, cooking and selecting of foods.

Good practices

This is when the pregnant mothers include fruits, vegetables, meat, milk and milk products in their diet at least once per day, and for frequency of four or more meals per day.

Poor practices

This is when the pregnant mothers did not practice food recommendation for pregnant women and for frequencies, less than once per day regarding fruits, vegetables, meat, milk, and milk products and meal frequency less than three times per day.

Ethical consideration

Ethical clearance was obtained from the Institutional Review Board of Addis Ababa University. Communication with different hospital administrators were made through formal letter obtained from Addis Ababa University. After the purpose and objective of the study have been informed, written and verbal consent was obtained from each study participant. Participants were informed that participation was on voluntary basis and they can withdraw from the study at any time if they were not comfortable about the questionnaire. In order to keep confidentiality, the information was maintained throughout by excluding names as identification in the questionnaire and kept their privacy during the observation by observing them alone.

RESULTS

A total of 322 pregnant mothers participated in the study, with 94.7% response rate. The mean age (0±SD) of the participants was 28.44 (0±4.199) years, while age range was 18 to 42. About 75% of the respondents were in the age range of 25 to 34 years (Table 1). From the participants, 27% had good knowledge about maternal nutrition during pregnancy (Figure 1). Regarding attitude of mothers about nutrition during pregnancy, 156 (48.4%) had favorable attitude. The highest positive attitude score were for preparing meals with iron-rich foods (91%) followed by preparing meals with iodized salt (90.7%) (Figure 2). Concerning micronutrient supply, 204 (63.4%) of women had iron tablets and took them correctly, but only 25 (7.8%) of women had folic acid supplies at three months before pregnancy and within three months after conception. In general, 34.5% of the pregnant mothers reported good practices regarding antenatal nutrition (Figure 3).

Factors associated with maternal nutrition knowledge during pregnancy in Addis Ababa public hospitals

The factors associated with nutritional knowledge during pregnancy include educational status of the women, family income, attitude and number of pregnancies (Table 2).

Factors associated with maternal nutrition attitude during pregnancy in Addis Ababa public hospitals

Knowledge was another factor associated with favorable nutritional attitudes during pregnancy (Table 3).

Factors associated maternal nutrition practice during pregnancy in Addis Ababa public hospitals

The husband's education, occupation, monthly income and knowledge were additional factors associated with nutrition practice during pregnancy (Table 4).

DISCUSSION

This study was conducted to investigate the level of

Table 1. Socio-demographic characteristics of pregnant mothers attending ANC (N=322).

Variable	Number	Percentage (%)	
Age	15-24	50 (15.5)	-
	25-34	244 (75.5)	-
	35-44	28 (8.7)	-
Marital status	Single	6 (1.9)	-
	Married	307(95.3)	-
	Divorced	1 (0.3)	-
	Widowed	3 (0.9)	-
	Separated	5 (1.6)	-
Religion	Orthodox Tewahido	210 (65.2)	-
	Muslim	73 (22.7)	-
	Protestant	36 (11.2)	-
	Catholic	1 (0.3)	-
	Others	2 (0.6)	-
Ethnicity	Amhara	128 (39.8)	-
	Tigrie	22 (6.8)	-
	Oromo	76 (23.6)	-
	Gurage	64 (19.9)	-
	Others	32 (9.9)	-
Family size	One	3 (0.9)	-
	Two	-	-
	Three	26 (8.1)	296 (91.9)
Others	Using salt to cook the main meal	238 (73.9)	84 (26.1)
	Habit of eating fresh citrus fruits/juice	77 (23.9)	245 (76.1)
	Habit of taking coffee or tea	61 (18.9)	261 (81.1)
	Iron Supply	204 (63.4)	118 (36.6)
	Folic Acid supply	25 (7.8)	297 (92.2)
	Frequency of meal per day	211 (65.5)	111 (34.5)
	Habit of taking snacks between meals	219 (68.0)	103 (32.0)
	Habit of eating carbohydrates b/n meals	204 (63.4)	118 (36.6)
	Eating protein daily	303 (94.1)	19 (5.9)
	Habit of eating fresh vegetables	87 (27.0)	235 (73.0)
	Drinking milk	101 (31.4)	221(68.6)
	Eating milk products	57 (17.7)	265 (82.3)
	Eating meat	21 (6.5)	301 (93.5)
	Following weight	259 (80.4)	63 (19.6)

nutritional knowledge, attitudes, and dietary practices of pregnant women during pregnancy and associated factors in Addis Ababa, Ethiopia. Based on this study, 27% of the mothers had knowledge about nutrition during pregnancy, which is lower than previous studies conducted in 2013 in East Wollega, Ethiopia which is 64.4%, and in 2012 in Malaysia it was 70% (Daba et al., 2013; Mitra et al., 2012). As the result showed there is a knowledge gap about nutrition during pregnancy among pregnant mothers in Addis Ababa. The difference might be due to sociodemographic differences and low attention for counseling about nutrition during pregnancy by considering the mothers as knowledgeable on it since the mothers are from capital city of Ethiopia.

In this study, the mothers' knowledge regarding the importance of milk and its products, protein, iron, source of vitamins, calcium and iron were 87(27%),86 (26.7%), 149 (49.4%), 171 (53.1%), 75 (23.3%) and 54 (16.8%)

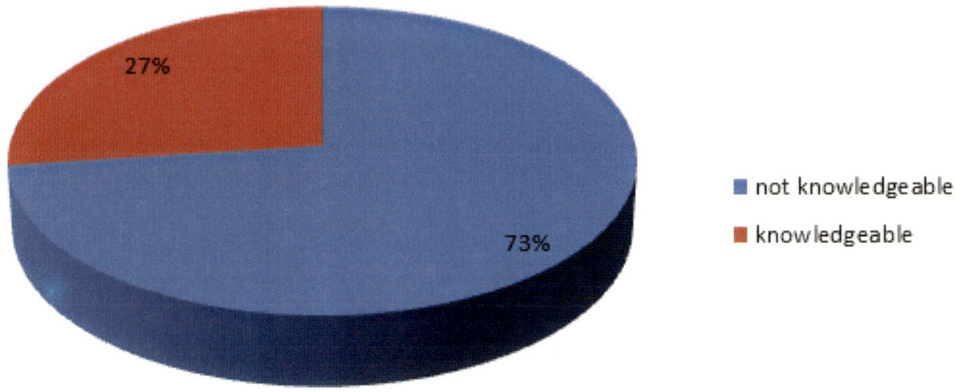

Figure 1: knowledge of pregnant mothers towards Nutrition during pregnancy in Addis Ababa, public hospitals, 2015

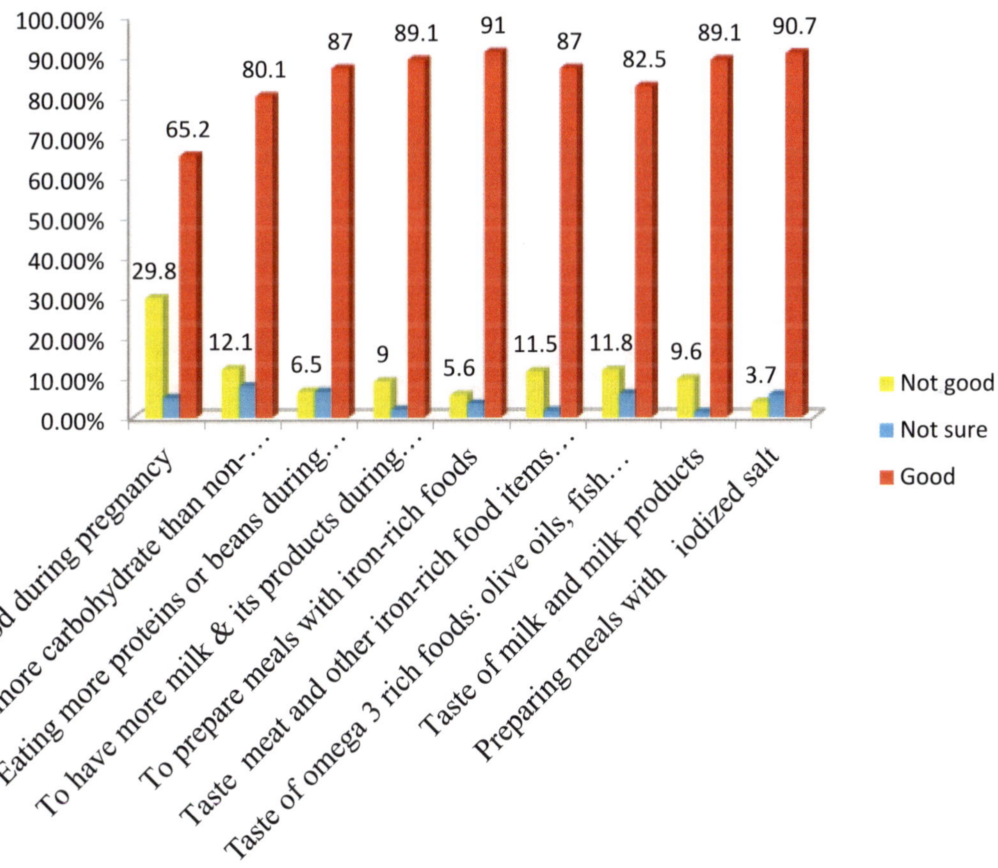

Figure 2: Attitude of mothers to wards nutrition during pregnancy in Addis Ababa, public hospitals, 2015

respectively. Which is lower than the study conducted in Ethiopia at district level (78.2, 68.5, 57.3, 62.9, 71.8%and 61.3% respectively) (Federal Democratic Republic of Ethiopia, 2013). The difference might be due to residence differences and giving attention for other milk substituting products, since they have different options. This study also revealed 147(45.7%) and 114 (35.4%) of pregnant mothers had knowledge about the danger of malnutrition on the mother and her fetus, respectively. This is similar with the study in East Wollega, which is 34.8% (Daba et al., 2013). Most of the pregnant mothers (280 (87%)) thought that eating more protein or beans during

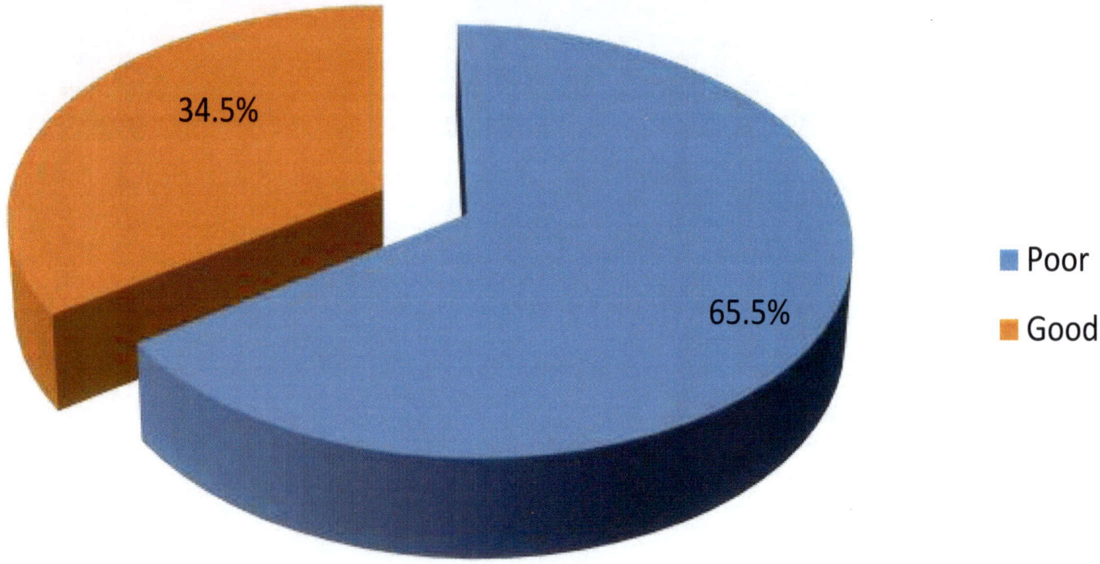

Figure 3. Nutrition practice level of pregnant mothers in Addis Ababa, public hospitals, 2015

Table 2. Factors associated with nutritional knowledge of pregnant mothers (N=322).

Variable		Knowledge			95% CI
		Yes (%)	No (%)	COR	AOR
Education	Diploma and above	55 (53.4)	48 (46.6)	19.5 (7.842-48.384)***	8.054 (2.843-26.130)**
	Secondary school	26 (23.4)	85 (76.6)	5.2 (2.045-13.222)**	3.047 (1.046-8.873)*
	Primary and no formal education	6 (5.6)	102 (94.4)	1	1
Husband education	Diploma and above	49 (48.5)	52 (51.5)	7.4 (3.464-15.996)***	1.276 (0.452-3.604)
	Secondary school	28(21.2)	104 (78.8)	2.1 (0.976-4.635)	1.015 (0.384-2.682)
	Primary and no formal education	10(11.2)	79 (88.8)	1	1
Occupation	Employee	28 (51.9)	26 (48.1)	4.2 (2.228-7.927)***	0.889 (0.378-2.094)
	Private business	1 8(26.9)	49 (73.1)	1.4 (0.756-2.719)	0.46 (0.200-1.040)
	House wives	41(20.4)	160 (79.6)	1	1
Monthly average income	> 3500	54(46.6)	62 (53.4)	13.4 (5.414-32.941)***	5.95 (2.025-17.480)**
	2000-3500	27(25.0)	81 (75.0)	5.1 (2.009-13.002)**	3.093 (1.076-8.890)**
	< 2000	6(6.1)	92 (93.9)	1	1
Obstetric score	Multigravida	71 (29.8)	167 (70.2)	1.807 (0.980-3.330)	2.175 (1.034-4.573)*
	Primigravida	16 (19.0)	68 (81.0)	1	1
Associated diseases	Yes	15 (41.7)	21 (58.3)	2.1 (1.039-4.337)*	0.655 (0.276-1.554)
	No	72 (25.2)	214 (74.8)	1	1
Attitude	Positive	67 (42.9)	89 (57.1)	5.496 (3.124-9.666)***	4.4 (2.315-8.299)***
	Negative	20 (12.0)	146 (88.0)	1	1

***= p<0.001, ** = p<0.01, *=p<0.05, COR= Crude Odds Ratio, AOR= Adjusted Odds Ratio

Table 3. Factors associated with nutritional practices of pregnant mothers (N=322).

Variable		Attitudes		95% CI	
		Positive (%)	Negative	COR	AOR
Education	Diploma and above	68 (66.0)	35 (34.0)	3.437 (1.952-6.054)***	0.826 (0.275-2.482)
	Secondary school	49 (44.1)	62 (55.9)	1.398 (0.813-2.406)	0.721 (0.320-1.621)
	Primary and no formal education	39 (36.1)	69 (63.9)	1	1
Husband education	Diploma and above	62 (61.4)	39 (38.6)	3.289 (1.810-5.978)***	1.572 (0.529-4.671)
	Secondary school	65 (49.2)	67 (50.8)	2.007 (1.147-3.512)*	1.994 (0.943-4.215)
	Primary and no formal education	29 (32.6)	60 (67.4)	1	1
Occupation	Employee	34 (63.0)	20 (37.0)	2.139 (1.153-3.971)*	1.569 (0.421-3.452
	Private business	33 (49.3)	3 4(50.7)	1.221 (0.702-2.125)	0.681 (0.296-1.569)
	House wives	89 (44.3)	112 (56)	1	1
Monthly average income	> 3500	68 (58.6)	48 (41.4)	2.667 (1.529-4.651)**	2.237 (0.905-5.530)
	2000-3500	54 (50.0)	54 (50.0)	1.882 (1.074-3.300)*	0.975 (0.447-2.127)
	< 2000	34 (34.7)	64 (65.3)	1	1
Previous delivery	Abnormal	57 (60.0)	38 (40.0)	1.825 (1.070-3.113)*	1.184 (0.630-2.225)
	Normal	60 (45.1)	73 (54.9)	1	1
Knowledge	Knowledgeable	67 (77.0)	20 (23.0)	5.496 (3.124-9.666)***	5.5 (2.411-12.650)***
	Not knowledgeable	89 (37.9)	146 (62.1)	1	1

***= p<0.001, ** = p<0.01, *=p<0.05, COR= Crude Odds Ratio, AOR= Adjusted Odds Ratio.

Table 4. Factors associated with nutritional practices of pregnant mothers (N=322).

Variable		Practices		95% CI	
		Good (%)	Poor (%)	COR	AOR
Age	35-44	12 (42.9)	16 (57.1)	4.607 (1.542-13.767)**	0.639 (0.121-3.377)
	25-34	92 (37.7)	152 (62.3)	3.718 (1.606-8.610)**	0.901 (0.225-3.619)
	15-24	7 (14.0)	4 3(86.0)	1	1
Education	Diploma and above	58 (56.3)	45 (64.0)	9.419 (4.686-18.934)**	1.202 (0.308-4.695)
	Secondary school	40 (36.0)	71 (64.0)	4.117 (2.050-8.267)**	1.837 (0.598-5.643)
	Primary and no formal education	13(12.0)	95(88.0)	1	1
Husband education	Diploma and above	64 (63.4)	37 (36.6)	7.892 (4.015-15.511)***	6.375 (1.798-22.605)**
	Secondary school	31 (23.5)	101 (76.5)	1.400 (0.714-2.748)	1.905(0.661-5.491)
	Primary and no formal education	16 (18.0)	73 (82.0)	1	1
Occupation	Employee	28 (51.9)	26 (48.1)	3.341 (1.791-6.231)***	1.522 (0.505-4.581)
	Private business	34 (50.7)	33 (49.3)	3.196 (1.795-5.692)***	1.229 (0.491-3.074)
	House wives	49 (24.4)	152 (75.6)	1	1
Husband occupation	Employee	41 (49.4)	42 (50.6)	2.357 (1.412-3.935)**	2.896 (1.256-6.675)*
	Not employee	70 (29.3)	169 (70.7)	1	1
Monthly average income	> 3500	70 (60.3)	46 (39.7)	13.391 (6.310-28.419)***	3.073 (1.010-9.350)*

Table 3. Cond.

	2000-3500	31 (28.7)	77 (71.3)	3.543 (1.631-7.695)**	1.459 (0.501-4.249)
	< 2000	10 (10.2)	88 (89.8)	1	1
Previous delivery	Abnormal	45 (47.4)	50 (52.6)	2.425 (1.392-4.226)**	1.632 (0.776-3.432)
	Normal	36 (27.1)	97 (72.9)	1	1
Knowledge	Knowledgeable	55 (63.2)	32 (36.8)	5.494 (3.237-9.325)***	2.675 (1.138-6.288)*
	Not knowledgeable	56 (23.8)	179 (76.2)	1	1
Attitude	Positive	69 (44.2%)	87 (55.8%)	2.342 (3.237-9.325)***	1.577(0.728-3.414)
	Negative	42 (25.3%)	124 (74.7%)	1	1

***= p<0.001, ** = p<0.01, *=p<0.05, COR= Crude Odds Ratio, AOR= Adjusted Odds Ratio.

pregnancy is good for their pregnancy. This study also revealed that 87 (27%) and 101(31.4%) of pregnant mothers reported practices of eating fresh vegetables and daily milk consumption respectively.

The practice is lower than the study conducted in America (58.9 and 42.7%) respectively (Federal Democratic Republic of Ethiopia, 2013). Therefore, Addis Ababa pregnant mothers needs to improve utilization of fresh vegetables and milk consumption. The difference might be due to cultural, socio economic differences and access to nutritious food. Of the mothers surveyed, 209 (65%) reported having four or more meals per day. More than 219 (68%) of the respondents reported eating snacks between meals. This means the remaining 32% of the mothers do not have good meal practice based on the recommended meal practice.

204 (63.4%) reported eating more carbohydrates between meals during their pregnancy, which was higher than the study conducted in East Wollega (33.9%) (Berg et al., 2011). This study uncovered that, 303(94.1%) of the pregnant mothers had the habit of eating either plant or animal protein daily. This finding was greater than the study conducted in Ethiopia at district level (42.7%) (Federal Democratic Republic of Ethiopia, 2013). The difference may be accessibility of variety of foods in cities than districts. Majority of the mothers in this study, 204 (63.4%) had a good iron supply during pregnancy, which is similar with the study conducted in Western Kenya (62%) (Perumal et al., 2013). This study revealed that, 111(34.5%) of the pregnant mothers had good nutritional practices, which is similar to the study conducted in the East Wollega (Berg et al., 2011).

Conclusion

Most pregnant women in this study reported poor level of knowledge and practices about nutrition and balanced diet during pregnancy. Monthly income, educational level and attitude were the significant factors affecting nutritional knowledge of mothers during pregnancy. Monthly income, husband education and occupation were significant predicting factors for nutritional practices during pregnancy. Good knowledge about maternal nutrition usually affects nutritional attitudes during pregnancy.

RECOMMENDATION

Since pregnant women in this study reported poor knowledge and nutritional practices during pregnancy, health care providers should introduce strategies for providing health education about proper and balanced maternal nutrition during ANC visits.

CONFLICT OF INTERESTS

The authors have not declared any conflict of interests.

REFERENCES

Abdella A (2010). Maternal mortality trend in Ethiopia. Ethiopian Journal of Health Development 24(1).

Berg KC, Torgersen L, Von Holle A, Hamer RM, Bulik CM, Reichborn-Kjennerud T (2011). Factors associated with binge eating disorder in pregnancy. International Journal of Eating Disorders 44(2):124-133.

Collins S (2007). Treating severe acute malnutrition seriously. Archives of disease in childhood 92:453-461.

Daba G, Beyene F, Fekadu H, Garoma W (2013). Assessment of Knowledge of Pregnant Mothers on Maternal Nutrition and Associated Factors in Guto Gida Woreda, East Wollega Zone, Ethiopia. Journal of Nutrition and Food Sciences 3(235).

Edris M, Tekle H, Fitaw Y, Gelaw B, Engedaw D, Alemu T (2005). Maternal nutrition for the Ethiopian health center team. Addis Ababa, Ethiopia.

Federal Democratic Republic of Ethiopia (2013). Central Statistical Agency Population Projection of Ethiopia for All Regions at Wereda Level from 2014-2017. August 2013.

Federal Democratic Republic of Ethiopia MoH (2010). Health Sector Development Programme IV 2010/11–2014/15, 2010.

IYCN (2011). Infant & Young Child Nutrition Project; Literature Review Prepared for the Message and Materials Development Workshop produced through support provided by the United States Agency for International Development (USAID), Addis Ababa, Ethiopia, 2011. Available at: http://www.iycn.org/files/IYCN-Ethiopia-Literature-review-122810.pdf

Marías YF, Glasauer P (2014). Guidelines for assessing nutrition-related knowledge, attitudes and practices. Food and Agriculture Organization of the United Nations (FAO).

Mitra M, Wan A, Manan W, Affizal A, Mohd S (2012). Dietary Knowledge and Behaviors in a Sample of Malay Pregnant Women; UMT 11th International Annual Symposium on Sustainability Science and Management 09th –11th July 2012, Terengganu, Malaysia, 2012.

Perumal N, Cole DC, Ouédraogo HZ, Sindi K, Loechl C, Low J, Levin C, Kiria C, Kurji J, Oyunga M (2013). Health and nutrition knowledge, attitudes and practices of pregnant women attending and not-attending ANC clinics in Western Kenya: a cross-sectional analysis. BMC pregnancy and childbirth 13(1):146.

Shekar M, Heaver R, Lee YK (2006). Repositioning nutrition as central to development: A strategy for large scale action. World Bank Publications.

Subarnalata S, Panda B (2006). A study of nutritional status of pregnant women of some villages in Balasore district, Orissa. Journal of Human Ecology 20(3):227-232.

12

Women autonomy and maternal healthcare services utilization among young ever-married women in Nigeria

Awoleye Abayomi F, Victor Chima* and Alawode Oluwatobi A

Department of Demography and Social Statistics. Obafemi Awolowo University, Ile-Ife, Nigeria.

In Nigeria, the lifetime risk of death from pregnancy or childbirth complications is 1 in 30. Maternal healthcare utilisation addresses the risk of maternal mortality and morbidity but its utilisation is influenced by varying factors of which autonomy has been neglected especially for young married women. Therefore, this study examined the relationship between young married women's level of autonomy and maternal health care utilisation in Nigeria. Secondary data from the 2013 Nigeria Demographic and Health Survey was analysed (n=4996) with consideration of young ever married women (age 15 to 24), who had at least one live birth in the last five years preceding the survey. The binary logistic regression models were fitted into the data. Findings revealed that only 30% of women aged 15 to 24 delivered at a health facility while 44% of the total pregnant women had four or more antenatal care visits before delivery. Also, young women with low autonomy were less likely to meet the minimum requirement of four antenatal visits (OR=0.35: CI: 0.29-0.43) and less likely to deliver at a health facility (OR=0.32: CI: 0.27-0.39). The study underscores the need to empower young women to achieve higher levels of autonomy due to its obvious implication on their health and to encourage integrated interventions that considers engaging household and community structures on the benefits of women autonomy and its importance for mother and child's health. Policy and program considerations that would enable the removal of socio-cultural/demographic barriers towards women autonomy in Nigeria should be encouraged.

Key words: Maternal healthcare utilization, antenatal, postnatal, place of delivery, women autonomy

INTRODUCTION

Maternal mortality refers to the death of a woman during pregnancy or within 42 days after the termination of a pregnancy, from any cause related to the pregnancy or its management but not from accidental causes (PRI, 2013). On a global scale, developing countries account for almost all maternal deaths (99%) of the world maternal deaths (WHO, 2015), while in Nigeria, one woman dies every thirteen minutes from preventable causes related to pregnancy or childbirth making the country to account for 14% of the global total maternal deaths second only to India (APHRC, 2017). It is however interesting to note that it has been established in literature that most of these deaths and health consequences faced by women are preventable (Anya et

*Corresponding author. E-mail: chimavictor1@yahoo.com.

al., 2008; APHRC, 2017).

The challenge of reducing maternal mortality remains a major health problem in Nigeria and recent statistics from national surveys show that in 2008 the estimated maternal mortality ratio (MMR) was 545 /100,000 live-births while in 2013 it estimated to be 576 /100,000 live births implying that the ratio increased between that five-year period and Nigeria did not achieve the millennium development goal 4 of improving maternal health (WHO, 2015). Literature has established utilisation of maternal health care services such as antenatal care visits, place of delivery (delivery at health facility) and postnatal care received from skilled health workers as veritable and effective way of reducing the risk of maternal mortality and morbidity (Bayu et al., 2015; Deo et al., 2015; Hagos et al., 2014; Ochako et al., 2011; Situ, 2013).

The world currently has the highest number of young people in all of human history, with about 1.2 billion people aged 15 to 24 as at the year 2017 (PRB, 2017). This large numbers of young people are faced with numerous challenges which threaten their health and social wellbeing including their sexual and reproductive life. Many of these young people especially girls in less developed countries get married at young ages, fall victim of adolescent or teenage pregnancies and so on.

Adolescent girls who get pregnant in Nigeria have been reported to be at heightened risk of maternal mortality as report has been found that they are less likely to use maternal healthcare services compared to older women (APHRC, 2017). Another study showed that most of these young women due to their uniqueness (Banke-Thomas et al., 2017), neither benefited from these services nor derive any joy of motherhood, as a result of their young age, lack of autonomy and inexperience (Baral et al., 2010). Studies have examined the relationship between women's autonomy and utilisation of any or all of the maternal health care services, and have found association between them (Asweto et al., 2014; Baral et al., 2010; Bhandari et al., 2017; Hagos et al., 2014; Lowe et al., 2016; Speizer et al., 2014; Thapa, 2012; Tiruneh et al., 2017). Other factors such as age, education, employment or labour force participation and wealth quintile have also been found to be associated with maternal healthcare utilisation (Acharya et al., 2017; Adhikari, 2016; Asweto et al., 2014; Banke-Thomas et al., 2017; Baral et al., 2010; Dahiru and Oche, 2015; Deo et al., 2015; Fawole and Adeoye, 2015; Kamiya, 2010; Okeshola and Sadiq, 2013; Sebayang et al., 2017; Sharma et al., 2007; Situ, 2013; Tarekegn et al., 2014; Teklehaymanot et al., 2017; Tiruneh et al., 2017; Urbaeva, 2015; Woldemicael, 2007a, 2007b; Workineh and Hailu, 2014; Yaya et al., 2017).

Umar (2017) submitted that the ability of a young woman to make independent decisions and take appropriate actions on her reproductive desire is dependent on her level of autonomy especially in a society like Nigeria where in some cultures young girls are married off to older men. Further, owing to their inexperience, the married female adolescent need to seek permission from their mother-in-law or husband before taking steps on health matters including maternal healthcare services and that of their babies because they lack the needed autonomy or decision-making power to seek health services (Baral et al., 2010).

However, most, if not all of these studies have focused on the full reproductive age spectrum of 15 to 49 years while little attention has been paid to how young married women's autonomy influence their utilisation of maternal health care services in Nigeria especially the married ones, as increasing the autonomy of these young women could be an effective strategy to maximize the use of maternal healthcare services in developing countries if research findings and recommendations are put in place, and this would give these women the much needed "voice" to be able to seek health care services.

Hence, this study seeks to examine the relationship between autonomy and utilisation of maternal health care services among young ever-married women in Nigeria.

MATERIALS AND METHODS

The study utilized secondary data from the 2013 Nigeria Demographic and Health Survey (NDHS) with a total sample size of 4996 young married women aged 15 to 24 who had at least one child in the last five years preceding the survey. Sampling for the survey involved the use of a nationally representative two-stage cluster sampling design with stratification for rural and urban residence. The outcome variable was utilisation of maternal health care service using place of delivery and number of antenatal care visits. Each of the outcome variables were dichotomized; those who delivered their babies in government hospital, government health center, government health post, other public sectors, private health center and other private sector were coded as (1) while those who delivered their babies at respondent home, other home and others are coded as (0). The number of antenatal care visits was also dichotomized as (0) less than four visits, (1) four visits and above.

Further, the principal explanatory variable was women's autonomy which was measured using women decision on large household purchase, decision on visits to relative/family and decision on woman's own health care. In these three indicators an overall composite score was created to reflect number of decision women participate either alone or jointly. This was achieved by generating a new variable by adding the 3 variables measuring women's autonomy. This produced a minimum of 0 and a maximum of 3. Respondent who had scored between 2 to 3 were classified as "high autonomy" and respondent who scored between 0 to 1 classified as "low autonomy". Other important socio-demographic variables included in the analysis were; wealth index, employment status, highest level of education, religion, place of resident, marital status and age of respondents.

Data was analysed at the univariate, bivariate and multivariate levels. At the univariate level, simple frequencies were obtained, test of associations were conducted between the dependent and independent variables at the bivariate level while variables were fitted into the binary logistic regression in the multivariate level analysis and these variables fitted into the logistic regression were those that were found to be associated with the dependent variable at the bivariate level. For the model specification, in an experiment with possible outcomes as either success or failure, coded 1 or 0 respectively representing a binary outcome, the rate of change in the outcome of interest with respect to explanatory variable(s) can be achieved examining its log odds as shown in the binary logistic model below;

$$\ln p/1-p = \beta 0+\beta 1X1 + \beta 2X2+ \beta 3X3+\ldots +\beta nXn$$

Where $\ln p/1-p$ represents the log odds of using maternal healthcare services, β0 represents the maternal healthcare service utilisation risk without interplay with any explanatory variable, and β1X1 + β2X2+ β3X3+... +βnXn represents the fraction by which the use of maternal healthcare services is altered by a unit change in the respective explanatory variables X1, X2, X3, ...Xn, which in this case includes women autonomy and selected women's socio-demographic characteristics of these young women.

RESULTS

Background of respondents

Table 1 presents the socio-demographic characteristics of the study respondents. Youths of age 20 to 24 years made up three-quarter of the study respondents. Approximately 76% of the respondents were either in the poorest or poor categories of wealth status, with 53% of the respondents reported to be currently working. Exactly 9 in 10 respondents were married, slightly more than half (54 percent) had no education and more than two-thirds of the respondents reported Islam as their religion, with almost the same proportion residing in rural areas.

Utilization of maternal health care services

Table 2 presents the selected intervening variables and their frequency distributions among study respondents. Exposure to mass media was reported by 61% of the women. Almost all women in the study reported having either high or average level of autonomy in their households. Further analysis revealed that the proportion of women who reported average autonomy tripled the proportion with high autonomy while less than one percent reported having low autonomy in the household. On household decision making, more than 70% of the women reported that their husbands alone make decision on the women's health and large household purchases while less than 25% stated these decisions are made jointly. Only 3% of these women reported making decisions alone on their health and on large household purchases. Slightly more than three-fifth of the women (62%) reported that their husbands make decision alone on visit to family or relatives while a small proportion (4%) stated that they make decision on visit to family or relatives alone.

Tables 3 and 4 shows the relationships between the independent, intervening variables and maternal health care utilisation among the respondents. It was revealed that increasing age amongst married youths lead to increase in number of antenatal care visits and facility delivery.

The chi-square statistics indicated significant association between respondents' age, antenatal care ($\chi 2=66.27$, $p<0.05$) and place of delivery ($\chi 2=46.7$, $p<0.05$). The chi-square statistics also confirmed the significant association between the respondents' wealth status, antenatal care ($\chi 2=975.15$, $p<0.05$) and place of delivery ($\chi 2=1044.26$, $p<0.05$). Women in the poorest wealth quintile were found to have attended less antenatal care and least utilized facility delivery. Further results showed that the higher the wealth status of respondents the higher the utilisation of maternal health care services.

Respondents who reported being employed had four or more antenatal care visits and also utilized facility delivery than their counterparts who were unemployed. The Chi-square statistics showed a significant association between respondents' employment status and antenatal care visit ($\chi 2=59.14$, $p<0.05$) and place of delivery ($\chi 2= 56.47$, $p<0.05$). Findings revealed that the higher the respondents level of education, the higher the utilisation of maternal health care services. Respondents with higher education had four or more antenatal care and utilized facility delivery in comparison with other educational levels. The Chi-square test showed significant association between respondents' level of education and antenatal care ($\chi 2=930.89$, $p<0.05$) and place of delivery ($\chi 2= 1,138$, $p<0.05$). Examining religious affiliation, Christians reported four or more antenatal care visits and utilized facility delivery than their counterparts and the Chi-square statistics revealed that respondents' religion is significantly associated with antenatal care ($\chi 2=329.92$, $p<0.05$) and place of delivery ($\chi 2= 634.29$, $p<0.05$). Results show respondents who reside in urban area had four or more antenatal care and utilized facility delivery in comparison to rural residents, with the Chi-square statistics also showing that place of residence is significantly associated with antenatal care ($\chi 2=452.33$, $p<0.05$) and place of delivery ($\chi 2= 541.85$, $p<0.05$).

Women who reported taking decisions alone on her health, large household purchases and visit to relatives reported attending four or more antenatal visits and utilized facility delivery than other women. The Chi-square statistic showed significant association between decision on health and number of antenatal visit ($\chi 2=224.17$, $p<0.05$) and place of deliver ($\chi 2= 290.0$, $p<0.05$); Also, decision on large household purchase was found to be significantly associated with antenatal care ($\chi 2=230.31$, $p<0.05$) and place of delivery ($\chi 2=326.36$, $p<0.05$), and this was also the case between women who make decision alone on visit to relative and antenatal care visits ($\chi 2=232.79$, $p<0.05$) and place of delivery ($\chi 2=285.95$, $p<0.05$).

Analysis of the influence of autonomy on antenatal visits and facility delivery revealed that an increasing level of autonomy lead to increase in number of antenatal visits

Table 1. Distribution of respondents by selected socio-demographic characteristics.

Variable	Frequency (4996)	Percentage (%)
Age of respondent		
15-17 years	338	6.8
18-19 years	851	17.0
20-24 years	3.807	76.2
Wealth index		
Poorest	1.338	26.8
Poorer	1.384	27.7
Middle	993	19.9
Richer	812	16.3
Richest	468	9.4
Employment status		
Not working	2.332	47.0
Working	2.632	53.0
Level of education		
No Education	2.720	54.4
Primary	811	16.2
Secondary	1.383	27.7
Higher	83	1.7
Religion		
Catholic	334	6.7
Other Christians	991	20.0
Islam	3.595	72.5
Traditional	39	0.8
Place of residence		
Urban	1.313	26.3
Rural	3.682	73.7
Marital status		
Married	4.850	97.1
Widowed	19	0.4
Divorced/Separated	127	2.5

Source: 2013 NDHS.

and facility delivery. The Chi-square statistic revealed that women's level of autonomy is significantly associated with antenatal care ($\chi 2=239.33$, $p<0.05$) and place of delivery ($\chi 2=332.48$, $p<0.05$). Exposure to mass media also had a positive influence antenatal visit and facility delivery with the Chi-square test showing a significant association ($\chi 2=397.82$, $p<0.05$) and ($\chi 2=306.20$, $p<0.05$) for antenatal and place of delivery respectively.
Distance to health facility was assessed and it was found that respondents who reported that distance to health facility was not a big problem had four or more antenatal care visits and utilized facility delivery than their counterparts with the Chi-square test showing a significant association between distance to health facility and antenatal care visit ($\chi 2=306.50$, $p<0.05$) and place of delivery ($\chi 2=195.10$, $p<0.05$).

Multivariate analyses

Table 5 presents results of the influence of independent variables on antenatal care visits and place of delivery. In model I, results show that women in the highest wealth quintile are 6 times more likely to attend four or more antenatal care visits than those in the poorest quintile (OR= 6.91, $p< 0.05$). Women who are employed are 3 times more likely to attend antenatal care than the

Table 2. Distribution of respondents by women's level of autonomy, household decision making and healthcare utilization.

Variable	Frequency (4.996)	Percentage (%)
Level of autonomy		
High	1.057	21.9
Average	3.761	77.7
Low	20	0.4
Exposure to mass media		
Not exposed	1.921	39.0
Exposed	3.005	61.00
Distance to health facility		
Big problem	1.749	35.1
Not a problem	3.233	64.9
Number of antenatal care visits		
Less than four visits	2744	56.0
Four visits and above	2.159	44.0
Place of last delivery		
Health facility	1.490	29.9
Home	3.496	70.1
Decision on own health		
Respondent alone	164	3.4
Respondent and husband	1.145	23.7
Husband alone	3.510	72.5
Others	22	0.5
Decision on large household purchase		
Respondent alone	155	3.2
Respondent and husband	1.069	22.1
Husband alone	3.591	74.2
Others	24	0.5
Decision on visit to family or relative		
Respondent alone	233	4.8
Respondent and husband	1.572	32.5
Husband alone	3.018	62.4
Others	18	0.4

Source: 2013 NDHS.

unemployed and a woman's level of education was found to significantly influence antenatal care visit as women with secondary or higher educational level were more than 3 times likely to attend antenatal care than those who had no education (OR=3.94, $p<0.05$). Further results at the multivariate level showed that there was no significant relationship between respondents' religion and antenatal care visit but residence played an important role in antenatal care visit as rural residents were 27% less likely to attend antenatal care in comparison to their counterparts who reside in urban areas.

The inclusion of intervening variables in model II alters the nature of the relationship between respondents' socio-economic determinants and antenatal care visit. In the model, results show that respondents who are in the highest wealth quintile are more than 5 times likely to attend 4 or more antenatal visit. Likewise, educated women were 2 times more likely to attend antenatal care in comparison to those who had no formal education.

Results further revealed a significant relationship

Table 3. Cross tabulation of maternal health care utilization and independents and intervening variables.

Variable	Antenatal care		Place of delivery	
	4 visits and above	< 4 visits	Health facility	Home
Age of respondents				
15-17 years	92 (27.4)	244 (72.6)	62 (18.3)	276 (81.7)
18-19 years	308 (36.9)	527 (63.1)	200 (23.5)	649 (76.5)
20-24 years	1.759 (47.1)	1.973 (52.9)	1.229 (32.3)	2571 (67.7)
Statistic	χ^2=66.27 DF=2	p<0.05	χ^2=46.7 DF=2	p<0.05
Wealth index				
Poorest	243 (18.3)	1.081 (81.7)	95 (7.2)	1.240 (92.9)
Poorer	441 (32.4)	921 (67.7)	248 (17.9)	1.133 (82.1)
Middle	523 (53.8)	450 (46.2)	372 (34.5)	620 (62.5)
Richer	567 (71.6)	225 (28.5)	429 (52.9)	383 (47.1)
Richest	386 (85.2)	67 (14.8)	346 (74.20)	120 (25.8)
Statistic	χ^2=975.15 DF=4	p<0.05	χ^2=1044.26 DF=4	p<0.05
Employment status				
Not working	872 (38.0)	1.420 (62.0)	569 (24.4)	1.760 (75.6)
Working	1.272 (49.3)	1.310 (50.7)	904 (34.4)	1.721 (65.6)
Statistic	χ^2=59.14 DF=1	p<0.05	χ^2= 56.47 DF=1	p<0.05
Level of education				
No education	667 (24.9)	2.016 (12.9)	306 (11.3)	2.408 (88.7)
Primary	424 (53.9)	363 (46.1)	256 (35.3)	523 (64.7)
Secondary	1000 (73.9)	353 (26.1)	824 (59.7)	556 (40.3)
Higher	69 (85.1)	12 (14.9)	75 (90.3)	8 (9.7)
Statistic s	χ^2=930.89 DF=3	p<0.05	χ^2= 1,138 DF=3	p<0.05
Religion				
Catholic	201 (61.6)	125 (38.4)	220 (66.0)	114 (34.0)
Other Christian	647 (67.7)	309 (32.3)	539 (54.5)	450 (45.5)
Islam	1.285 (36.2)	2.261 (63.8)	716 (20.0)	2.872 (80.0)
Traditional	15 (36.9)	25.0 (63.2)	7 (18.9)	32 (81.2)
Statistics	χ^2=329.92 DF=3	p<0.05	χ^2= 634.29 DF=3	p<0.05
Place of residence				
Urban	898 (70.0)	385 (30.0)	732 (55.7)	582 (44.3)
Rural	1.262 (34.9)	2.359 (65.2)	759 (20.7)	2.914 (79.3)
Statistics	χ^2=452.33 DF=1	p<0.05	χ^2= 541.85 DF=1	p<0.05
Mother marital status				
Married	2.085 (43.8)	2.676 (23.5)	1.429 (29.5)	3.412 (70.5)
Widowed	13 (73.5)	5 (26.5)	10 (55.0)	8 (45.0)
Divorce	62 (49.2)	64 (50.8)	51 (40.5)	75 (59.5)
Statistics	χ^2=7.21 DF=2	p<0.05	χ^2= 12.18 DF=2	p<0.05
Decision on respondent health				
Respondent alone	120 (75.9)	38 (24.1)	98 (59.4)	67 (40.6)
Respondent and husband	661 (59.0)	458 (41.0)	519 (45.4)	625 (54.6)
Husband alone	1.286 (37.3)	2.167	793 (22.7)	2.708 (77.3)
Others	14(65.1)	7 (34.9)	15 (68.1)	7 (31.9)
Statistics	χ^2=224.17 DF=3	p<0.05	χ^2= 290.0 DF=3	p<0.05

Table 4. Cross tabulation of maternal health care utilization and independents and intervening variables.

Variable	Antenatal care		Place of delivery	
	4 visits and above	< 4 visits	Health facility	Home
Decision on large household purchase				
Respondent alone	105 (70.5)	44 (29.5)	86 (55.6)	69 (44.4)
Respondent and husband	640 (61.40)	403 (38.0)	523 (49.0)	545 (51.0)
Husband	1.318 (37.3)	2.217 (62.7)	802 (22.4)	2.781 (77.6)
Others	16 (72.1)	6 (27.9)	14 (57.5)	10 (42.5)
Statistics	χ^2=230.31 DF=3	p<0.05	χ^2=326.36 DF=3	p<0.05
Decision on visits to relative				
Respondent alone	159 (69.7)	69 (30.3)	122 (52.4)	111 (47.7)
Respondent and husband	863 (56.0)	679 (44.0)	668 (42.6)	902 (57.5)
Husband	1.047 (35.3)	1.918 (64.7)	627 (20.8)	2.383 (79.2)
Others	11 (66.0)	5 (34.0)	9 (52.0)	8 (48.0)
Statistics	χ^2=232.79 DF=3	p<0.05	χ^2=285.95 DF=3	p<0.05
Women's level of autonomy				
High autonomy	674 (65.3)	358 (34.7)	553 (52.3)	504 (47.7)
Medium autonomy	1.394 (37.7)	2.304 (62.3)	860 (22.9)	2.891 (77.1)
Low autonomy	11(62.0)	7(3.0)	11 (29.5)	9 (44.0)
Statistics	χ^2=239.33 DF=2	p<0.05	χ^2=332.48 DF=2	p<0.05
Exposure to mass media				
Not exposed	489 (25.9)	1.398 (74.1)	293 (15.3)	1.624 (84.7)
Exposed	1.646 (55.8)	1.303 (44.2)	1.177 (39.2)	1.823 (60.8)
Statistics	χ^2=397.82 DF=1	p<0.05	χ^2=306.20 DF=1	p<0.05
Distance to health facility				
Big problem	465 (26.8)	1.268 (73.2)	302 (17.3)	1.442 (82.7)
Not a big problem	1.687 (53.4)	1.470 (46.6)	1.186 (36.7)	2.042 (63.3)
Statistics	χ^2=306.50 DF=1	p<0.05	χ^2=195.10 DF=1	p<0.05

between exposure to mass media, distance to health facility and utilisation of antenatal care services. Women with access to mass media were almost twice more likely to attend antenatal care than other women (OR=1.48, p<0.05), likewise those who reported that distance to health facility was not a problem (OR=1.98, p<0.05). Model III examined the relationship between the principal variable; women's level of autonomy and antenatal care. Respondents' with low level of autonomy were 65% less likely to attend antenatal care compared to their counterparts who had high level of autonomy (OR=0.35, p<0.05). The inclusion of intervening variables in model IV slightly changed the extent of relationship but women's autonomy still had significant influence on antenatal care with an increased odd ratio of 5% (OR=0-40, p<0.05).

Model V presents the relationship between respondents' socio-demographic determinants and facility delivery holding intervening variables constant. Result shows that respondents in the highest wealth index were 7 times more likely to deliver in facilities in comparison to

Table 5. Multivariate analysis of the selected independents, intervening and outcome variables.

Variable	Number of antenatal care visits				Place of delivery			
	Model 1	Model 2	Model 3	Model 4	Model 5	Model 6	Model 7	Model 8
	OR	OR	OR	OR	OR	OR	OR	OR
Wealth index								
Poorest	1.00	1.00	-	-	1.00	1.00	-	-
Poorer	1.62*	1.45*	-	-	1.84*	1.81*	-	-
Middle	2.87*	2.28*	-	-	3.53*	3.30*	-	-
Richer	4.21*	3.20*	-	-	4.42*	4.10*	-	-
Richest	6.91*	5.16*	-	-	7.01*	6.44*	-	-
Employment status								
Not working	1.00	1.00	-	-	1.00	1.00	-	-
Working	1.3*	1.31*	-	-	1.29*	1.26*	-	-
Level of education								
No education	1.00*	1.00	-	-	1.00	1.00	-	-
Primary	2.15*	2.11*	-	-	1.92*	1.87*	-	-
Secondary	3.18*	2.88*	-	-	3.03*	2.88*	-	-
Higher	3.94*	3.28*	-	-	13.97*	12.63*	-	-
Religion								
Catholic	1.00	1.00	-	-	1.00	1.00	-	-
Other Christian	1.17**	1.22**	-	-	0.48*	0.46*	-	-
Islam	1.00**	0.97**	-	-	0.27*	0.25*	-	-
Traditional	1.00**	1.27**	-	-	0.28*	0.29*	-	-
Place of residence								
Urban	1.00	1.00	-	-	1.00	1.00	-	-
Rural	0.73**	0.81**	-	-	0.60*	0.63*	-	-
Marital status								
Married	1.00	1.00	-	-	1.00	1.00	-	-
Widowed	2.66**	2.55**	-	-	1.78**	1.68**	-	-
Divorced/Separated	0.97**	0.96**	-	-	1.33**	1.37**	-	-
Exposure to mass media								
Not exposed	-	1.00	-	-	-	1.00	-	-
Exposed	-	1.48*	-	-	-	1.62**	-	-
Distance to health facility								
Big problem	-	1.00	-	-	-	1.00	-	-
Not a problem	-	1.98*	-	-	-	0.62*	-	-

Table 5 Cont'd

Women's level of autonomy								
High autonomy	-	-	1.00	1.00	-	-	1.00	1.00
Low autonomy	-	-	0.35*	0.40*	-	-	0.32*	0.38*
Exposure to mass media								
Not exposed	-	-	-	1.00	-	-	-	1.00
Exposed	-	-	-	3.02*	-	-	-	2.95*
Distance to health facility								
Big problem	-	-	-	1.00	-	-	-	1.00
Not a problem	-	-	-	2.75*	-	-	-	2.31*

*p<0.05, **p>0.05.

women in other wealth quintile (OR=7.01, p<0.05). Being employed was another positive factor as women who were working were 29% more likely to deliver in facilities in comparison to the unemployed. Considering respondents' level of education, respondents' who had a higher level of education were more than 13 times likely to have health facility delivery compared to women who did not have formal education (OR=13.97, p<0.05), that is, the higher the respondents' level of education the higher the utilisation of facility delivery. Respondents' who reside in the rural area were 40% less likely to deliver in health facilities compared to urban residents. Introduction of intervening variables in model VI revealed that there is a significant relationship between wealth index, employment status, level of education, religion, place of residence, distance to health facility and place of delivery.

Results further showed that women who were in the richest category were more than 6 times likely to deliver at health facilities than women in the reference category (OR=6.44, p<0.05). Result pattern reveal an increasing proportion of facility delivery with increasing wealth quintile and occupation (OR=1.26, p<0.05).

In addition, holding intervening variables constant, a significant relationship was observed between women's level of autonomy and place of delivery. Women who reported low level of autonomy were 68% less likely to deliver at health facility compared to other women (OR=0.32, p<0.05). Introduction of the intervening variables revealed a significant relationship between women's level of autonomy, exposure to mass media, distance to health facility and place of delivery; with women who were exposed to mass media approximately 3 times more likely to deliver at health facility than other women (OR=2.95, p<0.05). With respect to distance to health facility, women who reported distant to health facility not being a problem are more than 2 times likely to deliver at health facility other women (OR=2.31, p<0.05) (Table 5).

DISCUSSION

The study objective was to examine the relationship between young women's socio-demographic characteristics, level of autonomy and maternal health care utilisation among young ever married women in Nigeria. It was found that more than half (56%) of young women had less than four antenatal visits while pregnant while the required standard by the World Health Organization (WHO) was a minimum of 4 antenatal visit and as much as 8 visits. It was also found that less than 40% women deliver at a health facility. This study found significant relationships between women autonomy, antenatal care visits and health facility delivery. The findings of this study are consistent with the findings of (Asweto et al., 2014; Baral et al., 2010; Bhandari et al., 2017; Deo et al., 2015; Fawole and Adeoye, 2015; Woldemicael, 2007b), who found that maternal healthcare utilisation is influenced by women autonomy. Also, the findings of this study are in agreement with the findings of Sharma et al., (2007) where it was stated that women with greater autonomy irrespective of physical and financial resources are able to manage their own children's health care and make fertility decisions too. Furthermore, other findings including those of Kamiya

(2010); Tarekegn et al., (2014); Teklehaymanot et al., (2017); Thapa, (2012); Workineh and Hailu, (2014) and Deo et al. (2015) found that significant associations between women autonomy and utilisations of maternal healthcare services and specifically stated that women with higher level of autonomy were nearly three times more likely to have at least 4 antenatal care visits. Speizer et al. (2014) highlighted the role of community norms in institutional delivery but stated that women autonomy played a major role in ensuring these deliveries are facility based. This was also the case in Ethiopia as found by Tiruneh et al. (2017)

Findings on the relationship between women autonomy and maternal healthcare utilisation is explained by the fact that younger women in marriages are not as educated as older women, don't have the financial wherewithal to make decisions that have financial implications and follow through, don't have adequate information to ensure evidence-based decision making and also perceive that they are inexperienced to make decisions on issues related to motherhood and pregnancy, hence the dependence of their mother in-laws but this is in contrast to the findings of Hagos et al. (2014) in Ethiopia and Lowe et al. (2016) in Gambia where it was found that women who had autonomy in decision making about place of delivery were less likely to deliver in a health facility and that at the time of delivery, the decision to receive care by trained personnel was often beyond the women's control, resulting in birth-related complications respectively.

Socio-demographic determinants strongly influencing maternal healthcare utilisation identified in this study include employment status, educational level, exposure to mass media and household wealth index. These has also been established in other studies as Okeshola and Sadiq (2013) stated that there is a close relationship between household wealth index and maternal healthcare utilisation among young women in Nigeria; that is, the richer the family, the higher the likelihood of a young woman using maternal healthcare services. Also, in Kenya, Ochako et al. (2011) established that household wealth is significantly associated with the use of maternal healthcare services among young women as also highlighted by the studies of Bhandari et al. (2017), Fawole and Adeoye (2015), Hagos et al. (2014) and Tarekegn et al. (2014) and summarised that households with more financial strength have more access to healthcare generally and not just maternal healthcare, hence, women in these households should ordinarily attend maternal healthcare services more than women from households in the lower wealth quintiles.

Education was also found to be significantly associated with the use of maternal healthcare services and this is consistent with the findings of Furuta and Salway (2006), Sipsma et al. (2014), Adeoye (2015), Bhandari et al. (2017), Fawole and Tiruneh et al. (2017), Duah and Adisah-Atta (2017). This finding can be explained by the fact that better educated women have access to more information either through the mass media or social media compared to less educated women. Employment status or labour force participation was also found to have a significant association with maternal healthcare services and this is supported by the findings of Sebayang et al., (2017), where it was found in Myanmar that adolescent mothers with a high level of labour force participation had higher odds of attending ante-natal care services compared to older women. This might probably be due to the fact that women who are engaged in labour force are better exposed to information from colleagues at work on the importance of maternal healthcare services or that they have the financial capability to cater for financial costs associated with receipt of health services.

Conclusion

This study examined the relationship between women autonomy and utilization of maternal healthcare services (antenatal care and facility delivery) among young ever-married women in Nigeria. The findings of the study have revealed low level of maternal healthcare utilization among young ever-married women in Nigeria, with a high proportion of young women not attending antenatal visits while pregnant and not using the health facilities for delivery of their children. Women autonomy was found to be significantly associated with use of maternal healthcare services among young ever-married women in Nigeria. Other factors revealed that household wealth index, employment status, level of education, place of residence, distance to health facility and exposure to mass media also contributes to antenatal care use and facility delivery. Based on these findings, it is recommended that women should be empowered financially and educationally to ensure they possess the knowledge of the benefits of maternal healthcare and have the financial strongholds to back decisions to use such services. Also, sensitization programs should be targeted to household and community structures to enhance knowledge of the benefits of maternal healthcare and facility delivery as this will ensure household and community barriers such as permission from husband or mother in-laws and other community norms are addressed. Finally, government and programs should adopt strategies that encourage women to utilise maternal healthcare services; this could be in the form of active referrals using community resource persons, social protection schemes such as provision of transportation vouchers and integrated community outreaches by skilled health workers.

Ethical consideration

The Nigerian Demographic and Health Survey (DHS)

data used for the study was downloaded from the website of MEASURE DHS after a written request was submitted to the DHS ICF MACRO and permission was granted to use

ACKNOWLEDGEMENT

The authors wish to appreciate the measure of DHS for providing and granting them the approval to use the data for the study.

CONFLICT OF INTERESTS

The authors have not declared any conflict of interests.

REFERENCES

Acharya P, Adhikari TB, Neupane, D, Thapa K, Bhandari PM (2017). Correlates of institutional deliveries among teenage and non-teenage mothers in Nepal. PLoS ONE 12(10):e0185667.

Adhikari R (2016). Effect of Women's autonomy on maternal health service utilization in Nepal: a cross sectional study. BMC Women's Health 16(26):7.

African Population and Health Research Center (APHRC) (2017). Maternal Health in Nigeria: Facts and Figures *Fact Sheet*. African Population and Health Research Center.

Anya SE, Hydara A, Jaiteh LE (2008). Antenatal care in The Gambia: Missed opportunity for information, education and communication. Pregnancy and Childbirth, 8(1):9.

Asweto CO, Ouma JO, Aluoch JR, Obonyo CO (2014). Women Empowerment and Skilled Attendance/Facility Delivery in a Rural Community of Western Kenya. Education 5000(62):48-53.

Banke-Thomas OE, Banke-Thomas AO, Ameh CA (2017). Factors influencing utilisation of maternal health services by adolescent mothers in Low-and middle-income countries: a systematic review. BMC Pregnancy and Childbirth 17(65).

Baral YR, Lyons K, Skinner J, Van Teijlingen ER (2010). Determinants of skilled birth attendants for delivery in Nepal. Kathmandu University Medical Journal 8(31):325-332.

Bayu H, Fisseha G, Mulat A, Yitayih G, Wolday M (2015). Missed opportunities for institutional delivery and associated factors among urban resident pregnant women in South Tigray Zone, Ethiopia: a community-based follow-up study. Global Health Action 8(1):28082.

Bhandari TR, Kutty VR, Sarma PS, Dangal G (2017). Safe delivery care practices in western Nepal: Does women's autonomy influence the utilization of skilled care at birth? PLoS ONE 12(8):e0182485.

Dahiru T, Oche OM (2015). Determinants of antenatal care, institutional delivery and postnatal care services utilization in Nigeria. Pan Afrian Medical Journal 21(321).

Deo KK, Paudel YR, Khatri RB, Bhaskar RK, Paudel R, Mehata S, Wagle RR (2015). Barriers to utilization of antenatal care services in eastern Nepal. Frontiers in Public Health 3(197):1-7.

Duah HO, Adisah-Atta I (2017). Determinants of Health Care Decision Making Autonomy among Mothers of Children under Five Years in Ghana: Analysis of 2014 Ghana Demographic and Health Survey. International Journal of Women's Health and Wellness 3(4).

Fawole OI, Adeoye IA (2015). Women's status within the household as a determinant of maternal health care use in Nigeria. African Health Sciences 15(1):217-225.

Furuta M, Salway S (2006). Women's Position Within the Household as a Determinant of Maternal Health Care Use in Nepal. International Family Planning Perspectives 32(1):17-27.

Hagos S, Shaweno D, Assegid M, Mekonnen A, Afework MF, Ahmed S (2014). Utilization of institutional delivery service at Wukro and Butajera districts in the Northern and South Central Ethiopia. BMC Pregnancy and Childbirth 14(178).

Kamiya Y (2010). Endogenous Women's Autonomy and the Use of Reproductive Health Services: Empirical Evidence from Tajikistan *OSIPP Discussion Paper: DP-2010-E-010*: Osaka School of Inernational Public Policy, Osaka University.

Lowe M, Chen DR, Huang SL (2016). Social and Cultural Factors Affecting Maternal Health in Rural Gambia: An Exploratory Qualitative Study. PLoS ONE 12(9):e0163653.

Ochako R, Fotso JC, Ikamari L, Khasakhala A (2011). Utilization of maternal health services among young women in Kenya: Insights from the Kenya Demographic and Health Survey, 2003. BMC Pregnancy and Childbirth 11(1).

Okeshola FB, Sadiq IT (2013). Determinants of Home Delivery among Hausa in Kaduna South Local Government Area of Kaduna State, Nigeria. American International Journal of Contemporary Research 3(5):78-85.

Population Reference Bureau (PRB) (2017). 2017 World Population Data Sheet with a Special focus on Youth. https://www.prb.org/2017-world-population-data-sheet/

Population Research Institute (PRI) (2013). Definitions of Maternal Mortality. In: P. R. Institute (Ed.), USA (pp. 5). https://www.pop.org/definitions-of-maternal-mortality/

Sebayang SK, Efendi F, Astutik E (2017). Women's Empowerment and the Use of Antenatal Care Services in Southeast Asian Countries DHS Working Paper No. 129. Rockville, Maryland, USA: ICF.

Sharma SK, Sawangdee Y, Sirirassamee B (2007). Access to health: women's status and utilization of maternal health services in Nepal. Journal of Biosocial Science 391(5):67.

Sipsma H, Ofori-Atta A, Canavan M, Udry C, Bradley E (2014). Empowerment and use of antenatal care among women in Ghana: a cross-sectional study. BMC Pregnancy and Childbirth 14(364).

Situ KC (2013). Women's Autonomy And Maternal Health Care Utilization In Nepal. (Mater of Public Health), University of Tampere.

Speizer IS, Story WT, Singh K (2014). Factors associated with institutional delivery in Ghana: the role of decision-making autonomy and community norms. BMC Pregnancy and Childbirth 14(398).

Tarekegn SM, Lieberman LS, Giedraitis V (2014). Determinants of maternal health service utilization in Ethiopia: analysis of the 2011 Ethiopian Demographic and Health Survey. BMC Pregnancy and Childbirth 14(161)

Teklehaymanot A, Niguse D, Tesfay A (2017). Early Postnatal Care Service Utilization and Associated Factors among Mothers Who Gave Birth in the Last 12 Months in Aseko District, Arsi Zone, South East Ethiopia in 2016. Journal of Women's Healthcare 6(1). Available at: https://www.omicsonline.org/open-access/early-postnatal-care-service-utilization-and-associated-factors-among-motherswho-gave-birth-in-the-last-12-months-in-aseko-distric-2167-0420-1000358.php?aid=86510

Thapa DK, Niehof A (2013). Women's autonomy and husbands' involvement in maternal health care in Nepal. Social Science and Medicine 93:1-0.

Tiruneh FN, Chuang KY, Chuang YC (2017). Women's autonomy and maternal healthcare service utilization in Ethiopia. BMC Health Services Research 17(718).

Umar AS (2017). Women Autonomy and the Use of Antenatal and Delivery Services in Nigeria. MOJ Public Health 6(2):00161. Available at: http://medcraveonline.com/MOJPH/MOJPH-06-00161.pdf

Urbaeva Z (2015). Women's Autonomy and Utilization of Prenatal Services in Armenia and Azerbaijan: Analysis of Demographic and Health Surveys 2005-2006. (Doctor of Philosophy), Arizona State University.

World Health Organisation (WHO) (2015). Trends in Maternal Mortality: 1990 to 2015 Executive Summary: World Health Organisation.

Woldemicael G (2007a) Do Women with Higher Autonomy Seek More Maternal and Child Health-Care? Evidence from Ethiopia and Eritrea. *Vol. MPIDR WORKING PAPER WP 2007-035* (pp. 27).

Woldemicael G (2007b) Do women with higher autonomy seek more maternal and child health-care? Evidence from Ethiopia and Eritrea. MPIDR Working Paper WP 2007-035. Max Planck Institute for Demographic Research. Available at:

https://www.demogr.mpg.de/en/projects_publications/publications_1904/mpidr_working_papers/do_women_with_higher_autonomy_seek_more_maternal_and_child_health_care_evidence_from_ethiopia_and_2745.htm
Workineh YG, Hailu DA (2014). Factors affecting utilization of postnatal care service in Jabitena district, Amhara region, Ethiopia. Science Journal of Publci Health 2(3):169-176.
Yaya S, Bishwajit G, Ekholuenetale M (2017). Factors associated with the utilization of institutional delivery services in Bangladesh. PLoS ONE, 12(2):e0171573.

Care of postpartum women following complicated labour and delivery at the University Teaching Hospital, Lusaka, Zambia: Self- reported practices by midwives

Priscar Sakala Mukonka*, Patricia Katowa Mukwato, Concepta Namukolo Kwaleyela and Margaret Maimbolwa

School of Nursing Sciences, University of Zambia, Zambia.

Although childbirth is considered to be a normal physiological process, complications leading to postpartum maternal mortality and morbidity may arise in 20% of the cases; it can affect the mother, foetus or both and may be long or short term. The aim of the study was to assess practices of midwives on the care of postpartum women who experienced complicated labour and delivery from time of admission to the postnatal wards until their discharge. A descriptive cross sectional survey was conducted at the University Teaching Hospital – Women and Newborn in Lusaka. 51 midwives working in postnatal wards participated in the study. Data were collected using a self administered questionnaire with a 4 point likert scale and some closed and open ended questionnaires. SPSS version 20 statistical package was used to analyze data, expressed as descriptive summary measures. Majority of the midwives (78.9%) reported that the care they provided to postpartum women who had complicated labour and delivery was not comprehensive and satisfactory due to shortage of staff and high workload, inadequate materials and equipment to use and midwives' lack of motivation and bad attitude. Midwives scored themselves high in observing and assessing the postpartum women while they rated themselves low in performing for the women self-care activities. There is need to improve the care rendered to the postpartum women with complicated labour and delivery in order to promote good health and to prevent postpartum complications.

Key words: Postpartum mothers/women, postnatal care, complicated labour and delivery, self- reported practices, midwives, hospital care.

INTRODUCTION

Although childbirth is considered to be a normal physiological process, complications may arise in 20% of the cases (Hoque and Klein, 2011; Dippenaar and Da Serra, 2013). Complicated labour and delivery is any process of labour and delivery affected by any conditions or disorders that adversely affect women and their foetal health (Hoque and Klein, 2011). The postpartum period is particularly important for women, as during this period they may develop serious, life-threatening complications. There is evidence that a large

*Corresponding author. E-mail: pmukonka@yahoo.com.

proportion of maternal and neonatal deaths occur during the postpartum period, with postpartum heamorrhage being an important cause; therefore, comprehensive postnatal care of postpartum mothers (PPM) is very essential as failure to do so may result in short or long term postpartum maternal morbidities and mortalities. Although the postnatal period is the most critical period, it is also the most neglected phase for providing quality care for mothers and babies because essential postnatal care and attention to their overall wellbeing may not be available or accessible by the mothers (MOH, 2011; Saleem et al., 2014).

It is estimated that 340 000 maternal deaths occur worldwide each year in low-income countries and 61% of these maternal deaths occur during the first six weeks after birth, and nearly half of those deaths take place during the first week after delivery (Lohela, 2012; WHO, 2013; Saleem et al., 2014). In the Sub-Saharan Africa including Zambia, many women do not have access to health care during early postnatal period putting them at high risk of illness and death (Warren, 2015; Ngozi et al., 2016).

The Zambia's safe motherhood guidelines recommend that women receive at least four postnatal checkups, the first within six hours of delivery, the second on the second day following delivery, the third on the sixth day following delivery, and the last within six weeks after delivery (MoH, 2011).

According to the Zambia Demographic Health Survey (2013-2014) (ZDHS), only 63% of women received postnatal care within the critical first two days following delivery broken down as: Forty-eight percent of women received postnatal care within four hours of delivery, 14% received care within 4-23 hours, and 2% were seen 1-2 days following delivery. Twenty-eight percent of women did not receive a postnatal checkup within the recommended time (CSO, 2014). In Lusaka Province, 17% of postpartum mothers did not receive postnatal care within the first critical 2 days after delivery. The ZDHS also indicates that 70% of postpartum women are cared for by either nurses or midwives. This is contrary to the antenatal care attendance which is at 96% and mothers received care from skilled health personnel (CSO, 2014). This makes postnatal care still to be a problem in terms of accessibility.

The University Teaching Hospital is the biggest referral hospital in Lusaka and the country as a whole with average total deliveries of 1,100 per month out of which more than 30% are complicated (UTH, 2017). Provision of quality care by skilled midwives to women who have complicated deliveries is very cardinal to prevent or reduce short and long term postpartum maternal morbidities and mortalities. The aim of this study was to assess the self reported practices of midwives in the postnatal wards at the UTH on the care of postpartum women who experienced complicated labour and delivery from time of admission to the postnatal wards until their discharge from the hospital. Improving health care performance is an increasing challenge globally; high quality service provision and enhanced patient experience are common elements of health care policy in many countries (Bick et al., 2011). Many studies have concentrated on using clients or postpartum women to rate the care they receive from health care providers including midwives, and most often the rating has been very negative. This has often been without consideration of many factors at hand such as staffing levels, availability of materials and equipment among others (Bick et al., 2011; Morrow et al., 2013).

Furthermore, many studies have focused on the utilisation of postnatal care services and not necessarily on the care midwives deliver to the mothers as seen from the midwives' perspective. Midwives' views on the value and role of the postnatal care they provide have received little attention, despite being a core element of the midwifery role since time in memorial (Bick et al., 2011).

There is limited literature that has considered Midwives as respondents in the care they provide to postpartum women, yet nurses and midwives are in an ideal position to report on the quality of care they provide to the clients in the various health settings (McHugh and Stimpfel, 2012) as they are the *de facto* surveillance system overseeing the patient care experience. The conceptual basis for using nurses as reliable and valid informants about the quality of care in the hospital in which they work is well grounded in organizational sociology (Aiken et al., 2000).

Therefore, nurses and midwives are in a much better position to rate their own care given the background of their work environment and further advocate for change or improvement. It is inherent in any profession to desire to do better and if given an opportunity be able to give a true picture of the situation and give sound recommendations for improvement. This study therefore used nurse-midwives as respondents in the care they rendered to postpartum women with complications of labour and delivery and admitted in postnatal wards

MATERIALS AND METHODS

A quantitative descriptive cross sectional survey was conducted at the University Teaching Hospital Women and Newborn (UTH-WN) in Lusaka District. The UTH-WN is a national public 3rd level specialist referral Hospital for maternal, reproductive and newborn health as well as a centre for teaching and research. The hospital has a total bed capacity of 453 (UTH-WN 2018). The study population was Midwives working at the hospital in the postnatal wards.

The hospital was purposively selected as a study site because it is the biggest referral hospital in the district of Lusaka and usually attends to different cases of complicated deliveries. All the four postnatal wards in the hospital were also purposively included in the study to enhance the numbers of the midwives to participate. Consecutive sampling technique was used to select a total of 51 midwives to participate in the study in August 2017. All the midwives who were found working in the postnatal ward in the month of August were included in the population sample. Midwives

Table 1. Demographic characteristic of respondents.

N – 51	N	(%)
Gender		
Male	0	0
Female	51	100
Participants' age (years)		
Below 20	2	3.9
20 – 29	7	13.7
30 – 39	21	41.2
40 – 49	10	19.6
50 and above	11	21.6
Participants' level of professional education		
Certificate	15	29.4
Diploma	34	66.7
Degree	2	3.9
Designation of participants		
Nursing Officers/ Ward In Charge	3	3.9
Registered Nurse Midwives	34	66.7
Certified /Enrolled Midwives	14	27.5
Participants' number of years working on the ward		
Less than 1	29	56.9
1 - 5	18	35.3
6 – 10	3	5.9
More than 10	1	2.0

asked to be given enough time to complete the questionnaire as they could not do it immediately because of the busy work schedules. The author, through the ward in charges and the nursing officers, distributed the questionnaires to the midwives who were found on duty in August 2017. This was done in order to maximize the numbers of participation by midwives. There was a 100% response rate as all the questionnaires were completed by the midwives and brought back to the nursing sister. The author collected the completed questionnaires from the office of the nursing sister.

Data were collected using a self administered questionnaire, which contained a 4 point Likert scale questions (Always – 3. Sometimes – 2, Rarely – 1 and Never - 0) and also some closed and open-ended questions to assess midwives' practices of caring for postpartum women who had complicated labour and delivery. The areas covered were: demographic data, whether care was comprehensive or satisfactory, care during hospitalization which included observations and assessment of the mothers and Information, Communication and Education (IEC) during hospitalization. After the data collection instrument was developed, it was subjected for scrutiny by the supervisors who checked the questions whether they were valid enough to yield the intended responses and advised on the necessary revisions to be made. The questionnaire was then pre-tested at a General Hospital within Lusaka. Midwives working in the postnatal ward completed the questionnaires. Pretesting of the instrument helped establish reliability of the instrument in that after analyzing the questionnaires, areas of inconsistencies were established, revised and retested. The revision of the questionnaires involved removing some repeated questions, and those which were unclear or ambiguous and also rephrasing some questions. The revision of the questionnaire also ensured that questions were clear, concise, appropriate and consistent. The proposal was approved by the Biomedical Research Ethics Committee of the University of Zambia; written permission was granted by the National Research Council under the Ministry of Health and the Senior Medical Superintendents at the UTH and the General Hospital. Privacy, anonymity and confidentiality were maintained and participation in study was purely voluntary.

Collected data were securely kept in a locked cupboard and only accessible to the researcher. Data were entered in a computer and analysed using SPSS version 20 computer statistical package. The demographic variables (age, parity, level of education) were summarized using descriptive summary measures and inferential statistics: expressed as frequencies and percentages/proportions for continuous and categorical variables. Results were presented as frequency distribution tables. Likert scale results were summarised in frequency distribution tables with 'Always' scoring the highest mark (3) and 'Rarely' the lowest mark (1). A score of 'Never' did not attract any mark (0). An average score for each category of care has also been computed on the 4 point likert scale. The following variables assessed the different aspects of care from the time the mothers were admitted to the postnatal wards until their discharge from the hospital: demographic characteristics, whether care was satisfactory and comprehensive, observations and assessment of mothers, self deficit care and IEC.

Table 2. Reasons why Midwives thought the care they provided to Postpartum mothers who had complicated labour and delivery was not comprehensive and satisfactory.

N=37	N	%
Low staffing levels and too much work	24	64.9
Inadequate medical and surgical supplies	5	13.5
Lack of medical equipment	2	5.4
Others (No Motivation, bad attitude, erratic	6	16.2
Water supply, no blood for severe cases of anaemia)		%

RESULTS

Demographic characteristic of respondents

There were a total of 51 midwives who participated in the study and all of them 51 (100%) were females 21(41.2%); aged between 30 -39 years and 11(21.6%) were 50 and above years. On level of education, 34(66.7%) had diplomas, 15(29.2%) had certificates and only 2(3.9%) had Bachelors' degree in nursing. As regards the designation of the respondents, 34(66.7%) were Registered Nurse-Midwives, 14(27.5%) were certified or enrolled midwives and 3(3.9%) were either Nursing officers or ward in charges. Majority of the respondents 29(56.9%) had worked for less than one year in the postnatal wards followed by 18 (35.3%) respondents who had worked between 1- 5 years in the postnatal wards (Table 1).

Whether care of postpartum mothers (PPM) who had complicated labour and delivery was comprehensive and satisfactory

Respondents were asked whether the care they provided to the postpartum mothers who had experienced complicated labour and delivery was comprehensive and satisfactory. Majority of the respondents 40(78.4%) stated that the care they rendered to postpartum mothers with complicated labour and delivery was not comprehensive and satisfactory and only 11(26.6%) felt that the care they provided to the women was comprehensive and satisfactory.

Reasons why midwives thought the care they provided to postpartum mothers who had complicated labour and delivery was not comprehensive and satisfactory

A total of 37(92.5%) midwives out of 40(100%) who had said that the care they provided to the postpartum women with complicated labour and delivery was not comprehensive and not satisfactory gave the following reasons why they thought the care was not comprehensive and satisfactory. 24(64.9%) out of a total of 37(100) respondents stated that low staffing levels and too much work were the main reasons for care to postpartum mothers not being comprehensive and satisfactory "(*Sometimes especially night duty only two nurses get overwhelmed with patients, 50 patients to 2 nurses, can't observe or do what they need to do on each mother and baby)"*; 5(13.5%) stated that inadequate medical and surgical supplies were the main reason and 6(16.2%) stated other reasons such as no motivation for staff "(*frustrations, no promotions as to what someone deserves – no appointment for specialized training achieved)"*; bad attitude by nurses "(*Sometimes even when staffing is good, do not carry out care*)"; erratic water supply and inadequate blood for severe cases of anaemia. 2(5.9%) stated that lack of necessary equipment to carry out care as one of the reasons for the care not being comprehensive and not satisfactory as well (Table 2).

Care of postpartum women who had complicated labour and delivery during hospitalization in the postnatal wards

To assess the postpartum care of women with complicated labour and delivery during hospitalization to postnatal wards, midwives were asked to score themselves on how often they performed caring activities using a 4 point likert Scale which had 'always -3, sometimes - 2, rarely - 1 and never - 0". Respondents scored themselves as ALWAYS carrying out the caring activities in the following areas: Out of a total of 51 respondents, 47(92.2%) always checked the vital signs, 43(84%) always provided clean environment, 43(84.3%) always administered medicines, 33(64.7%) always assisted with early ambulation, 31(60.8%) always checked for vaginal bleeding, 24(47.1%) always checked the episiotomy/laceration site for healing or signs of infection, 17(33.3%) always examined the abdomen for involution and 15(29.4%) always performed breast examination. The total average score on the 4 point likert scale (always - 3, sometimes – 2, rarely – 1 and never – 0) was 2.5 (Table 3).

Table 3. Likert scale rating of respondents' responses on care of postpartum women with complicated labour and delivery during hospitalization to postnatal wards.

N	(%)	Average score on likert scale	
Provided clean and ventilated environment			
Always	43	84	2.8
Sometimes	7	13.7	
Rarely	0	0	
Never	1	2.0	
Check vital signs 4 hourly or as necessary			
Always	47	92.2	2.9
Sometimes	3	5.9	
Rarely	3	5.9	
Never	0	0	
Check vaginal bleeding			
Always	31	60.8	2.6
Sometimes	19	37.3	
Rarely	1	2.0	
Never	0	0	
Breast examination			
Always	15	29.4	2.1
Sometimes	25	49.0	
Rarely	10	19.6	
Never	1	2.0	
Assist in early ambulation			
Always	33	64.7	2.4
Sometimes	11	21.6	
Rarely	7	13.7	
Never	0	0	
Check episiotomy/laceration site			
Always	17	33.3	2.1
Sometimes	24	47.1	
Rarely	9	17.6	
Never	1	2.0	
Check abdomen for involution			
Always	24	47.1	2.5
Sometimes	26	51.0	
Rarely	1	2.0	
Never	0	0	
Administer drugs			
Always	43	84	2.8
Sometimes	6	11.8	
Rarely	2	3.9	
Never	0	0	
Average performance			
Always	253	62	2.5

Table 3. Cont.

Sometimes	156	41
Rarely	33	8.0
Never	3	0.7

Midwives performing self care activities for postpartum mothers who had complicated labour and delivery during time of hospitalization in postnatal wards

In order to assess whether midwives performed nursing care activities for the postpartum women who had complicated labour and delivery while admitted to the postnatal wards, respondents were asked to rate their performance on a 4 point likert scale (always - 3, sometimes – 2, rarely – 1 and never – 0) on how often they performed or assisted the women in the various self care activities while admitted to the postnatal wards. Out of a total of 51 respondents, the following rated themselves as ALWAYS performing or assisting with the caring activities in the following areas: 5(9.8%) always performed or assisted with bed bath, 3(5.9%) always helped women with sitz baths and dressing up and 1(2.0%) always performed or assisted with either oral toilet or grooming for the women. The average total score on the 4 point likert scale (always - 3, sometimes – 2, rarely – 1 and never – 0) was 1.6 points (Table 4).

Information, education and communication (health education) to postpartum mothers who had complicated labour and delivery while admitted in postnatal ward

In order to assess how often respondents delivered IEC to postpartum mothers while admitted in the postnatal wards, respondents were asked to rate themselves on a likert scale (always - 3, sometimes – 2, rarely – 1 and never – 0) on the various IEC (health education) items they gave to the postpartum women who had complicated labour and delivery while admitted to the postnatal wards. Out of a total of 51 (100%) respondents, the following rated themselves as ALWAYS performing the IEC activities to the women as follows: 36(70.6%) always gave IEC on general hygiene, 23(45.1%) on perineal toilet, 19(37.1%) on how to detect excessive bleeding, 32(62.7%) on the importance of early ambulation, 15(29.4%) on involution of the uterus, 5(9.8%) on care of the breasts including management of breast problems, 21(41.25) on importance of exclusive breastfeeding, 16(31.2%) on types of medicines given, relevance and administration, 26(50.9%) on importance of good nutrition, 16(31.4%) on importance of rest and 3(5.9%) on postnatal exercises. The average total score on the 4 point likert scale (always - 3, sometimes – 2, rarely – 1 and never – 0) was 2.2 points (Table 5).

DISCUSSION

Improving healthcare performance is an increasing challenge globally. High quality service provision and enhanced patient experience are a common element of healthcare policy. Postnatal care especially for women who have had complicated labour and delivery is very critical for prevention of complications in the postpartum period. The aim of this study was to assess the self reported practices of midwives in the postnatal wards on the care of postpartum women who experienced complicated labour and delivery from time of admission to the postnatal wards until their discharge from the hospital.

Midwives assessed their own practices on various aspects of care on the postpartum women who had complicated labour and delivery admitted to the postnatal wards at the University Teaching Hospital – Women and Newborn in Zambia. From the background characteristics, it could be deduced that midwifery is still predominantly female driven as all the respondents were females though qualified at different levels. The scenario may be similar in other parts of the world such as the United Kingdom where sex discrimination was abolished in 1975 which also allowed males to train as midwives; yet the male midwives still make up 0.4% of the entire midwifery population under the National Health System (Jones, 2017).

Facility based postnatal care is very important especially for mothers who have had complicated labour and delivery as mothers are observed and monitored to enhance quick recovery and also to prevent postpartum complications. A number of studies have however found that the care provided to postpartum mothers does not equal to their needs. In a study conducted in Germany, midwives felt that they could not live up to the quality of midwifery care they aspired for, they were disappointed with themselves as they thought that the women were underserved and also disappointed with the care they received. Midwives attributed this situation to them being overwhelmed with work (Lohmann et al., 2018). Similar findings were obtained in a study in which majority of the professional nurses reported that the quality of care for postnatal women had deteriorated meaning that patient care was poor in the public hospitals (Somahela et al., 2015; Pallangyo et al., 2017; Dlamini et al., 2017).

However, some participants in the same study reported

Table 4. Respondents' responses on performing self care activities for postpartum mothers who had complicated labour and delivery during time of hospitalization in postnatal wards.

N	(%)	Average Score on likert scale	
Bed bath			
Always	5	9.8	1.7
Sometimes	22	52.9	
Rarely	11	21.6	
Never	8	15.7	
Big bath			
Always	5	9.8	1.7
Sometimes	27	52.9	
Rarely	17	33.3	
Never	2	3.9	
Oral care			
Always	1	2.0	1.2
Sometimes	15	29.4	
Rarely	18	35.8	
Never	8	15.7	
Sitz baths			
Always	3	5.9	1.7
Sometimes	23	5.1	
Rarely	17	33.3	
Never	17	33.3	
Grooming			
Always	1	2.0	1.5
Sometimes	23	45.1	
Rarely	20	39.2	
Never	7	13.7	
Dressing up			
Always	3	5.9	1.7
Sometimes	31	60.8	
Rarely	12	23.5	
Never	5	9.8	
Average performance			
Always	18	5.9	1.6
Sometimes	146	47.6	
Rarely	95	31.0	
Never	47	15.3	

that the quality of care had remained the same (Somahela et al., 2015). Other studies also revealed that health care providers felt the same way and they cited similar reasons as in this study for the state of care provided to postpartum women (Raynner, 2010; Mannava et al., 2015). A study conducted in Victoria, Australia revealed that hospital postnatal care was complex and characterized by multiple barriers which impact on the provision of quality postnatal care (Rayner 2013). Midwives in this study felt in a similar way as in many other studies that the care they provided to postpartum mothers who had complicated labour and

Table 5. Information, education and communication to postpartum mothers following complicated deliveries while admitted in postnatal ward.

N =51	N	(%)	Average Score
General purpose hygiene			
Always	36	70.6	2.7
Sometimes	13	25.5	
Rarely	1	2.0	
Never	1	2.0	
Perineal toilet/hygiene			
Always	23	45.1	2.4
Sometimes	26	51.0	
Rarely	1	2.0	
Never	1	2.0	
Detecting excessive bleeding			
Always	19	37.3	2.1
Sometimes	17	33.3	
Rarely	5	9.8	
Never	10	19.6	
Early ambulation			
Always	32	32.7	2.6
Sometimes	17	33.3	
Rarely	0	0	
Never	2	3.9	
Involution of the uterus			
Always	15	29.4	2.1
Sometimes	29	56.9	
Rarely	7	13.7	
Never	0	0	
Care of breast/mgt of problems			
Always	5	9.8	2.1
Sometimes	45	88.2	
Rarely	0	0	
Never	1	2.0	
Importance of colostrums/exclusive BF			
Always	21	41.2	2.1
Sometimes	19	37.3	
Rarely	1	2.0	
Never	2	3.9	
Types of medicine/relevance/Admin			
Always	16	31.4	2.3
Sometimes	33	64.7	
Rarely	0	0	
Never	2	3.9	
Nutrition			
Always	26	50.9	2.1

Table 5. Contd.

Sometimes	21	41.2	
Rarely	3	5.9	
Never	1	1.9	
Importance of rest			
Always	16	31.4	2.1
Sometimes	30	58.8	
Rarely	5	9.85	
Never	0	0	
Postnatal exercises			
Always	3	5.9	1.7
Sometimes	32	62.7	
Rarely	10	19.6	
Never	6	11.8	
Nutrition			
Always	209	37.3	2.1
Sometimes	291	52	
Rarely	33	5.9	
Never	26	4.7	

delivery admitted to the postnatal wards was unsatisfactory and not comprehensive to meet the needs of the mothers due to a number of factors. This study therefore agrees with other studies that health care providers including midwives are aware of the care they provide to their clients/patients and thus capable to give a clear and unbiased situation of the care they provided to the postpartum women who had complicated labour and delivery. All studies cited low staffing levels as the main reason for their dissatisfaction with the care they provided to the postpartum mothers.

A study on improving inpatient postnatal services, midwives' views and perspectives of engagement in a quality improvement initiative which also sought to find out the timing when midwives performed observations and examinations on postpartum mothers in postnatal wards revealed low percentages such as, on first contact (7- 13%), at most times (33 -89%) and whenever it was necessary (3 -33%) (Bick et al., 2011).

Midwives in this study scored themselves low in breast examination and postnatal exercises. Another study conducted in Dedza District in Malawi, revealed that only 22% nurse-midwives conducted full postnatal examination on mothers and neonates on discharge and 63% of midwives discharged mothers without checking their vital signs (Chimtembo et al., 2013). The inadequacy in postnatal health care could be attributed to differing priorities and perceptions among health care staff as well as patients themselves and because of this discrepancy, the needs of the postpartum mothers are not adequately provided for (Fogel, 2017). However, in another study, midwives scored themselves high (85%) on checking the observations on postpartum mothers (Rayner, 2010).

In this study, the average score on always performing observations and examination on mothers was 62% which was not too different from other studies. A study on what prevents quality midwifery care uncovered a number of barriers to the provision of quality care by midwifery personnel. The barriers were grouped into three broad areas as social, economic and professional with all the three resulting in moral distress and burnout (Filby et al., 2016). Midwives provide the majority of care for women before and during pregnancy, labour and delivery and in the postpartum period but most of the times their views on matters of service delivery may be underplayed.

After enduring a complicated delivery, women may not be in a position to undertake self care activities and it is the duty of the midwives to assist the women depending on the level of independence. Midwives were asked to score themselves on how often they performed caring activities on the postpartum mother who had complicated deliveries in relation to self care deficits (Table 4). Self care nursing activities are those activities which individuals may not be able to perform for themselves because of illness or any other condition but they would be able to do so if they were in good condition (https://en.wikipedia.org/wiki/Self-care_deficit_nursing_theory).

The overall performance was very low as only 5.9% of the midwives scored themselves as 'Always' performing the self care activities for the postpartum women who had experienced complicated deliveries. Similar findings have been reported in many studies where health care providers reported not to be able to provide quality of care to postpartum women due to the same reasons cited in this study. However, there are also studies where quality care has been provided by health care providers (Aiken et al., 2000; Mannava, 2015; Lohmann et al., 2018).

Midwives caring for postpartum women with complicated deliveries help in the prevention of complications and enhances quick recovery (Çapik, 2015). A literature view on midwifery in the postpartum period revealed that postpartum mothers who delivered by cesarean section expressed concern that the care and assistance they received was not what they had expected as midwives were uncaring, neglectful and disappointing. Midwives were expected to engage in care of the somatic or physical needs such as relief of pain and the need for mobilization while admitted to postnatal wards (Panagopoulou et al., 2017). A postpartum woman should be cared for as a whole, with all the aspects of care being considered.

Information, Education and Communication (IEC) to postpartum women is a very important component of postnatal care as this ensures continuation of care after discharge from the hospital. Postpartum mothers are educated on various aspects of puerperium and how to care for themselves and their newborn babies to prevent complications that may arise during and after hospitalization. Midwives were asked to score themselves on how often they educated or advised postpartum mothers on various aspects of postnatal care. Only an average of 37.8% of midwives reported as 'Always' giving IEC to postpartum women while admitted in the postnatal wards.

A study conducted in Kenya revealed that the overall adequacy of health information given by health workers to postpartum women was 16% on voiding and pelvic exercises. However, the same study revealed that 92% of health workers gave adequate health information on breast feeding (Kamau, 2014). Another study from Dedza District in Malawi also found that majority of the midwives gave health education to the mothers (Chimtembo et al., 2013).

On the other hand, a literature review on midwifery in the postnatal period indicated that midwives did not give advice to postpartum mothers as the women lacked information and knowledge concerning postpartum care and that there was noticeable lack or inconsistent advice regarding breastfeeding, both in relevance to the importance for the infant or the appropriate technique (Panagopoulou et al., 2017). Women further stated that advice related to their own self care needs and their role in the postpartum period was highly valued.

IEC to postpartum mothers is very important as it empowers mothers to take responsibility of their own health and that of the newborn baby and to prevent postpartum complications which may result in morbidities and maternal mortalities.

IMPLICATION FOR PRACTICE, POLICY AND NURSING PROGRAMMES

This study has proved that health care providers such as midwives could be engaged to evaluate their own care they provide to the mothers during the postpartum period. As professionals, midwives would give a true reflection of the current situation as they desire to improve on the care they provide to the clients. Midwives' indication that the care they provide to postpartum mothers who had complicated labour admitted to the postnatal ward was not comprehensive and satisfactory gives an indication that the situation needs to be quickly addressed. There are a number of reasons advanced for the current state of care given to postpartum women which should be taken into consideration such as improvement in staffing levels to cater for the increased workload, increased supply of medical and surgical supplies including provision of necessary equipment. The other reasons such as low motivation, bad attitude, erratic water supply and inadequate blood for severe malaria clients may seem less important, but they are all very cardinal to the provision of quality care to the postpartum mothers. A true turning point comes with self- realization of one's own inadequacies and a deep desire to do something about it to change the situation. This study has just done that and it is hoped that policy makers will take this opportunity to provide the necessary requisites and challenge the midwives to improve their practice.

CONCLUSION AND RECOMMENDATIONS

This study has revealed that generally postnatal care to postpartum women who had experienced complicated labour and deliveries is low in a number of areas and therefore needs to be improved. Midwives scored themselves according to the care they provided to the postpartum women admitted to postnatal ward up to the time they were discharged. It is therefore recommended that ward managers should ensure that staffing levels are adequate to match the workload and also provide all the necessary materials and equipment for provision of care. It is also recommended that human resources issues that concern the motivation of midwives such as promotions should be looked at as demotivated workers though given all the requites may still have low output. Situations which make midwives helpless and discouraged such as unavailability of water and blood for anaemic patients should be avoided. The hospital management should always make such provisions to ease up the work of midwives. Ward managers should also make efforts and step up their supervisory skills to ensure that more midwives always undertake the necessary required care for the postpartum women who had experienced complicated labour and delivery in order to enhance maternal wellbeing and prevent ill health during the postpartum period.

LIMITATION OF THE STUDY

Although several studies have proved that nurses and midwives are reliable and valid informants on the care they provide in the hospital, a bias may still exist which may be over rating or under rating themselves. A study in which postpartum women are informants should be undertaken so that comparisons could be made on the care provided to postpartum women who have complicated labour and deliveries.

CONFLICT OF INTERESTS

The authors have not declared any conflict of interests.

ACKNOWLEDGEMENTS

We would like to acknowledge the financial support provided by the Norwegian Agency for Development (NORAD) through the NORHED QZA-0848 QZA-MW-13/00032 Grant

REFERENCES

Aiken L, Patrician P (2000). Measuring organizational traits of hospitals: The revised nursing work index. Nursing Research 49(3):146-153.

Bick DE, Rose V, Weavers A, Wray J, Beake S (2011). Improving inpatient postnatal services: midwives views and perspectives of engagement in a quality improvement initiative. BMC Health Services Research 11(1):293.

Çapik A, Nazik E, Özdemir A, Apay SE (2015). The effect of the care given using orem's Self – Care Model on the postpartum self – evaluation. International Journal of Caring Science 8(2):393

Central Statistical Office (CSO) (2014). Ministry of Health (MOH) [Zambia], ICF International (2014). Zambia Demographic and Health Survey 2013-14. Rockville, Maryland, USA: Central Statistical Office, Ministry of Health, and ICF International.

Chimtembo LK, Maluwa A, Chimwaza A, chirwa E, Pindani M (2013). Assessment of quality of postnatal care services offered to mothers in Dedza district, Malawi. Open Journal of Nursing 3(04):343.

Dippenaar J, Da Serra D (2013). Seller's midwifery.2nd Edition. Lansdowne: Juta.

Dlamini BR, Sandy PT, Gule WP (2017). The extent of midwives' knowledge and practices during the provision of immediate postnatal care in Swaziland. Journal of AIDS and Clinical Research 8(3).

Filby A, McConville F, Portela A (2016). What prevents quality midwifery care? A systematic mapping of barriers in low and middle income countries from the provider perspective. PLoS chimwazaONE 11(5):e0153391.

Fogel N (2017). The inadequacies in postnatal health care. Current Medicine Research and Practice 7(1):16-17.

Hoque M, Klein MC (2011). Incidence of obstetric and foetal complications during labor and delivery at a community health centre, midwives obstetric unit of durban, South Africa. ISRN obstetrics and gynecology, 2011.

Jones D (2017). Male midwives: How men are changing the rules. https://www.totaljobs.com/insidejob/male- midwives-men-changing-rules/ accessed on 3/10/2018

Kamau WI (2014). Assessment of postnatal care education given to mothers pre-discharge in health facilities in Nairobi county.

Lohela TJ, Campbell OMR, Gabrysch S (2012). Distance to Care, facility delivery and early neonatal mortality in Malawi and Zambia. PLoS One 7(12):

Lohmann S, Mattern E, Ayerl GM (2018). Midwives' perceptions of women's preferences related to midwifery care in Germany: A focus group study. Midwifery 61:53-62.

Mannava P, Durrant K, Fisher J, Chersich M, Luchters S (2015). Attitudes and behaviours of maternal health care providers in interaction with clients: A systematic review. Globalization and health 11(1):36.

McHugh MD, Stimpel AW (2012). Nurse reported quality of care: A measure of hospital quality. Research in Nursing and Health 35(6):566-575.

Ministry of Health (MOH) (2011). National Health Strategic Plan 2011-2015. Lusaka, Zambia.

Morrow J, Mclachlan H, Newton M, Forster D, Davey MN (2013). Redesigning postnatal care: exploring the views and experiences of midwives. Midwifery 29(2):159-166

Ngozi J, Tornes YF, Mukasa PK, Salongo W, Kabakyenga J, Sezalio M, Wouters K, Jacqueym Y, Geertytuyden JV (2016). Puerperal sepsis, the leading cause of maternal deaths at a Tertiary University Teaching Hospital in Uganda. BMC Pregnancy and Childbirth 16(1):207.

Pallangyo EN, Mbekenga C, Källestål C, Rubertsson C, Olsoon P (2017). "If really we are committed things can change, starting from us": Healthcare providers' perceptions of postpartum care and its potential for improvement in low-income suburbs in Dar es Salaam, Tanzania. Sexual and Reproductive Healthcare 11:7-12

Panagopoulos V, Hancock J, Tziaferi S (2017). Midwifery in the postnatal period: A systematic review of the literature. Nosileftiki 56(2).

Rayner AJ, Mclachlan HL, Peters L, Forster DL (2013). Care providers' views and experiences of postnatal care in private hospitals in Victoria, Australia. Midwifery 29(6):622-627

Rayner JA, Malachlan H, Foster DA, Peters L, Yelland J (2010). A state review of postnatal care in private hospitals in Victoria, Australia. BMC Pregnancy and Childbirth 10(1):26.

Saleem S, McClure EM, Goudar SS (2014). A prospective study of maternal, foetal and neonatal deaths in low and middle income countries. Bulletin of the World Health Organization 92:605-612.

Somahela KJ, Yako EM, Khumalo T (2015). Professional nurses perceptions on quality of patient care. African Journal for Physical Health Education, Recreation and Dance 21(2):176-211.

University Teaching Hospital (2017). Integrated Provincial Meeting Report. Lusaka.

University Teaching Hospital –women and Newborn (2018). Integrated Provincial Meeting Report. Lusaka.

Warren CE (2015). Exploring the quality and effect of comprehensive postnatal care models in East and Southern Africa. International Centre for Reproductive Health.

World Health Organisation (2013). Recommendations on postnatal of the Mother and Newborn, WHO library cataloguing in publication data.

14

Practice of child spacing and its associated factors among women of child bearing age (15 to 49 years) in Illubabor zone, South West Ethiopia

Dereje Tsegaye*, Muluneh Shuremu and Kebebe Bidira

Department of Public Health, Faculty of Public Health and Medical Sciences, Mettu University, Mettu, Ethiopia.

Optimal birth spacing refers to resting period between pregnancies that allows the mother time to recuperate from pregnancy, labor and lactation. Long time period between births allows the next pregnancy and birth to be at full gestation and growth for years. This study aimed to assess practice of child spacing and its associated factors among women of child bearing age in Ilubabor Zone of Oromia National Regional State, South West Ethiopia, from January to June 2016. A community based cross sectional quantitative study design was used. A stratified multistage sampling procedure and face to face interview with Afan Oromo and Amharic version was done by administering questionnaire on 826 women of child bearing age. Women from rural areas were about 3 times more likely to have short birth interval than their urban counterparts [AOR =3.39 (95% CI: 1.13, 4.10)]. Respondents with no formal education were 2.56 times more likely to practice short birth interval than those with higher education [AOR = 2.56, 95% CI (1.60, 3.42)]. As compared to mothers whose husbands were employee, women whose husbands were farmers were more likely to have short birth interval [AOR = 3.50, 95% CI (1.29, 4.42)]. Mothers who breast fed their child for less than 12 months were 5 times more likely to practice short birth interval than those who breast fed for 24 months or more [AOR = 5.36, 95% CI ((3.43,6.34)]. Women who were not using contraceptives were 4.42 times more likely to give birth within short period of time than contraceptive users [AOR = 4.12 (95% CI: 2.71, 5.82)]. Women with fourth wealth quartile were 3.18 times more likely to have short birth interval than those with the lowest wealth quartile [AOR = 3.18(95% CI: 1.75, 4.56)]. Birth interval was short in this study. Therefore, greater attention should be given to contraceptive use and paternal education in addition to infant and child mortality prevention.

Key words: Birth spacing, knowledge, contraceptive, women.

INTRODUCTION

Scholars defined optimal birth spacing as resting period between pregnancies that allows the mother time to recuperate from pregnancy, labor and lactation. Longer time period between births allows the next pregnancy and birth to be at full gestation and growth for years. Family planning programs support two years intervals between

*Corresponding author. E-mail: deretsegaye@gmail.com.

births for infant and child health and survival (RamaRao et al., 2006; Orji et al., 2004). But recent studies recommend that birth intervals of 3 to 5 years are safer for mothers and babies as compared to birth intervals of two years or less (Yohannis et al., 2003; Orji et al., 2004).

Inter birth interval (IBI) has significant effect on the health status of the mother and her child (Cleland et al., 2008). It was indicated to be linked with increased risk of maternal morbidity and mortality, preterm birth, low birth weight, small for gestational age (SGA), labor dystocia, premature rupture of membranes, third-trimester bleeding, anemia and puerperal sepsis (USAID, 2005; WHO, 2005).

According to the Ethiopian Demographic and Health Survey (EDHS, 2014) report, with the exception of first birth, there is an inverse relationship between the length of the preceding birth interval and proportion of child who are stunted. The shorter the interval, the higher the proportion of children stunted. In Ethiopia, 40% of children under age five are stunted, and 18% of children are severely stunted. In general, the Central Statistical Agency (CSA) provide the prevalence of stunting increases as the age of a child increases, with the highest prevalence of chronic malnutrition found in children age 24-35 months (52%) and lowest in children between age six and eight months (9% percent) (CSA, 2014).

Besides the health implication, closely spaced birth intervals accelerate the population growth and challenge the development efforts of a country. By limiting women contribution to economic development, it makes difficult for them to become productive members of society. Moreover, when a newborn baby comes, that family will invest more of its limited resources to care for the newborn, while the other children will be left behind to receive insufficient share of the resources (USAID, 2005). On the contrary, optimal birth spacing (OBS) yields the greatest health, social and economic benefits for the family. Although, previous research findings advocate an interval length of 2 years between two consecutive births for a better maternal and child health (WHO, 2005), current evidence shows that births should be spaced at three to five years apart to ensure the greatest health benefits for mothers, newborns and older children (WHO, 2005; USAID, 2005).

Davanzo et al. (2004) attributes the adverse consequences of a short birth interval for infant and child survival and maternal mortality to the biological effects related to the "maternal syndrome "or more generally, the women not fully recovering from one pregnancy before supporting the next one (which may lead, for e.g., to anaemia and premature rupture of membranes).

Ethiopia is one of the countries with the highest maternal mortality ratios in Africa and the world, estimated at 673 per 100,000 live births in 2011. This is associated with the low levels of antenatal care and birth attendance by health professionals in Ethiopia, especially among the poor-as well as early age at marriage and first birth. Among the 20 to 35 years old, about 30% of all female adult deaths are from maternal deaths at birth (CSA, 2006 cited in World Bank, 2007).

Addressing these issues is vital because short birth interval is a modifiable risk factor and is potentially within the control of individuals and couples. Birth spacing is a public health intervention that can use available modern contraceptive methods and technologies. The birth spacing programs, using contraception in combination with revised and strengthened birth spacing education and counseling messages, can be mainstreamed into existing health and non-health programs in both clinical setting and community setting. Therefore, understanding practice of birth interval and its associated factors among women of reproductive age is critical for countries like Ethiopia with a population policy aiming at reducing fertility.

MATERIALS AND METHODS

Study design

A community based quantitative cross-sectional study design was used. All married women in reproductive age group (15 – 49 years) having at least two children available at their household during the data collection period were included in the study.

Sample size determination

The sample size was determined using the formula for single population proportion and considering 36.8% proportion of optimal birth interval in Lemo District, Southern Ethiopia (Yohannes et al., 2011), 95% CI 5% margin of error, design effect of 2 and 10% non response rate yielding the total sample size of 826.

An attempt was made to adopt a three stage sampling technique. The first stage involved the selection of districts by simple random sampling technique. The second stage was selection of Kebeles from the selected districts again using simple random sampling technique. Then, the third stage was selection of households using systematic random sampling technique.

Data collection procedures

The data were collected using pre-tested interview guided semi-structured questionnaire. The questionnaire was prepared in English and translated to Amharic and Afan Oromo versions. It was checked for its consistency and then translated back to English by different individuals. The translations were made by those who are well oriented with the stated languages (language professionals). The instrument was adopted from different literatures developed for similar purpose by different authors and tools designed by various organizations.

Data analysis

The data were double entered onto EPI data version 3.1 and exported to SPSS (SPSS Inc. version 20.0, Chikago, Illiois) computer software for further analysis. Errors related to inconsistency of data such as missing values and outliers were checked and well thought-out during data cleaning. Descriptive statistics were used to give clear picture of the dependent and independent variables. Frequency distributions of the variables were worked out using tables and figures. Logistic regression model fitness was checked by using Hosmer Lemshow test of significance and omnibus test.

A two-step logistic regression (bivariate and multivariable) analysis was done to see the effect of independent variables on practice of child spacing in married women of child bearing age (15-49 years). In the first step, bivariate analyses were done to assess the association between each independent variable and the outcome variables. All variables with p-value less than or equal to 0.25 in the bivariate logistic regression model were entered into the multivariable logistic regression model using backward elimination method to control for all possible confounders. At this step, odds ratio along with 95% CI was estimated to identify factors associated with optimum child spacing.

Data quality control

The appropriateness of the questionnaire in terms of content, consistency, language and organization was checked meticulously and was modified in line with standards, guidance and suggestion from peer reviewers. A pretest was employed in Bedele 01 kebele on a total of 42 (5%) of respondents five days prior to the actual data collection. Findings were discussed among data collectors and supervisors in order to ensure the quality of data.

Based on the pretest, questions were revised, edited and those found to be unclear or confusing were modified. Finally, structured closed ended Afan Oromo and Amharic version questionnaire were used for data collection.

Supervisors and data collectors were trained on the data collection process, accuracy and completeness for three consecutive days. The overall activity was closely monitored by principal investigators of the study during data collection. To reduce non-response rate and unwanted confusion, necessary information and description was given to the study participants before initiating the interview. The data quality was controlled by designing ideal data collection tools and close supervision with aggressive monitoring. The information obtained was checked and cleaned up before and after data entry.

RESULTS

Socio-demographic characteristics

Out of 811 study population, 582 (71.8%) were rural residents and the rest 229 (28.2%) were urban residents. One-third (32.2%) were in the age ranges of 25-29 years. About three-fourth (72.6%) were Muslim. Out of the total participants, nearly two-third (61.4%) cannot read and write, whereas 52.7% of the respondent's husband attended primary education. About one third of the participants (66.5%) were from Oromo ethnic group. Greater parts of the respondents (84.0 %) were housewives and 72.7% of the respondent's husbands were farmers. More than half, 472 (58.2%) were in the third wealth quartile (Table 1).

Knowledge of birth spacing

Almost all (97.7%) of the respondents have ever heard about optimal birth interval between two successive live births. Among those who have the awareness, less than one-fifth (16.4%) reported the optimal birth interval between two consecutive births to be between 36 and 60 months. The results showed that almost all (98.2%) of the respondents, reported the presence of health advantages of birth spacing.

Birth history of the respondents

More than one-third (36.3%) of the respondents gave birth to live child. The intention to become pregnant before the conception of the last child was asked. Accordingly, 321 (41.2%) of the respondents wanted to become pregnant then and 459 (56.6%) desired to postpone the pregnancy to sometime later. Sex and status of the last child was also asked. Accordingly, 588 (72.5%) of the mothers had male and 764 (94.2%) of the children were alive.

Practice of birth spacing

More than half (51.2%) of the study subjects had short birth interval. More than one-third (34.9%) respondents had optimum birth interval and the remaining had long birth interval (Figure 1).

Breast feeding practices

The study revealed that 366 (45.1%) of the respondents breast fed their children for 24 months or more and the reason for stopping breast feeding for about three–fourth (72.5%) of the respondents was the child was too old.

Use of contraceptives

More than half (55.1%) of the respondents have not been using contraceptive methods before conception of the last child. Nearly three–fourth of the respondents reported that the reason for not using contraceptive was desire for more children.

Predictors of birth interval

In the multivariable logistic regression analysis, women from rural residents were 3.39 times more likely to have short birth interval than their urban counterparts [AOR =3.39 (95% CI: 1.13, 4.10)]. Respondents who cannot read and write were 2.56 times more likely to practice short birth interval than those with secondary education and above [AOR = 2.56, 95% CI (1.60, 3.42)]. As compared to mothers whose husbands were employee, women whose husbands were farmers more likely to

Table 1. Socio-demographic characteristics of the respondents in Illubabor Zone, South West Ethiopia, 2016.

Variable	Categories	Frequency (n=811)	Percent
Residence	Rural	552	68.1
	Urban	299	31.9
Maternal age	20 - 24	122	15
	25 - 29	262	32.2
	30 - 34	201	24.8
	35 - 39	102	12.6
	40 - 44	124	15.3
Marital status	Married	768	94.7
	Divorced	18	2.2
	Widowed	25	3.1
Religion	Protestant	61	7.5
	Orthodox	161	19.9
	Muslim	589	72.6
Ethnicity	Oromo	539	66.5
	Amhara	272	33.5
Maternal education	Cannot read and write	489	61.4
	Primary	192	23.7
	Secondary and above	121	14.9
Husband's education	Cannot read and write	294	36.3
	Primary	427	52.7
	Secondary and above	90	11.1
Maternal occupation	Employee	60	7.4
	Housewife	681	84.0
	Merchant	30	3.7
	Others	40	4.9
Husband's occupation	Employee	130	16.0
	Merchant	30	3.7
	Farmer	590	72.7
	Others	61	7.5
Wealth Index	Lowest quartile	92	11.3
	Second quartile	148	18.2
	Third quartile	472	58.2
	Highest quartile	99	12.2

have short birth interval [AOR = 3.50, 95% CI (1.29, 4.42]. Mothers who breast fed their child for less than 12 months were more likely to practice short birth interval than those who breast fed for 24 months or more [AOR = 5.36, 95% CI ((3.43,6.34)]. Women who were not using contraceptives were 4.42 times more likely to give birth within short period of time than contraceptive users [AOR = 4.12 (95% CI: 2.71, 5.82)]. Women with fourth wealth

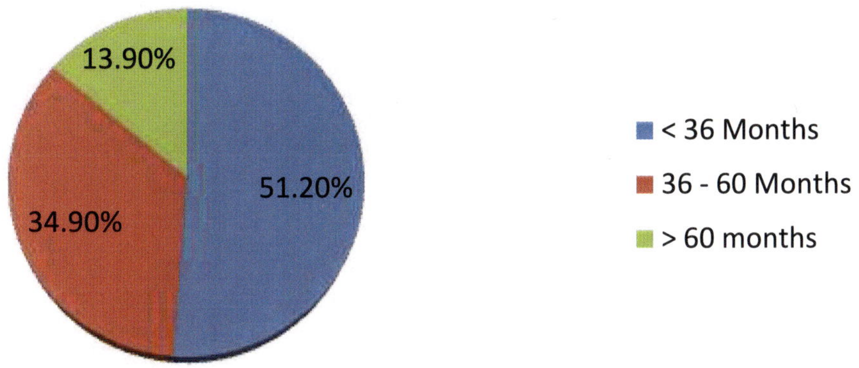

Figure 1. Proportion of birth interval among women of reproductive age (15 - 49 years) in Illubabor Zone, South West Ethiopia, June, 2016.

quartile were 3.18 times more likely to have short birth interval than those with the lowest wealth quartile [AOR = 3.18(95% CI: 1.75, 4.56)]. (Table 2)

DISCUSSION

This study tried to assess the practice and determinants of child spacing among women of child bearing age in Illubabor Zone, South West Ethiopia. More than half (51.2%) of the respondents had short birth interval. Place of residence, maternal education, husband's occupation, wealth quartile, duration of breast feeding, contraceptive use and status of index child, were independent predictors of child spacing among women of reproductive age.

A study conducted in Southern Ethiopia in 2010 indicated that more than half (57.6%) of the study subjects had short birth interval. Two hundred ninety (35.8%) respondents had optimum birth interval and the remaining had long birth interval (Yohannes et al., 2011). This study also revealed similar result in that more than half, 415 (51.2%) of the study subjects had short birth interval. Two hundred and eighty three (34.9%) respondents had optimum birth interval and the remaining had long birth interval.

Similarly, the study conducted in Southern Ethiopia revealed that rural women were more likely to have short birth interval than urban women (Yohannes et al., 2011). This study also revealed similar result that rural women were more likely to have short birth interval than urban women. This study found out that respondents who cannot read and write were 2.56 times more likely to practice short birth interval than those with secondary education and above. This finding is also consistent with a study conducted in Northern Iran in 2007, where with increase in maternal education level, the birth interval significantly increased (Hajian-Tilaki et al., 2009).

The study conducted in Dabat district showed that women whose husbands were farmers had about 2.3 times more likely to have subsequent birth after the index child as compared to women whose husbands were employees (Tessema et al., 2013). This study also found out those women whose husbands were farmers had high chance of having short birth interval.

Women with the fourth wealth quartile were more likely to have short birth interval than those with the lowest wealth quartile. This finding is similar to a study conducted in Southern Ethiopia that revealed women with highest wealth quartile were more likely to have short birth interval than those with lowest wealth quartile (Yohanes et al., 2011). The reason might be women with the lowest wealth quartile might be busy on their daily earning to fulfill their basic needs which might have resulted in delay of becoming pregnant.

Mothers who breast feed their children for less than 12 months were more likely to practice short birth interval than those who breast feed their children for 24 months or more. This finding is again consistent with a study conducted in Northern Iran that showed, with increased duration breast feeding, the mean birth interval increased significantly (Hajian-Tilaki et al., 2009).

In a study in Southern Ethiopia, women who were not using contraceptives were more likely to give birth within short period of time than users (Yohannes et al., 2011). The finding of this study is consistent with this similar finding that showed women who were not using contraceptives were more likely to give birth within short period of time than contraceptive users.

In Ethiopia, different studies showed significant higher risk of a conception in the months following the death of an index child, even after controlling for postpartum amenorrhea and breastfeeding status. Most Ethiopian women are more eager to replace a dead child when they are close to their desired family size (Lindstrom and Kiros, 2007). This study also revealed that mothers whose index chid were alive were more likely to have long birth interval than mothers whose index child died. It is alleged that the difference in the birth interval is related to the desire of parents to replace a dead child as well as

Table 2. Multivariable logistic regression analysis indicating factors associated with birth spacing among respondents in Illubabor Zone of Oromia National Regional State, 2016.

Characteristics	Birth interval		AOR 95% CI
	Optimal N (%)	Sub optimal N (%)	
Residence			
Urban	30(13.1)	199(86.9)	1.00
Rural	283(43.5)	328(56.5)	3.29 (1.13, 4.10)
Maternal education			
Cannot read and write	167(33.6)	330(66.4)	2.56(1.60, 3.42)
Primary education	55(28.6)	137(71.4)	0.79(0.55, 1.14)
Secondary and above	61(50.4)	60(49.6)	1.00
Education of husband			
Cannot read and write	68(23.2)	225(76.8)	2.53(0.82, 3.53)
Primary education	185(43.3)	242(56.7)	1.65(0.49, 2.77)
Secondary and above	30(33.3)	60(66.7)	1.00
Occupation of husband			
Employee	74(51.0)	71(49.0)	1.00
Farmer	178(31.0)	396(69.00	3.50 (1.29, 4.42)
Others*	31(34.10	60(65.9)	0.49(0.28, 1.850
Wealth quartile			
Lowest quartile	26(28.30)	66(71.7)	1.00
Second quartile	509(34.00)	979(66.0)	1.31(0.74, 2.310
Third quartile	1729(36.40)	300(63.60	1.45(0.89, 2.370
Fourth quartile	35(35.40)	64(64.6)	3.18(1.75, 4.56)
Duration of breast feeding (months)			
0 - 6	29(15.8)	154(84.20)	2.36(0.37, 4.06)
7 - 12	40(30.8)	90(69.2)	5.36(3.43, 6.39)
13 - 23	30(22.90	101(77.1)	1.57(0.89, 2.78)
≥24	1849(50.3)	182(49.7)	1.00
Contraceptive use			
Yes	61(37.20	103(62.8)	1.00
No	10(15.2)	56(84.8)	4.12(2.71,5.82)
Status of index child			
Alive	19(41.3)	27(58.7)	1.00
Dead	264(34.6)	500(65.4)	3.75(1.41, 4.37)

*Merchants, students, daily laborers; AOR =adjusted odds ratio, CI = confidence interval. The bolded values are the variables in the final model.

to the loss of fertility delaying effects of breastfeeding.

Readers shall take into contemplation, the following limitations when interpreting the findings of this study. First, the cross-sectional nature of the study had made it impossible to reach at causal relationship between different independent variables and birth interval. Second, the source of data for this study was based on the self-report of respondents, and provided no validation of obtaining information with objective source such as health facility cards. But it is logical to assume that biasis are less likely in delivery related events as compared to sensitive issues such as sexual behavior and drug abuse and respondents were informed about the importance of giving accurate responses and also assured confidentiality of their responses.

CONCLUSION AND RECOMMENDATIONS

Almost all the respondents have ever heard about optimal birth interval between two successive births. However, more than half (57%) of the participants in the reproductive age group have been practicing short birth interval below the recommended duration of optimal birth spacing. Place of residence, maternal education, husband's occupation, wealth quartile, duration of breast feeding, contraceptive use and status of index child, were independent predictors of optimal child spacing among women of reproductive age.

Hence, in the interventions designed to address optimal birth spacing, use of contraceptive methods and maternal education should be given greater attention in addition to prevention of infant and child mortality.

CONFLICT OF INTERESTS

The authors declare that there is no conflict of interest.

ACKNOWLEDGEMENTS

The authors thank Mettu University for coordinating as well as granting fund to the project and also appreciate the University Research and Technology Transfer Directorate, Faculty of Public Health and Medical Sciences staff. They also thank IlluAbabor Zone Health Office and acknowledge the data collectors, supervisors and participants for their genuine dedication and participation during the study.

REFERENCES

Central Statistical Agency of Ethiopia (CSA) (2006). Ethiopian demographic and health Survey, Addis Ababa, Ethiopia and Calverton, Mary land USA.

Central Statistical Agency of Ethiopia (CSA) (2014). Ethiopian demographic and health survey Addis Ababa, Ethiopia and Calverton, Mary land USA.

Cleland J, Bernstein S, Ezeh A, Faundes A, Glasier A, Innis J (2006). Family planning: the unfinished agenda. Lancet 368(9549):1810-1827.

Davanzo J, Razzaque A, Rahman M, Hale L (2004). The Effects of Birth Spacing on Infant and Child Mortality, Pregnancy Outcomes, and Maternal Morbidity and Mortality in Matlab, Bangladesh. Available at: http://s3.amazonaws.com/academia.edu.documents/41477680/RAND_WR198.pdf?AWSAccessKeyId=AKIAIWOWYYGZ2Y53UL3A&Expires=1497866961&Signature=EhcvHYZxJhOPz88t6TBca2PbD8c%3D&response-content-disposition=inline%3B%20filename%3DThe_effects_of_birth_spacing_on_infant_a.pdf

Ethiopia Mini Demographic and Health Survey (EDHS) (2014). Ethiopia Mini Demographic and Health Survey 2014. Central Statistical Agency Addis Ababa, Ethiopia. Available at: https://www.unicef.org/ethiopia/Mini_DHS_2014__Final_Report.pdf

Hajian-Tilaki KO, Asnafi N, Aliakbarnia-Omrani F (2009). The patterns and determinants of birth intervals in multiparous women in babol, Northern Iran. Southeast Asian J. Trop. Med. Public Health. 40(4):852-60.

Lindstrom DP, Kiros GE (2007). The impact of infant and child death on subsequent fertility in Ethiopia. Popul. Res. Policy Rev. 26(1):31-49.

Orji E, Shittu A, Makinde O, Sule S (2004). Effect of prolonged birth spacing on maternal and prenatal outcome. East Afr. Med. J. 81(8):388-391.

RamaRao S, Townsend J, Askew I (2006). Correlates of inter-birth intervals: implications of optimal birth spacing strategies in Mozambique. Frontiers in Reproductive Health, Population Council. Available at: http://pdf.usaid.gov/pdf_docs/PNADG133.pdf

Tessema GA, Zeleke BM, Ayele TA (2013). Birth interval and its predictors among married women in Dabat District, Northwest Ethiopia: A retrospective follow up study. Afr. J. Reprod. Health 17(2):39-45.

USAID (United States agency for International Development) (2005). Strengthening family planning policies and programs in developing countries: An Advocacy Toolkit, USA. Available at: http://www.policyproject.com/pubs/manuals/Family%20Planning%20Toolkit%20final.pdf

World Health Organization (WHO) (2005). Report of a WHO technical consultation on birth spacing: Geneva, Switzerland, 13-15 June 2005. Geneva: WHO. Department of Making Pregnancy Safer. Department of Reproductive Health and Research. Available at: http://apps.who.int/iris/bitstream/10665/69855/1/WHO_RHR_07.1_eng.pdf

Yohannes S, Wondafrash M, Abera M, Girma E (2011). Duration and determinants of birth interval among women of child bearing age in Southern Ethiopia. BMC Pregnancy Childbirth 11:38.

Yohannis F, Yemane B, Alemayehu W (2003). Differentials of fertility in rural Butajira. Ethiop. J. Health Dev. 17(1):17-25.

15

Evidence based nursing practice and associated factors among nurses working in Jimma zone public hospitals, Southwest Ethiopia

Dawit Hoyiso[1], Abinet Arega[2*] and Terefe Markos[3]

[1]Department of Nursing College of Health Science Hawassa University, Ethiopia.
[2]Department of Health Education and Behavioral Sciences, Jimma University, Jimma, Ethiopia.
[3]Department of Epidemiology, Jimma University, Jimma, Ethiopia.

In spite of all the various programs and strategies to promote the use of research finding, there is still gap between theory and practice. A number of studies from various countries have reported that nurses' experience of evidence-based practice is low. In Ethiopia, there is an information gap on the extent of evidence based nursing practice and its associated factors. The study aims to assess the implementation of evidence based nursing practice and associated factors among nurses in Jimma zone public hospitals. Institution based cross-sectional study was conducted from March 1-30/2015. A total of 333 sampled nurses for quantitative and 8 in-depth interview of key informants were involved in the study. Semi-structured questionnaire was adapted from funk's BARRIER scale and Friedman's test. Pretest was done on 17 nurses of Bedele hospital. Multivariable linear regression was used to determine factors of evidence based nursing practice. Of 333 distributed questionnaires, 302 were completed, giving 90.6% response rate. Of 302 participants, 245 were involved in EBP activities different levels. About 45 (18.4%) had implemented evidence based practice to low level, 42% had implemented evidence based practice to medium level and 39.6% of the respondents had implemented evidence based practice to high level. The first greatest perceived barrier was setting characteristic. Knowledge about research evidence was positively associated with implementation of evidence based nursing practice. Similarly, place of graduation was positively associated with implementation of evidence based nursing practice. Small number of participants had implemented EPB frequently. Evidence-based nursing practice was positively associated with knowledge of research, place where respondents graduated, and the availability of information resources. Organizational factors were found to be the greatest perceived barrier. Intervention programs on awareness creation, training, resource provision, and curriculum issues to improve implementation of evidence based nursing practice by stakeholders are recommended.

Key words: Evidence based practice, nursing practice, research utilization Ethiopia.

INTRODUCTION

Evidence based practice (EBP) is the use of best research finding (evidence) to answer a burning clinical question together with one's own clinical expertise generated from outcome management or quality improvement projects and patient preference and values. Researchers generate new knowledge through rigorous research (external evidence) and EBP provides clinicians the tools to translate the evidence into clinical practice and integrate it with internal evidence to improve the quality of health care and patient outcomes (Melnyk and Fineout-Overholt, 2004).

Its basic principles are that practical decision made should be based on research studies and that these research studies are selected and interpreted according to some specific norms and characteristic for EBP. EBP utilizes the most up to date methods of providing care, which have been proven through appraisal of high quality studies and statistically significant research finding (Wikipedia, 2014).

Health care that is evidence-based and conducted in a caring context leads to better clinical decision and patient outcomes. Gaining knowledge and skill in the EBP process provides nurses and other clinicians the tools needed to take ownership of their practice. There are five sequential steps to the EBP process. Step 1: Asking the clinical questions in the Patient/Population, Intervention/Issue of interest, Comparison, Outcome and Time frame (PICOT) format to get more effective evidence. Step 2: Searching for the best evidence to select. Step 3: Critically appraising the evidence. Step 4: Addressing the sufficiency of the evidence to implement or not to implement, and evaluating the outcome of the evidence implementation (Fineout-overholt et al., 2005).

In spite of all the programs and strategies to promote the use of research finding, there is still a gap between theory and practice (Penagiari, 2008). And there are many practices that are being implemented in healthcare that have no or little evidence to support their use (e.g. double-checking of pediatric medication, routine assessment of vital signs every 2 or 4 h in hospitalized patients (Melnyk and Fineout-Overholt, 2004).

Difference in outcomes, health inequalities, and poorly performing health service continue to present a challenge to all nurses. Poorly informed decision-making is one of the main reasons to service can fail to be delivered in an optimal way and can also contribute variation in practice which makes less efficient, ineffective, and inequitable. Half of the world's death could be prevented with simple cost effective interventions; not enough is known about how to make these more widely available to the people who need them. Changing practice is difficult, wastes time and can have unexpected outcome. However, change can be exciting and motivating. Understanding and planning how to take evidence into practice, to action knowledge, is important. This area because it is so critical, has been the subject of an increasing amount of research itself (International Council of Nurses, 2012).

All over the world, there is a growing appreciation of the importance and difficulty of evidence based nursing practice (EBNP). As part of international efforts to facilitate the dissemination of EBNP, research has focused on identifying barriers to utilization of EBNP. Identifying such barriers can help international efforts to develop strategies to overcome these. One of these barriers was found to be lacking the knowledge and skills to evaluate research finding (Eizenberg, 2011).

A number of studies from various countries have reported that nurses practice EBP and distinct EBP activities to low extent (Bostrom et al., 2013).

Researchers have argued that daily practice in nursing care is influenced more by tradition, intuition, and experiences and less by scientific research. Reviews in literature focus on the difficulty that exists trying to apply research finding into practice. The major barriers to the utilization of research finding were found to be the work organization (setting), the adopter (nurse), and presentation of research findings (Eizenberg, 2011).

Even though evidence based health care has been shown to be an efficient and much needed practice worldwide, developing countries have difficulties in accessibility of existing evidence and medical resources than in developed countries.

In Africa, EBP implementation is late as compared to developed world. Incorporating evidence-based health care (EBHC) into the African context means setting priorities, developing evidence summaries, and guidelines and implementing research finding relevant for African countries to support health care for all. Contextualizing evidence relates to several issues, including the lack of evidence available for an African setting. The effectiveness of an intervention in Africa may be different from that found in studies elsewhere because of factors such as: later presentation, co-infections, malnutrition, higher levels of self-medication and use of traditional, reduced level of resources, including human resource for basic health care and political instability. In addition, effective interventions, as determined by many systematic reviews, may not be available or affordable in most African settings. This means that Africa needs valid African-specific research and that authors of systematic reviews should consider this by avoiding overgeneralization when making conclusion (Forland et al., 2013).

In Ethiopia, the federal ministry of health lacks skilled health professionals who could help to synthesize evidence for policy-making. Moreover, at all levels of the health systems there is little culture or tradition of trusting or using evidence (Gautham et al., 2014).

Also in Ethiopia as well as in the study area there is a gap of shortage of research articles published concerning

*Corresponding author. E-mail: vmdzomeku@gmail.com

EBP utilization. This study seeks to explore level of EBP implementation and will give information concerning factors, which hinder implementation of EBP among nurses working in Jimma zone public hospitals.

METHODOLOGY

Study setting and design

Institution based cross-sectional study was conducted from in four public hospitals found in Jimma zone, Oromia Regional State from March 1-30, 2015. Jimma is the town of Jimma zone, which is one of the Oromia Regional States, which is 352 km away from Addis Ababa, the capital city of Ethiopia, in southwestern part of the country.

Study populations

Three hundred and two nurses who were present at work in Jimma Zone public hospitals.

Sample size and sampling procedures

The sample size was determined based on the single population proportion formula and an assumption of 50% was taken, since level of evidence based practice utilization is not known. Assuming a 10% non-response rate, a total sample size of 333 nurses were required.

Overall sample was proportionally allocated to each hospital and systematic sampling was used to select participants of the study. All sampled nurses working in four public hospitals of Jimma zone during data collection period were included in the study. Those nurses who were having work experience less than 6 months were excluded.

Data collection

The data was collected using pre-tested semi-structured questionnaire adapted version of Funk's BARRIERS scale to measure nurse's perceived barrier of research utilization and Friedman's test was used to measure knowledge of respondents (Eizenberg, 2011).

This questionnaire included the 29-item barrier scale to research utilization. This scale asked the nurses to rate the extent to which they supposed each item as barrier to nurse's use of research evidence to change or improve their practice.

The questionnaire was prepared in English language. The first part of the questionnaire contained items, which measure socio-demographic characteristic of the respondents. The second part of the questionnaire contained questions about awareness and knowledge of evidence based nursing practice. The third part of the questionnaire contained questions about the evidence practice activities. The fourth part of the questionnaire contained questions about source of information and availability of information resources. Part five of the questionnaire contained the 'BARRIER' scale, which measured the nurse's perception on barriers of research evidence utilization. The 'BARRIER' scale was divided into four parts (subscales): characteristic of the adopter (nurse's value, skills, and awareness), characteristic of the organization (setting, barriers and limitation), characteristic of the innovation (qualities of the research) and characteristic of the communication (presentation and accessibility). The subscales Cronbatch's alpha values were 0.85 for presentation scale, 0.79 for nurse subscale, 0.82 for setting subscale and 0.86 for research (innovation) subscale.

Study variables: Dependent variables implementation of evidence based practice

The scale that measured implementation of EBP in this study includes seven items with minimum score of 7 and maximum score of 35. Moreover, the score on implementation of evidence based nursing practice (EBNP) was transformed into Tertian classification. The higher the score the higher the implementation of EBNP. The independent variables include: socio-demographic factors (age, sex, marital status, qualification, position in the organization and level of hospital), organizational factors (administration support, colleague support, time availability, and incentive for staff), characteristic of individual (communication character, awareness on best evidences, knowledge on research evidence, salary, place of graduation), and characteristic of research evidence (way of presentation, understandability of research report, availability, and accessibility of research reports).

Statistical analysis

The data were carefully entered into Epidata V3.1, edited and cleaned for inconsistencies and missing values. Data was analyzed using SPSS version 16.0. Descriptive statistic was used to summarize data. Bivariate and multivariable linear regression was used to assess the association between dependent variable and independent variables. The variable with p-value less than 0.05 was taken as having significant association.

Ethical considerations

Ethical clearance was obtained from ethical committee of JU (IRB), College of Public Health and Medical Science. A formal letter, from the College of Public Health and Medical Science of Jimma University was obtained and summited to Jimma zone health office and concerned bodies to obtain their cooperation. The purpose of the study was explained to the participants at the time of data collection and written consent was obtained from the participants to confirm whether they will participate or not. The participants of the study were informed that the participation was voluntary based. Confidentiality of the response was ensured throughout the study.

RESULTS

Socioeconomic and demographic characteristics

Out of 302 respondents, 57% were male. The mean age was 27 years (SD±6.154), minimum age is 19 and maximum age is 58 years old. Majority were single 178 (58.9%). About 177 (58.6%) of the respondents were diploma holders. About 145 (48.0%) of the respondents were graduate from government higher institution and the rest were graduated from private institutions. About 274 (90.7) were in staff nurses and the rest 28 (9.3%) were in different managerial position (Table 1).

Awareness and knowledge about evidence-based practice

When the respondents were asked how familiar they

Table 1. Distribution of respondents by socio-demographics characteristic, in Jimma zone public hospitals, Jimma, southwest Ethiopia, 2015.

Characteristics		N	%
Sex	Male	172	57.0
	Female	130	43.0
Qualification	Diploma	177	58.6
	B.Sc. nurse	121	40.1
	Masters	4	1.3
Marital status	Ever Married	124	41.1
	Single	178	58.9
working hospital	JUSH	253	83.8
	Shenen-Gibe	16	5.3
	Limmu-Genet	19	6.3
	Agaro	14	4.6
Place of graduation	Government institutions/universities	145	48.0
	Private institutions/universities	157	52.0
Position in the hospital	Staff Nurses position	274	90.7
	Managerial position	28	9.3

were with concept, about 190 (62.9%) were familiar with the concept of EBP. When the respondents asked knowledge questions concerning research concept and research terms about 82 (27.2%) of respondents scored low level, about 78 (25.8%) of respondents scored medium level and about 92 (30.5%) of respondents scored high level (based on Tertian classification).

Source of information and availability of the information resource

Concerning the source of information and availability of the information resource, when asked how they evaluate the availability of information resource in the hospital, only 85 (28.1%) said that online resource were available and 76 (25.2%) said that print material were available. Major source of information that respondents usually find evidence for their nursing care practice was internet 118 (39.1%).

When asked how often they look for information from the given sources, about 135 (44.6%) were using reference book, about 40 (13.2%) were using research report, about 36 (11.9%) were using journal article and about 41 (13.5%) were using hospital library on the regular bases.

Level evidence based practice activity

From the total 302 participants, 245 (81.1%) had involved in different EBP activities to different level (from seldom to often). Total score was computed for individuals total score in EBP and Tertian classification was done on the total score of EBP activity measurements. Accordingly, about 45 (18.4%) of the respondents implemented EBP to low level (sometimes), about 103 (42%) of the respondents implemented EBP to medium level and about 97 (39.6%) of respondents implemented EBP to high level (Table 1).

Perceived barriers to research utilization

The top 5 perceived barriers reported in this study were (1) ‘physician doesn’t not cooperate with implementation of new evidences’; (2) ‘the nurse is isolated from knowledgeable colleagues with whom to discuss new findings’; (3) ‘there is no incentive for clinical practice development’; (4) ‘the nurse feels the benefit of changing practice is minimal’; and (5) there is resistance to make change in the work setting. Since 60% of this perceived barrier is from setting origin, the largest perceived barrier was organizational factors (mean =26.60, ±7.08).

Factors associated with implementation of evidence based nursing practice

Factors associated with implementation of EBNP were assessed and the significant association was found between knowledge about EBP and implementation of EBP. Knowledge about EBP was positively associated with EBNP implementation (β=0.76, P=0.008). For a unit

Table 2. Distribution of respondents by involvement in EBP activities, Jimma zone public hospitals, Jimma, Southwestern Ethiopia, 2015.

Activities	Never		Seldom		Occasionally		Regularly		Often	
	N	%	N	%	N	%	N	%	N	%
Asked clinical question r	119	39.4	24	7.9	80	26.5	54	17.9	25	8.3
Look for(searched) evidence	157	52	45	15	79	26	8	2.6	13	4.3
Read any evidence	107	35.4	29	9.6	68	22.5	71	23.5	27	8.9
Critically appraised evidence	122	40.4	40	13.2	53	17.5	57	18.9	30	9.9
Used current evidence	122	40.4	35	11.6	58	19.2	60	19.9	27	8.9
Evaluated the outcome	117	38.7	43	14.2	61	20.2	50	16.6	31	10.4
Teaching new evidence to others	120	39.7	50	16.6	62	20.5	44	14.6	26	8.6

Table 3. Multivariable linear regression final model.

Model	Unstandardized Coefficients		P	95% Confidence Interval for B	
	B	Std. Error		Lower Bound	Upper Bound
Knowledge score	0.762	0.285	0.008**	0.201	1.322
Sex					
Male	0.123	0.901	0.892	-1.652	1.897
Female (Ref.)					
Place of graduation					
Public	2.270	1.137	0.047*	0.031	4.510
Private (Ref.)					
Familiarity to EBP	1.124	1.104	0.310	-1.051	3.298
nurse subscale	0.090	0.074	0.227	-0.056	0.236
Level Nurse Education	0.528	1.165	0.651	-1.768	2.823
Availability of resource	0.675	0.244	0.006**	0.195	1.156

Maximum VIF = 1.882, adjusted R^2 = 0.084.

increase in knowledge about research, implementation of EBNP increases by 0.762. Similarly, place where the respondent graduated was positively associated with evidence based practice (β=2.270, P=0.047). Graduating from public universities increases evidence based practice by 2.270. Another positively associated variable is extent of resources availability such as internet services (online resource), print materials and other information resources (such knowledgeable colleagues) (β =0.67, P= 0.006). Availability of information resource such internet access increases the utilization of EBP by 0.67 (Table 3).

DISCUSSION

Participants in this study were involved in each activity of EBP with different levels of involvement, but for simplicity the score was summed up and transformed into Tertian classification. Accordingly, about 45 (18.4%) of the respondents had implemented EBP to low level (sometimes), about 103 (34.1%) of the respondents had implemented EBP to medium level (usually) and 97 (32.1%) of the respondents implemented EBP to high level (always).

This finding was consistent with the study done in Sweden by Bostrom et al, 2013 in which (60%), approximately similar level of EBP implementation was reported (19% asked clinical questions and performed searches in data bases, 56% used information sources, 31% appraised the literature, 30% participated in practice development, and 34% participated in evaluating clinical practice to high extent) (9, 13). Also finding from this study was analogous with the study conducted in South Africa, in which 35.6, 32.9, and 31.5% use EBP frequently, moderately and rarely, respectively. Even though in this study small numbers of respondents were frequently involved in EBP about (18.4 %), the finding is similar with finding from South Africa.

On the other hand the finding from this study is higher than the study done in Tikur Anbesa hospital in Addis Ababa, in which 57.6% participants applied EBP. Of them, 64 (52.8%), 38 (31.4%) and 19 (15.7%) applied EBP sometime, usually and always respectively (Hadgu et al., 2015).

This could be due the sample size difference. In this study, the sample is somewhat higher than the study done in Tikur Anbesa hospital. The other possible justification may be in Jimma University specialized hospital; there is nursing care standardization program that may increase nurses' application of new research evidence in their nursing care practice.

Concerning perceived barriers to research utilization from the top 5 reported barriers, 3 were setting related barriers, that is, about 60% were from organizational factors. Therefore, the greatest perceived factor was organizational factors (mean=26.60, SD±7.08). This finding was similar with studies done in USA, China, Iran, Maldives, German, and Australia. In addition, organizational factor has been consistently reported as greatest perceived factor. On the other hand, when we compare top 5 perceived barriers to research utilization with seven other studies except this study, most of the studies reported that 'insufficient time to read and implement new idea' was the most reported barrier (Eizenberg, 2011; Uysal et al., 2010; Heydari et al., 2014; Umarani, 2014; Dalheim et al., 2012; Gravel et al., 2006; Retsas, 2000; Schoonover, 2006; Shifaza et al., 2014).

In this study, knowledge about EBP was positively associated with EBP implementation ($\beta=0.76$, $P=0.008$). This finding was similar in pattern with study done in USA where nurses who reported having greater knowledge of EBP also reported a greater extent of evidence-based care ($r=0.42$, $p<0.0001$) (Melnyk et al., 2004). Similarly, the study done in Iran is in line with this finding where nurses who knew the definition of evidence-based nursing were more likely to utilize research findings in clinical practice than those who did not know (Pearson $\chi^2 = 23.912$, $P = 0.02$) (Heydari et al., 2014).

Similarly, in our country, one study that was conducted in Tikur Anbesa hospital reported that those nurses who have knowledge were 3 times more likely to practice EBP than those who do not have knowledge (Hadgu et al., 2015).

IMPLICATION FOR PRACTICE, POLICY AND NURSING PROGRAMS

In this study, small number of nurses applied EBP to high level (frequent basis). This means most of the nurse in Jimma zone public hospital uses traditional way of practice, that means depend on the expert opinion and school training, which may be out to date way of practice, which delays the latest way of patient care approach, which enhances the progress of patient outcomes. Since the use of evidence-based practice delivers the positive patient care outcomes nurse in Jimma zone public hospitals should implement EBP in their nursing care practice to positive patient care outcomes. It is very much important to consider nursing care policy and nursing curriculum issues so that curriculum planners should strictly emphasize on EBP philosophy during program preparation. Nursing care policy should empower nurse so that nurses autonomously implement EBP during nursing care practice. Other area that should be considered is educational preparation for nurse particularly in private institutions or colleges. Private nursing college should comply all the issue incorporated in Ethiopia nursing education programs so that graduate from private institution be competent in implementation of research findings in the nursing care practice.

LIMITATION OF THE STUDY

Since this study was based on self-report, the response on the EBP practice may be inflated due to social desirability bias of respondents.

CONCLUSIONS AND RECOMMENDATIONS

This study concluded that small number of nurses applied EBP to high level. Organizational factors were found to be the greatest perceived barrier. The implementation of evidence-based practice was associated with knowledge on research, place of graduation, and the availability of information resources. The level of perception and level of EBP implementation was not associated.

There has to be intervention program to facilitate the implementation of evidence in nursing practice by the respective stakeholders (Ethiopian Federal Ministry of Health, Oromia Regional Health Bureau, educators of nursing education and hospital administration of Jimma zone public hospitals).

Training should be conducted for nurses on implementation of evidence-based practice by Jimma zone public hospitals in collaboration with NGOS, Ethiopian Federal Ministry of Health and Oromia Regional Health Bureau.

Resources necessary to implement evidence based nursing practice should be provide by hospital administration of Jimma zone public hospitals in collaboration with Ethiopian Federal Ministry of Health, Oromia Regional Health Bureau and other NGOs

Intervention programs concerning organizational communication with issue on evidence based practice implementation should be done together with nurses and physician to create supportive staff by hospital administration of Jimma zone public hospitals.

Since there is gap of awareness on evidence based nursing practice curriculum planners should take into consideration to include the principle of evidence based nursing practice in Ethiopian nursing education programs especially in the undergraduate nursing education curriculum. Private nursing colleges should incorporate principles of evidence based practice in their nursing education programs so that graduates from private nursing college should be competent.

CONFLICT OF INTERESTS

The authors have not declared any conflict of interests.

ACKNOWLEDGEMENTS

The authors would like to thank the respondents who participated in the study. They are also grateful to Jimma University for funding the study.

REFERENCES

Bostrom AM, Rudman A, Ehrenberg A, Gustavsson JP, Wallin L (2013). Factors associated with evidence-based practice among registered nurses in Sweden: a national cross-sectional study. BMC Health Services Research, 13(1):165.

Dalheim A, Harthug S, Nilsen RM, Nortvedt MW (2012). Factors influencing the development of evidence-based practice among nurses: a self-report survey. BMC Health Services Research, 12(1):367.

Eizenberg MM (2011). Implementation of evidence-based nursing practice: nurses' personal and professional factors?. Journal of Advanced Nursing, 67(1):33-42.

Fineout-Overholt E, Melnyk BM, Schultz A (2005). Transforming health care from the inside out: advancing evidence-based practice in the 21st century. Journal of Professional Nursing, 21(6):335-344.

Forland F, Rohwer AC, Klatser P, Boer K, Mayanja-Kizza H (2013). Strengthening evidence-based healthcare in Africa. BMJ Evidence-based Medicine, 18(6):204-206.

Gautham M, Berhanu D, Umar N, Ghosh A, Elias N, Spicer N, Becker A, Schellenberg J (2014). Panel discussion: The challenges of translating evidence into policy and practice for maternal and newborn health in Ethiopia, Nigeria and India. BMC Health Services Research, 4(2):7.

Gravel K, Légaré F, Graham ID (2006). Barriers and facilitators to implementing shared decision-making in clinical practice: a systematic review of health professionals' perceptions. Implementation Science, 1(1):16.

Hadgu G, Almaz S, Tsehay S (2015). Assessment of Nurses 'Perceptions and Barriers on Evidence Based Practice in Tikur Anbessa Specialized Hospital Addis Ababa Ethiopia, 4(3):73-83.

Hadgu G, Almez S, Tsehay S (2015). Assessment of nurses' perceptions and barriers on evidence based Practice in Tikur Anbessa Specialized Hospital Addis Ababa Ethiopia. American Journal of Nursing Science, 4(3):73-83.

Heydari A, Zeydi AE (2014). Barriers to and Facilitators of Research Utilization among Iranian Nurses: a Literature Review. Journal of Caring Sciences, 3(4):265-275.

International Council of Nurses (ICN) (2012). Closing the gap from evidence to action 2012. Available at: http://www.icn.ch/publications/2012-closing-the-gap-from-evidence-to-action/

Melnyk BM, Fineout-Overholt E (2011). Evidence-based practice in nursing & healthcare: A guide to best practice. Lippincott Williams & Wilkins.

Melnyk BM, Fineout-Overholt E, Fischbeck Feinstein N, Li H, Small L, Wilcox L, Kraus R (2004). Nurses' perceived knowledge, beliefs, skills, and needs regarding evidence-based practice: Implications for accelerating the paradigm shift. Worldviews on Evidence-Based Nursing, 1(3):185-193.

Panagiari D (2008). Barriers and Facilitators for implementing evidence-based practice among German nurses working in a general hospital (Master's thesis, University of Twente). Available at: http://essay.utwente.nl/59157/1/scriptie_D_Panagiari.pdf

Retsas A (2000). Barriers to using research evidence in nursing practice. Journal of Advanced Nursing, 31(3):599-606.

Schoonover HD (2006). Barriers to research utilization among registered nurses working in a community hospital. Available at: https://research.libraries.wsu.edu/xmlui/bitstream/handle/2376/459/H_Schoonover_033106.pdf?sequence=1

Shifaza F, Evans D, Bradley H (2014). Nurses' perceptions of barriers and facilitators to implement EBP in the Maldives. Advances in Nursing, 1-7.

Umarani J (2014). Perceived barriers to Evidence Based Practice among Registered Nurses. Asian Journal of Biomedical and Pharmaceutical Sciences, 4(32):15-19. Avaialable at: https://www.alliedacademies.org/articles/studies-on-in-vitro-antioxidant-potential-of-pod-and-seed-parts-of-bauhinia-malabarica-roxb.pdf

Uysal A, Temel AB, Ardahan M, Ozkahraman S (2010). Barriers to research utilisation among nurses in Turkey. Journal of Clinical Nursing, 19(23-24):3443-3452.

Wikipedia (2014). Evidence-based practice. Available at: https://en.wikipedia.org/wiki/Evidence-based_medicine

16

Determinants of satisfactory facility-based care for women during childbirth in Kumasi, Ghana

Veronica Millicent Dzomeku[1*], Brian van Wyk[2], Lucia Knight[3] and Jody Rae Lori[4]

[1]Department of Nursing, Kwame Nkrumah University of Science and Technology, Kumasi, Ghana.
[2]School of Public Health, University of the Western Cape, South Africa.
[3]School of Public Health, University of the Western Cape, South Africa
[4]School of Nursing, University of Michigan, USA.

The majority of deaths of women and infants during pregnancy and childbirth occur in Africa. Although many pregnant women seek antenatal care, in Ghana they do not all continue to seek facility-based care for childbirth. Complications that lead to mortality often occur around childbirth and these are not always possible to predict during antenatal care. This makes facility-based childbirth imperative for reduction in maternal and infant mortality. Satisfaction with childbirth care is recognized as a key influence for future utilization of the facility for pregnant women. This paper explores what women in Kumasi, Ghana perceive as satisfactory facility-based childbirth care. An exploratory qualitative study that enrolled 56 consenting women attending either antenatal or postnatal care in four public health facilities in Kumasi was conducted. Data were collected using in-depth individual interviews which were audio recorded and transcribed verbatim. Content analyses led to the emergence of themes that reflected participants' conceptualizations of satisfaction with facility-based childbirth care. Four themes emerged related to women's satisfaction with facility-based childbirth, namely: (i) receiving courteous and dignified care; (ii) having a consistent caregiver during childbirth; (iii) experiencing a positive birth outcome; and (iv) having a skillful care practitioner. Nurses and midwives should update their clinical skills and also be trained to provide patient-centered care to meet the expectations of women during childbirth in Kumasi, Ghana.

Key words: Satisfaction, childbirth, facility-based childbirth, Kumasi-Ghana.

INTRODUCTION

Worldwide, in 2015 an estimated 303,000 women died from pregnancy-related causes during the third trimester and 2.6 million babies were stillborn (Alkema et al., 2006; United Nations Maternal Mortality Estimation Inter-Agency Group Collaborators and Technical Advisory Group, 2016; Blencowe et al., 2016; Lancet Stillbirth Epidemiology Investigator Group, 2016). It is noteworthy that more than half of these deaths occurred in Africa, and more so, that they could have been prevented by quality health care during pregnancy, labor, and delivery

*Corresponding author. E-mail: vmdzomeku@gmail.com

(WHO, 2014). Most of the complications that lead to maternal mortality occur during delivery and these are not easily predictable during the antenatal period (Crissman et al., 2012). Professional nursing care offers an opportunity to communicate with and support women and families during childbirth. It is argued that this leads to the development of a trusting relationship leading to satisfaction with care (WHO, 2014; Eghdampour et al., 2013; National Institute of Clinical Excellence (NICE), 2007; Birkhäuer et al., 2017). Satisfactory childbirth care may also positively affect a woman's bonding relationship with her child with subsequent implications for neonatal wellbeing (Baas et al., 2017).

The satisfaction of women with their facility-based childbirth care is a significant factor in their subsequent use of the facility for future childbirth and compliance with care (Oikawa et al., 2014; Tayelgn et al., 2011; Mehata et al., 2017). Moreover, experiences of disrespect and abuse during childbirth care have the potential to reduce women's satisfaction with health facilities (Magil-Cuerden, 2007; Kujawski et al., 2015; Moyer et al., 2013). Satisfactory childbirth care should meet the woman's personal expectations of receiving maximum support during care and building a trusting provider-patient relationship (Mehata et al., 2017).

When women have their expectations of labor and birth met, they are likely to be satisfied with care. A study in the United States of America (USA) found that personal control during childbirth was an important childbirth care requirement amongst participating women (Rominski-Danielson et al., 2016). A similar study in Australia found that having familiar faces engaging in the care process was important to satisfaction with birth care (Goodman et al., 2004). Similarly, the immediate maternal condition after birth, waiting time and the availability of waiting areas, as well as care provider and measures taken to provide privacy during examination, are factors that determined satisfaction with care among women studied in Ethiopia (Tayelgn et al., 2011). These studies demonstrate that women value sensitive and respectful relationships with competent clinicians who recognize and strive to provide them with patient-centered care.

In many African countries, including Ghana, skilled care is available only in health facilities, as skilled birth attendants usually do not attend home births. In health facilities skilled care is provided by doctors and nurses or midwives. However, due to the treatment women receive from facility-based care providers in Africa, many women opt for home births without skilled attendants (Lewis et al., 2016; Morad et al., 2013; Okafor et al., 2015; McMahon et al., 2014). In Ghana, only 42% of women seek facility-based care during childbirth (Ghana Statistical Service, 2009b). In 2017, the WHO (2017) reported Ghana had a maternal mortality rate of 319/100,000 live births. Health workers were reported to create barriers to care-seeking by being unwilling to assist pregnant women, beating women in labor, acting rudely, and using abusive language (Dzomeku et al., 2017). A similar study in Lagos reported lack of sympathy and empathy, neglect, rudeness and verbally abusive behavior, inadequate attention from health care providers, and lack of privacy in skilled health care setting (Okafor et al., 2015). Some study participants explained that the midwife ought to hit women if they fail to push in labour to prevent the baby from dying (Rominsky et al., 2016). Poor treatment of women forms barriers to effective use of skilled childbirth care (Holmes and Goldstein, 2012) and suggests that there is a need for a patient-centered approach to health care provision, particularly childbirth care (The Health Foundation, 2014).

In patient-centered care, the health professionals work collaboratively with their clients and patients to ensure satisfaction with care (The Health Foundation, 2014). The benefit of the patient-centered health care approach is to involve patients in their care while enabling them to make informed decisions (The Health Foundation, 2014). Satisfaction with childbirth care is critical to avoid pregnant women feeling vulnerable at the time when they need health care most and to ensure continued use of health care services (Biringer et al., 2009). While we know its importance, there is a paucity of literature on what constitutes satisfactory facility-based childbirth care for Ghanaian women. This paper reports on the determinants of facility-based childbirth care for women in Ghana.

Guiding questions

1. What do women perceive as satisfactory in facility-based childbirth care?
2. What are women's expectations of a facility-based childbirth care?
3. What are women's experiences of facility-based childbirth care?

Definition of key terms

Women/midwifery clients: Antenatal or postnatal mothers who receive childbirth care from one of the four public health settings of this study.

Satisfaction: The desired expectations and experiences of women about their childbirth care from public health facilities.

Childbirth: the period from antenatal, labour and postnatal.

Patient-Centred care: An approach to care that meets patients' expectations of care

METHODOLOGY

Ghana has ten administrative regions, each with a regional capital.

This study was conducted in Kumasi. The Kumasi metropolis has 20 public health facilities that provide childbirth health care services. Four facilities, the only teaching hospital in the region, one district hospital, and two rural facilities, were selected for the current study based on these characteristics and to provide a perspective of women receiving care in both rural and urban settings. Midwifery clients receiving health care services at antenatal or postnatal clinics in these four public health facilities constituted the study population. Purposive sampling strategies were used to recruit participants, and only participants who gave written consent were interviewed. Inclusion criteria were antenatal or postnatal women with no complications with their current pregnancies, who are regular patients at the facilities in which they were approached, and were willing to participate in the study. Between 12 and 15 individual interviews were conducted in each of these facilities yielding a total of 56 participants for the study.

Using an exploratory qualitative research approach, an interview guide, with probing questions, guided the determinants of satisfactory facility-based care for women during childbirth in Kumasi, Ghana. Individual in-depth interviews were recorded with the consent of participants using an interview guide. The interview guide had questions such as; what were your experiences with facility-based childbirth care, what were your expectations of facility-based childbirth care, what made you satisfied with facility based childbirth care? The researchers conducted four interviews a day and allowed two-week intervals between data collection days, allowing adequate time for listening to the tapes several times, transcribing, reading the text, and identifying further probes. Each interview lasted for between 45 to 60 min. This process of simultaneous transcription allowed an opportunity for further exploration during the next set of interviews with other participants. Data collection ran from December, 2014 to April, 2015 for six weeks in each facility. Data collection ceased in each setting once data saturation occurred (Morse and Field, 1995). Interviews were conducted in Twi (a local language). They were translated and transcribed into English, and then back translated to ensure that content was accurate. Using content analysis, data was analyzed by first reading through the transcripts several times to familiarize with the text. Data was then coded and similar codes were put together to form themes.

Ethics

Permission to conduct the study was obtained from the ethics committees of the Kwame Nkrumah University of Science and Technology, Kumasi and Komfo Anokye Teaching Hospital. Informed consent was sought and obtained by explaining the study and their role to participants. Permission was also sought and obtained to record interviews. Only consenting participants were involved in the study after their verbal approvals were obtained. Trustworthiness of the study was ensured by accurately identifying participants who met the study inclusion criteria. Colleague researchers and participants were engaged in peer debriefing and member check throughout the data collection period in order to ensure the quality and integrity of research questions and transcripts.

RESULTS

Table 1 shows the biographic data of women in this study. Participants were between the ages of 18 and 46 years. Approximately 2% had a basic level education; 32% had junior high school education; 23% had senior high school education; 16% has tertiary level education, and approximately 27% had no formal education. 34% were unemployed, 48% had informal employment, and 18% had formal employment. Four themes, each illustrating participants' satisfaction with facility-based childbirth care emerged from the data and are presented below. The themes were based on participants' anticipations of and/or prior knowledge and experience of facility-based childbirth care, namely: (i) receiving courteous and dignified care, (ii) having a consistent caregiver during childbirth, (iii) experiencing a positive birth outcome, and (iv) having a skillful care practitioner.

Courteous and dignified care

Some participants in this study described the childbirth care provided by the facility-based midwives as thoughtful and the midwives as having 'good manners'. Patients attributed this courteousness and dignified care to professionalism. Participants were satisfied when they perceived midwives as having time for them. They recommended that midwives should not be in a hurry to dismiss them during an appointment, but take due care to address all their needs.

"The midwife had all the time for me to answer my questions, even though we were many [women in the facility]. She was calm and cool about her work. She is what a midwife should be". [Woman from Ksouth 7, aged 31].

The participants also were impressed by, or wanted to have, a reliable caregiver who was present and willing to help at all times.

"The midwife was ready to help me at all times, I like her". [Woman from Ayid, aged 27].

This willingness made women feel like they were being well treated. Not only was the midwifes' presence important to participants' satisfaction with care but also their willingness to offer help and when women felt they could relate to them.

"She was approachable, I could relate to her freely". [Woman from Ksouth, aged 26].

Some participants also reported that their midwives treated them cordially. Women found this when midwives greeted them and/or responded appropriately to their greetings.

"The midwives were nice to me, also friendly, patient, and treated me as if I was one of them. They were patient and responded to our greetings. They showed interest in me and ask about my health and wellbeing". [Woman from Apat, aged 25].

This also made women feel welcome at and comfortable

Table 1. Description of participants' characteristics

Parameter	Total	Percentages
Age (years)		
< 20	2	3.6
21-30	27	48
31-40	25	44.6
41-50	1	1.8
Unknown	1	1.8
Formal Education		
Basic	1	1.8
Junior High School(JHS)	18	32
Senior High School (SHS)	13	23
Tertiary	9	16
None	15	26.8
Employment status		
Formal	10	17.9
Informal	27	48
Unemployed	19	33.9

in the facility. Visitors are received warmly with a smile and a handshake, signifying acceptance, in a manner consistent with Ghanaian culture.

"I expect midwives to receive patients with a smile, it is what you expect when you go to someone's house". [Woman from Ayid aged 29].

Participants in this study also expected the midwives to show them similar welcoming gestures, as culture demands. It was key to women in this study that they received dignified care from providers; this is when their bodies are respected.

"The midwife should not just come to me and start asking me to part my legs for vaginal examination without any explanation and permission. It will not make me feel good at all". [Woman from KATH 2, aged 32].

Women expected particularly their genitalia to be protected and respected as much as possible.

"In my previous childbirth in the facility, I did not receive any explanations before vaginal examinations were done. I was not happy about that at all". [Woman from KATH, aged 40]

Participants expected to provide consent before any invasive procedures. As one woman argued, being asked permission would help her feel that she was part of the process.

"The midwife should tell me what she want to do and seek my opinion, then I will feel that I am part of what is going on" [Woman from Ayid, aged 28].

When women were informed, they felt that their bodies and their person were respected. Non-consensual vaginal examination made women feel vulnerable and potentially degraded during care.

"I don't imagine the midwife to walk up to my bed with a tray and think that I know that she is going to perform vaginal examination. I will be very helpless if that happens". [Woman from Ksouth, aged 42].

Non-consented care could also be experienced as an abuse leading to dissatisfaction with care. For satisfaction with care, participants said they desired a cordial relationship with their care providers and respect for their body particularly their genitalia. When respect was not forthcoming from the midwives, it leads to dissatisfaction with care.

Desire for consistent care from a provider

Women in this study reported feeling satisfied with care when it was provided consistently by a care provider that they were familiar with. The perception was that a familiar midwife would be more likely to ensure their safety, because the midwife would be more committed to their care and their baby's well-being.

"I was praying to see a familiar face that is a midwife whom I am accustomed to, or one that I have met during

my antenatal care earlier. The midwife I met when I came here in labor was not someone I had met before. I was so disappointed when I first met her, because I do not know her and how safe she can deliver my baby. But she did well, because she was patient and kind to me". [Woman from Ayid, aged 30].

Moreover, participants expected that the care provider should get to know them during antenatal clinic visits.

"Knowing the midwife before the childbirth I think will make a lot of difference." [Woman from Apart, aged 42].

Some participants felt that they did not belong when they met their midwife for the first time during childbirth.

"You feel like a total stranger in a facility you have always been when you meet a new midwife on each visit and in childbirth." [Woman from Ksouth, aged 37 years].

Having a familiar midwife appeared to contribute to a woman's satisfaction with the childbirth experience. Being with a familiar person also provided women with an opportunity to discuss their fears and anxieties ahead of childbirth, as seen below:

"One thing that I have always wished for is that I will be given one midwife that takes care of me throughout my pregnancy and birth. Then, I know she knows me well, I will not be anxious at all. That will be fulfilling!" [Woman from Ksouth, aged 26].

Participants in this study expected the healthcare system to offer them a consistent and familiar care provider with whom they can identify throughout their childbearing cycle.

Expected positive birth outcomes

Another theme relevant to women's satisfaction with childbirth was the experience of a positive birth outcome. Participants in this study considered having a safe vaginal birth, having a living and healthy baby, and being healthy mothers, as positive birth outcomes, leading to their satisfaction with care.

"I am expecting to deliver safely, have my baby alive and be in good health. I know that there are some women who have complications in birth which can threaten their own lives or the life of their babies". [Woman from KATH, aged 38].

Alternatively, having a caesarean birth, even when mother and baby were healthy, was considered to be a negative birth outcome. This is evident in the following comment:

"My co-tenant delivered a few weeks ago it did not go well with her because she had a caesarean section. I pray that I have a safe birth". [Woman from Ksouth, aged 25].

This statement reflects women's perception of a positive birth outcome.

"In our family all women have a good outcome, they deliver by themselves. It is not good to be helped to deliver." [Woman from Ksouth, aged 42].

Another participant's response shows her perception of the relationship between vaginal birth and her womanhood.

"In my previous childbirths, I delivered by myself and that makes me feel good as a woman, am expecting to deliver again without assistance." [Woman from Ayid, aged 36].

Women in this study perceived only a vaginal birth as a positive birth outcome leading to satisfaction with the childbirth experience and care. They considered only going through the natural process of childbirth as successful.

Skillful nursing practices

Generally, all midwives, throughout their training, learn critical skills for the management of reproductive health care issues, including the management of normal pregnancy, labor, and the puerperium. As part of their skills, they are able to detect abnormality and manage the birth process and/or refer to the relevant departments or personnel. Participants expect the professional knowledge of midwives to support them in order to have vaginal birth.

"In terms of birth or conducting of the birth process, midwives do just what they have to do. The baby was not coming out well and that was why I was brought here. With the midwives efforts, everything went well. I did not have any surgery. I am very happy." [Woman from *KATH*, aged 40].

Women trusted their midwives to ensure that they received what they perceived as safe care. Safe care meant having a vaginal birth with mother and baby in a good condition.

"When the midwife examines you and tells you something about your baby, be sure that it is exactly the case. After examining me, she said I will deliver in the next 5 hours and this is what happened". [Woman from Ksouth, aged 22].

Participants were very confident that midwives had the skill to help them through their childbirth in order for them to have a safe and natural birth. Another participant noted:

"The midwife is very skillful, I was bought to the hospital after a difficult labor at home, but the way she went about it, they have been trained. I will not stay at home anymore; I will rather come early to the hospital". [Woman from Apat, aged 34].

Participants had confidence in the midwives to see them through labor because of their training and expertise.

"The hospital is the last stop once you come, the midwives are able to help you. You know it's their job and they know it". [Woman from KATH, aged 40].

Yet another participant recounted having had an encouraging experience with her care during the puerperium.

"I gave birth to twins. After the first twin, I was so exhausted. They [the midwives] encouraged me to help myself so that they can support me and honestly they did well. They gave me an intravenous infusion and monitored me until the second twin came out. They afterwards monitored my blood pressure until I was completely stable. They cleaned me up and sent me to a neatly prepared bed to rest and breastfeed them". [Woman from Ksouth, aged 26].

As noted earlier, participants also appreciated the supportive skills of the midwife after they delivered.

"The midwife came to assist me to put my baby to breast, I was happy because I did not know how to do that". [Woman from Ayid Aged 38].

Participants in this study talked about needing skillful care throughout the childbirth period, including during the puerperium, and with the care of the baby. It appears from the results of our study that the experience of, and perceived skills of, the midwives were a strong factor for satisfaction with facility-based childbirth care.

DISCUSSION

This study identified that participating women in Kumasi expect to receive courteous and dignified facility-based childbirth care. Participants expected their interactions with the providers to be cordial, that their views and perspectives would be sought and respected by the health care providers, and that they would receive adequate responses to their queries, questions, and concerns, consistent with a patient-centered approach to care. The literature reports that seeing clients as individuals and considering their views during care provision equates to dignity in care as this leads to the physical, emotional, and spiritual needs of clients being attended to, which is patient-centered care (WHO, 2014). Midwifery clients require emotional, physical, and advocacy support, particularly during labor (WHO, 2014; Royal College of Midwives, 2012). Participants in this study wanted forms of support that build their confidence in their ability to go through the process of labor and also to manage their pain. Our findings concur with those other researchers who found that failure to include women directly in decision-making processes and refusing to make and maintain eye contact during conversation or examination decreased women's self-confidence and their satisfaction with care (Crissman et al., 2012; Morad et al., 2013; Doherty, 2010). Women in this study desired to be involved in the care process in order to ensure safe delivery, and this led to satisfaction with childbirth care. Meeting women's expectations about childbirth care leads to satisfaction with care.

In the context of this study, participants expected to have familiar midwives taking care of them throughout the maternal health care continuum. It was noted that having a familiar caregiver strengthened the relationship between the women and the midwives and made it possible to plan successfully for the future. This is supported by evidence that women desire predictability of provider during their pregnancy and childbirth care, and that women need to maintain client/midwife relationships (Doherty, 2010). This finding echoes the findings of other researchers who reported that having different care providers can lead to the dissatisfaction of women (Goberna-Tricasa et al., 2011). The relationship with a midwife who monitors childbirth helps build trust between the client and the provider. Most women preferred a trusting relationship with their care providers because they felt vulnerable and wanted to be comforted by a familiar person (Royal College of Obstetricians and Gynaecologists (RCOG), 2007). This implies the need for familiarity throughout pregnancy and labour. This form of familiarity in a low resourced country like Ghana will be challenging to provide because of the severe health manpower shortages (Naicker et al., 2009). Despite this difficulty, focused antenatal care can be provided as a component of patient-centered care, where the same team of care providers sees the woman through her pregnancy and delivery. This may provide some of this familiarity that women desire in childbirth care (RCM, 2012) and will require planning and changing nursing and midwifery care from the current task orientation to patient-centered care, in order to ensure satisfaction with care.

Participants in this study wanted support and attention during childbirth, something supported by the evidence (Royal College of Midwives (RCM), 2012). Best practice recommends that all women in labor should receive one-on-one patient/midwifery support in established labour (RCM, 2012). However, this may remain a wish in many

African countries because of the human resource challenges facing the systems in Africa where there are 2.3 providers per 1000 population compared to 24.8 providers per 1000 population in the USA (Naicker et al., 2009).

For women in this study, having a caesarean birth is not considered a satisfactory outcome. This finding is consistent with a study in Nigeria where 81% of women reported that they would refuse caesarean section if required, even to save the their own lives and those of their neonates. This is attributed to what the authors describe as inaccurate cultural perceptions of labor and caesarean section (Aziken et al., 2007). In certain African settings, women are expected to go through vaginal birth as a signifier of their womanhood, and interventions in childbirth mean this may be compromised.

Women in this study seemed to perceive that the midwives supporting them in childbirth were highly skilled. Women reported that midwives were able to intervene in difficult labors and assist them to deliver safely. Women appreciated the midwives' perceived skills particularly when they had been in labor with unskilled birth attendant without progress or had bad experiences in the past. These findings were supported by previous research showing that most clients are satisfied with the physical support and skills of midwives when in labour (Eghdampour et al., 2013; NICE, 2007). The findings also support observations by other researchers that dissatisfaction with facility-based childbirth care originates from the perceived lack of, or inadequacy of skillful care (Kujawski et al., 2015). Access to skilled care has been identified as a challenge to reducing maternal mortality; and overcoming this requires competent health providers as well as an environment in which they can perform effectively (Graham et al., 2001). Measures to improve skilled birth care is particularly important when 15% of all births are complicated by a potentially fatal condition that requires emergency care (WHO, 2014); and a skilled provider can recognize the onset of complications, perform essential interventions, start treatment and supervise the referral of situations beyond his/her capabilities and/or that of her facility (WHO, 2017). Women in this study perceived the skills of the midwives as contributing to their satisfaction and this affected their decision to choose facility-based childbirth care over birth at home. This finding is consistent with evidence that women's satisfaction with care during childbearing leads to repeat use of facility-based childbirth and to recommending it to others (Dzomeku et al., 2017; Institute of Medicine, 2012). This study demonstrates that, to consider childbirth care satisfactory, women require patient-centered care that meets their expectations and experience.

Implications for practice

We identify the need for midwives to:

(i) enforce the practice of focused antenatal care initiative to ensure increased familiarity with a provider;
(ii) provide friendly and patient-centered care to women during childbirth;
(iii) respect the dignity, womanhood, and individuality of all women during care;
(iv) approach women sensitively and receive consent for all invasive procedures;
(v) include and inform women in and about their care;
(vi) intensify education of women about indications for interventions such as caesarean section during childbirth;
(vii) provide continuous professional development for midwives to sharpen their skills and ensure they remain relevant.

Limitations

This study did not consider other factors that may affect satisfaction with care such as the educational and socio-economic backgrounds of participants, their parity, the availability of facilities, and the environment within the health facility.

Conclusion

The study revealed that multiple factors may influence women's satisfaction with facility-based childbirth care in Kumasi including courtesy and dignity in care, communication and involvement, familiarity with care providers, positive birth outcome, and the skills of the midwife. These factors reflect women's anticipation of and their understanding of facility-based childbirth care which ought to be considered in the provision of care by providers. Skilled providers offering patient-centered care services are pivotal to the reduction of maternal mortality, therefore attention should be given to both the hard and soft skills development of providers. This study has provided evidence for the need to further provide professional development to midwives.

CONFLICT OF INTERESTS

The authors have not declared any conflict of interests.

ACKNOWLEDGEMENTS

Authors thank the participants who shared their expectations with us and the Metro Director for Ghana Health Service who facilitated access to the hospitals for data collection. The support of the Kwame Nkrumah University of Science and Technology, Kumasi and the Social Innovation in Public Health Impulse (SIPHI) fellowship program, University of Western Cape, South Africa is appreciated. Finally, the efforts of the research assistants David Ameyaw, Thomas Hinni and Precious Duodu during data collection and transcription are highly appreciated; along with the Pre-Publication Support Services (PREPSS) of the University of Michigan who supported the development of this manuscript by providing pre-publication peer-review and copy editing.

REFERENCES

Alkema L, Chou D, Hogan D, Zhang S, Moller AB, Gemmill A, Fat DM, Boerma T, Temmerman M, Mathers C, Say L, United Nations Maternal Mortality Estimation Inter-Agency Group collaborators and technical advisory group (2006). Global, regional, and national levels and trends in maternal mortality between 1990 and 2015, with scenario-based projections to 2030: a systematic analysis by the UN Maternal Mortality Estimation Inter-Agency Group. Lancet. 387(10017):462-474.

Aziken M, Omo-Aghoija L, Okonofua F (2007). Perceptions and attitudes of pregnant women towards ceasarean section in urban Nigeria. Acta Obstetric Gynaecol. Scand. 86(1):42-47.

Baas CI, Wiegers TA, de Cock TP, Erwich JJHM, Spelten ER, de Boer MR, Hutton, EK (2017). Client-Related factors associated with 'less than Good' Experiences of midwives care during childbirth in the Netherlands. Birth-issues in Perinatal care. 44(1):58-67.

Birkhäuer J, Gaab J, Calnan MW (2017). Is having a trusting doctor-patient relationship better for patients' health? European Journal for Person Centered Healthcare. 5(1):145-147.

Biringer, A, Maxted J, Graves L (2009). Family medicine maternity care: Implications for the future. A discussion paper of the maternity and newborn care committee. The college of family physicians of Canada. Available at: https://pdfs.semanticscholar.org/1018/2496eea5c2ea3be5d75237d67ef956c9a3f9.pdf

Blencowe H, Cousens S, Jassir FB, Say L, Chou D, Mathers C, Hogan D, Shiekh S, Qureshi ZU, You D, Lawn JE, Lancet Stillbirth Epidemiology Investigator Group (2016). National, regional, and worldwide estimates of stillbirth rates in 2015, with trends from 2000: A systematic analysis. Lancet Glob Health 4:98-108.

Crissman H, Engmann CM, Adanu RM, Nimako D, Crespo K, Moyer CA (2012). Shifting norms: pregnant women's perspectives on skilled birth attendance and facility-based delivery in rural Ghana. Afr. J. Reprod. Health pp. 15-26.

Doherty ME (2010). Midwifery care: reflections of midwifery clients. J. Perinatal Educ. 19(4):41-51. Doi: 10.1186/1472-698X-13-49 accessed at: http://www.biomedcentral.com/1472-698X/13/49.

Dzomeku VM, van Wyk B, Lori J (2017). Experiences of women receiving childbirth care from public health facilities in Kumasi, Ghana. Midwifery 55:90-95. DOI: http://dx.doi.org/10.1016/j.midw.2017.09.010

Eghdampour F, Jahdie F, Kheyrkhah M, Taghizadeh M, Naghizadeh S, Hagani H (2013). The impact of Aloe vera primiparous women: A randomized clinical trial. J. Caring Sci. 2(4):279.

Ghana Statistical Service (GSS) (2009b). Ghana Health Service (GHS), and ICF Macro. Ghana Demographic and Health Survey 2008. Accra, Ghana: GSS, GHS, and ICF Macro.

Goberna-Tricasa J, Banús-Giménez R, Palacio-Tauste A, Linares-Sancho A (2011). Satisfaction with pregnancy and birth services: The quality of maternity care services as experienced by women. Midwifery 27(6):231-237.

Goodman P, Mackey MC, Tavakoli AS (2004). Factors related to childbirth satisfaction. J. Adv. Nurs. 46(2):212-219.

Graham WJ, Bell JS, Bullough C (2001). Can skilled attendance at delivery reduce maternal mortality in developing countries? In: De Brouwere V, editor; Van Lerberghe W, editor. (eds). Safe Motherhood Strategies: A Review of the Evidence. Studies in Health Services Organization and Policy. 17. Antwerp: ITG Press. pp. 97-130.

Institute of Medicine (2012). Meeting the Challenge in the Developing World. Washington, DC: The National Academies Press. https://doi.org/10.17226/10841.

Kujawski S, Mbaneku G, Freedman LP, Ramsey K, Moyo W, Kruk ME (2015). Abuse and disrespect are barriers to use of facility-based childbirth care. Matern. Child Health J. 19(10):2243-2250.

Lewis L, Hauck YL, Ronchi F, Crichton C, Waller L (2016). Gaining insight into how women conceptualize satisfaction: Western Australian women's perception of their maternal care experience. BMC Pregnancy and Childbirth 16(1):29.

Magil-Cuerden J (2007). Showing respect for women: another skill for midwives. Br. J. Midwifery P 126. https://doi.org/10.12968/bjom.2007.15.3.23021.

Mehata S, Paudel YR, Dariang M, Aryal KK, Paudel S, Mehta R, King S, Barnett S (2017). Factors Determining satisfaction among facility-based maternity clients in Nepal Suresh, BMC Pregnancy and Childbirth 17:319.

Morad S, Parry-Smith W, McSherry W (2013). Dignity in maternity care; Evidence Based Midwifery. 21:5-15.

Morse JM, Field PA (1995). Nursing research: The application of qualitative approaches. Nelson Thornes.

Moyer CA, Dako-Gyeke P, Adanu RM (2013). Facility-based delivery and maternal and early neonatal mortality in sub-Saharan Africa: a regional review of the literature. Afr. J. Reprod. Health. 17(3):30-43.

Naicker S, Plange-Rhule J, Tutt RC, Eastwood JB (2009). Shortage of healthcare workers in developing countries-Africa. Ethn. Dis. 19(1):60.

National Institute of Clinical Excellence (NICE) (2007). Intrapartum Care: care of healthy women and their babies during childbirth. London RCOG Press.

Okafor I, Ugwu EO, Obi SN (2015). Disrespect and abuse during facility-based childbirth in a low income country. Int J Gynaecol Obstet, 128(2):110-113.

Oikawa M, Sonke A, Faye EO, Ndiaye P, Diadhiou M, Kondo M (2014). Assessment of maternal satisfaction with facility-based childbirth care in the rural region of Tambacouda, Senegal. Afr. J. Reprod. Health 18(4):95-104.

Rominski-Danielson S, Lori JR, Moyer C, Dzomeku VM, Nakua E (2016). When the baby remains there for a long time it is going to die so you have to hit her small for the baby to come out": Justification of disrespectful and abusive care during childbirth among midwifery students in Ghana, Health Policy and Planning. 32(2):215-224.

Royal College of Midwives (2012). Evidence Based guidelines for Midwifery-Led care in Labour: Supporting Women in Labour.

Royal College of Obstetricians and Gynaecologists (RCOG) (2007). Safer Childbirth. Minimum standards for the organisation and delivery of care in labour. London: RCOG press.

Tayelgn A, Zegeye D, Kebede Y (2011). Mothers satisfaction with referral hospital delivery service in Amhara Region, Ethiopia. BMC Pregnancy and Childbirth. 24:11:78.

The Health Foundation (2014). Person-Centered care made simple, what everyone should know about person-centered care. ISBN 978-1-906461-56-0.

World Health Organization (WHO) (2017). WHO recommendations on antenatal care for a Positive Pregnancy experience. Geneva, Switzerland, [http://www.who.int/reproductivehealth/publications/maternal_perinatal_health/anc-positive-pregnancy-experience/en/]. Accessed 10 January 2017.

World Health Organization (WHO) (2014). The prevention and elimination of disrespect and abuse during facility-based childbirth: WHO statement.

Knowledge, attitude and practice of surgical site infection prevention among post-operative nurses in a tertiary health in stitution in north-central Nigeria

Oluwakemi Ajike Kolade[1], Salisu Abubakar[3], Sanusi R. Adejumoke[3], Hanson Victoria Funmilayo[2], and Adelani Tijani[3*]

[1]Department of Nursing, Ladoke Akintola University of Technology, Ogbomoso, Oyo State, Nigeria.
[2]Ras AL Khaimah Medical and Health Science University, RAKCON, United Arab Emirate.
[3]Department of Nursing Sciences, Bayero University, Kano State, Nigeria.

Surgical operations are vital procedures in the health care delivery system. Advancement in surgery has played a pivotal role in managing and treating complex health challenges requiring the process. However, the process and procedure involved in surgical operations could significantly endanger the life of the patient. Healthcare associated infections (HAI) pose grave danger to patients and health workers alike. Empirically establishing the level of knowledge, attitude and actual practices of surgical site Infections (SSIs) infection prevention among nurses is therefore an issue for research if the alarming rate of SSIs in developing countries is to be checked. The study adopted cross-sectional survey and the population comprised surgical ward nurses in University of Ilorin Teaching Hospital, Ilorin. Data were generated using self-developed questionnaire with a reliability estimate of 0.88 on the Cronbach alpha scale. These data were analyzed using descriptive statistics of frequency counts and percentages and inferential statistics of Pearson Product Moment Correlation Coefficient at 0.01 alpha. Findings showed that respondents demonstrated relatively high level of knowledge on SSIs prevention, relatively poor attitude towards SSIs prevention and unsatisfactory level of SSIs prevention. When associations among the variables were examined, findings showed that there is positive association between all the variables studies. Findings showed that there is positive and moderate correlation between knowledge and attitude towards SSIs prevention ($r = 0.695$, $p = 0.000<0.01$) as well as between knowledge and practice ($r = 0.570$, $p = 0.000<0.01$). High correlation was however found for attitude and practice of SSIs prevention ($r = 0.763$, $p = 0.000<0.01$). Nurses' level of knowledge does not translate to desired attitude and practices on SSIs prevention. Improving attitude and practice of SSIs through close supervision, patients' rights education, in-service training and provision of supplies and consumables were recommended.

Key words: Surgical site infections, knowledge, attitude, practices, prevention, nurses.

INTRODUCTION

Surgical operations are vital procedures in the health care delivery system and becoming one of the most frequent hospital procedures which is associated with post-operative morbidities (Weiser et al., 2008). Advancement in surgery has played a pivotal role in managing and treating complex health challenges requiring the process. However, the process and procedure involved in surgery before, during and after the operations could significantly endanger the life of the patient. Healthcare Associated Infections (HAI) pose grave danger to patients and increased workload on health workers which ultimately affect the quality of nursing care (Famakinwa et al., 2014). Surgical site infection (SSI) is one of the most occurring HAI with serious consequence for patients' general condition and survival after a successful surgical intervention (Famakinwa et al., 2014). An SSI can be superficial incisional, deep incisional or organ space infection.

SSI refers to infections that occur as a result of surgical procedure and within thirty days of the procedure or 365 days if there is an implant (Mangram et al., 1999). SSIs are leading cause of HAIs particularly in developing countries (CDC, 2016); the incidence varies from hospital to hospital just as it equally varies from country to country. Available statistics show that incidence is lower in the developed countries where incidence of 2.0 to 6.4% (Anderson et al., 2008) compared to developing countries where incidence has been estimated at between 5.5 and 25% (Lohsiriwat and Lohsiriwat, 2009). Notable consequences of SSIs include but not restricted to prolonged hospital stay, high cost of care, increased psychological stress and trauma for patients and their families, low quality of life, increased risk of morbidity as well as increased risk of death. While some factors associated with SSIs are modifiable, others like age are not thereby calling for increased care among care providers.

However, risks for SSIs are classified into intrinsic extrinsic factors Famakinwa et al. (2014). While the intrinsic factors include advanced age, malnutrition, metabolic diseases, smoking, obesity, hypoxia, immune-suppression, and length of preoperative. Pre-operative skin preparation and skin antiseptics, antibiotic prophylaxis, inadequate sterilization of surgical instruments, surgical drains, surgical hands scrubs, and dressing techniques formed the extrinsic factors. All efforts of infection control among health care providers notwithstanding, infections remain a major unwanted side effect of surgical operation. This unwanted event causes serious harm to patients in both developed and resource constraint countries. The classical statement of Johan Peter Frank, Director of the General Hospital in Vienna around 1800: *Can there be a greater contradiction than a hospital disease: An evil that one acquires where one hopes to loose one's own disease?* Is very much applicable to health care even in this century. The major problem is not the lack of effective surgical precautions and evidence-based guidelines, but possession of knowledge, development of the right attitude and intention to carry out these guidelines to prevent SSIs. Efforts to reduce the frequency and severity of surgical wound infection continue to focus on peri-operative issues, infection control practices in the operating room, surgical site preparation, timing and choice of antibiotics, and physiologic support of a patient during and immediately following the procedure.

The nurses are important members of the surgical care team that stays with the patient round the clock. It is imperative for the surgical nurses to understand the basics of pre and post-operative wound infection prevention and control. The implementation of quality measures including antibiotic prophylaxis, hair removal using a clipper, tight control of pre- and post-operative glucose levels and avoiding hypothermia are all recognized key quality measures in reducing infection (Wick et al., 2008). The timing of surgical prophylaxis and the appropriate use of antimicrobial prophylaxis is an agreed quality indicator and represents a significant intervention in preventing SSIs (Humphreys and Cunney, 2008). An array of studies reported significant drop in the rates of SSIs associated with increased awareness among healthcare workers (Joyce and Nanjaiah, 2009; Eskander et al., 2013). On the other hand, lack of infection prevention and control awareness was found to be associated with poor practices of standard precautions by surgical wards nurses (Mahmud and AbdulSahib, 2011).

Empirically establishing the level of knowledge, attitude and actual practices of SSIs prevention among nurses is therefore an important issue for inquiry. The present study aimed to investigate knowledge, attitude and SSIs prevention practices among nurses in north-central, Nigeria.

MATERIALS AND METHODS

Descriptive survey research design of the correlational type was adopted for this study. The population comprised nurses working at the surgical wards and operating theatres of the University of Ilorin Teaching Hospital Ilorin, Nigeria. A convenience sampling was used to select 250 nurses who were free and willing to participate in the study. Data was collected using a questionnaire with reliability of 0.88 estimated on the Cronbach alpha scale. Participants' knowledge was assessed by 10 question, 2 points were awarded for each correct answer; zero point for incorrect answer while no idea attracted zero point as well. Attitude was assessed using ten questions with the statement constructed along a 4-point scale (strongly disagree to strongly agree). Since the items were negatively worded, strongly disagree attracted 4 points while

*Corresponding author. E-mail: atijani.nur@buk.edu.ng.

strongly agree attracted 1 point with agree and disagree taking 2 and 3 points respectively. In the same vein, practice was assessed using a-ten item scale on a 4-point scale (very often to never). Two research assistants collected the data using on the spot administration technique. Respondents where requested to read and fill a consent form before given copies of the questionnaire which were filled and collected on the spot. The essence of this administration technique was to avoid the loss of questionnaire. Filled copies of the questionnaires were scrutinized for complete filling and coded into SPSS. The coded data were analysed using descriptive statistics of frequency and percentages and inferential statistics of Pearson product moment correlation coefficient at 0.05 alpha level.

RESULTS

The ages of the respondents ranged from 25 to 51 mean 36 ± 3.7 and 168 (70.6%) were female with Nursing Officer I forming majority (36.1%). The rest respondents were Nursing Officer II (30.3%), Senior Nursing Officer (14.3%), Principal Nursing Officer (13.4%) and Chief Nursing Officer 5.9%. The years of experience of the nurses ranged from 1 to 20 with a mean of 14 ± 3.2 years.

On the knowledge of respondents on prevention of SSIs, 68.1% of the respondents correctly identified contaminated personnel hands as major sources of SSIs in the hospitals, 97.9% also correctly identified the need to wash hands or sanitize the hands after handling soiled linen. On the place of jewelries preventing proper hand washing, only 40.3% of the respondents demonstrated this knowledge with 22.7% having no idea. Findings also showed that 55% of the respondents reported that shaving before surgery reduces the chance of surgical site infections, 25.6% reported that they do not have an idea. More so, 46.6% reported that antimicrobial soap use before operation could reduce SSIs. Again, 45.8% of the respondents also reported that risk of SSIs after shaving is lowest when done shortly before the operation with a higher percentage, 62.2% reporting that application of antibiotic cream to the entry site reduces the risk of infections. Good knowledge of SSIs prevention was demonstrated by 92.4% response that washing hands or sanitizing before simple surgery or caring of surgical wound is important to preventing SSIs. In the same vein, 86.1% of the respondent also reported the need to wash hands before commencing work at the surgery ward.

Respondents' views on prevention of SSIs are represented in Table 1. The results further showed a relatively high practice of surgical wound prevention guidelines as only 15.1% of the respondents reported not washing their visibly soiled hands sometimes. Findings also showed that 71.4% reported using sterile technique to change dressing often, although 28.6% reported this practice just sometimes. It was also revealed that nearly half of the respondents (45%) reported that they sometimes change damp sterile dressing as often as possible. Also, only 16% reported complying with surgical wound guidelines very often with 34% reporting complying with these guidelines often. Again, only 22.3 and 27.3% reported using hand gloves and other protective devices very often and often respectively while 34.9% reported washing their hands before and after caring for a surgical wound very often. Generally, being safety conscious while discharging care for surgical wounds was reported to be practiced very often by only 17.6% of the respondents although 30.7% reported being safety conscious often with 6.3% reporting being indifferent.

The result of the study as shown in Table 2 above revealed that there is positive associations between all the variables studies. Findings showed that there is positive and moderate correlation between knowledge and attitude towards SSIs prevention with an r value of 0.695 and the p value at 0.000<0.001 showed that this association is significant. Similarly, there is also positive and moderate correlation between knowledge and practice at an r value of 0.570 and p value at 0.000<0.01. When association between attitude and practice was tested, findings showed that there is a high level of correlation between the two variables at an r value of 0.763 and p value at 0.000<0.01.

DISCUSSION

The result of the study demonstrated that respondents reported a fairly high level of knowledge on prevention or SSIs. A major issue in prevention of deleterious health outcomes is translation of possessed knowledge into actions. This is especially the case with health care providers whose professional trainings expose them to a body of knowledge on critical health issues. The challenge is therefore the translation of this knowledge to needed actions aimed at preventing negative health outcomes like surgical site infections. Knowing what to do is one thing and actually doing what one knows to do is an entirely different thing. It is equally important to ensure that possessed knowledge is potent enough to stimulate needed attitude to help maximize the possibility of translating what is known into desirable actions. Taking the issue of hand washing as an example, over 68% of the respondents reported knowledge of infection transmission in the hospital through professionals or care providers unwashed hands. But when attitude towards hand washing was investigated in the second research question items only 31.9% demonstrated strong positive attitude towards frequent and correct hand washing. When taking down to actual practice, findings showed that only 8.8% of the respondents reported washing their hands as soon as they report for duties at the ward frequently. This goes down to confirm the assertion that knowledge does not necessarily translates into action. It is however important to state that the findings of the study corroborate earlier findings by Famakinwa et al. (2014) that equally reported relatively high level of knowledge on SSIs prevention among nurses in Obafemi Awolowo Teaching Hospital, Ile-Ife, Nigeria. The result of

Table 1. Attitude towards SSIs prevention.

Items	Strongly agree	Agree	Disagree	Strongly disagree
There is no proof of the importance of the guideline for care of surgical wounds	36 (15.1%)	110 (46.2%)	54 (22.7%)	38 (16.0%)
Guidelines for care of surgical wounds make my work harder	60 (25.2%)	102 (42.9%)	76 (31.9%)	-
Following the guidelines for care of surgical wounds takes too much time	54 (22.7%)	127 (53.4%)	36 (15.1%)	21 (8.8%)
I do not care about guidelines for care of surgical wounds since they are not very necessary	21 (8.8%)	147 (61.8%)	49 (20.6%)	21 (8.8%)
Guideline for surgical wounds makes patient care very cumbersome	80 (33.6%)	101 (42.4%)	45 (18.9%)	12 (5.0%)
We do not have enough sterile dressings so this affect compliance with guideline for surgical wounds care	15 (6.3%)	65 (27.3%)	116 (48.7%)	42 (17.6%)
Since some nurses do not follow the guidelines for surgical wound care, I feel it is not important for me to follow them	36 (15.1%)	63 (26.5%)	98 (41.2%)	41 (17.2%)
Washing of the hands before and after taking care of a surgical wound is stressful	39 (16.4%)	90 (37.8%)	92 (38.7%)	17 (7.1%)
Frequent changing of damp sterile dressing brings undue stress	36 (15.1%)	98 (41.2%)	45 (18.9%)	59 (24.8%)
Using sterile technique while changing incision wound increases nurse stress	33 (13.9%)	54 (22.7%)	98 (41.2%)	53 (22.3%)

Table 2. Associations between knowledge, attitude and SSIs prevention practices.

Practice		Knowledge	Attitude	Practice
Knowledge	Pearson correlation	1	0.695(**)	0.570(**)
	Sig. (2-tailed)		0.000	0.000
Attitude	Pearson correlation	0.695(**)	1	0.763(**)
	Sig. (2-tailed)	0.000		0.000
Practice	Pearson correlation	0.570(**)	0.763(**)	1
	Sig. (2-tailed)	0.000	0.000	

**Correlation is significant at the 0.01 level (2-tailed).

the study also showed relatively poor attitude towards SSIs prevention and this is suspected to affect practice. As earlier stated, knowledge does not translate into positive attitude. Although knowledge is important in shaping right attitude, it is however not certain that knowledge gained will translate into positive attitude. Many barriers and extraneous factors might come into play to whittle down the potency of acquired knowledge in bringing about desired attitude. Since attitude is much more likely to influence behavior than just knowledge, emphasis aimed at bringing about improved SSIs prevention practices might be targeted at helping nurses develop positive attitude towards SSIs prevention. Nurses with poor attitude towards SSIs prevention will be more likely to engage in SSIs prevention practices as equally confirmed by this study that showed a positive and high correlation between attitude and SSIs prevention practices. An important way of improving SSIs prevention practices could therefore be targeted at improving on the attitude of nurses towards the prevention guidelines as this improvement will result in improvement in SSIs prevention practices. This study confirms the findings of Brisibe et al. (2014) that reported similar results among health care providers working in selected tertiary health institutions in Port Harcourt, Nigeria. On the issue of actual practice of SSIs prevention guidelines, results showed worrisome percentage of respondents who demonstrated lackadaisical attitude and indifference towards the practice of these guidelines. The results showed that a poor percentage of the respondents reported carrying out critical steps in preventing SSIs only sometimes when these practices should be done almost always. This finding corroborates the work of Brisibe et al. (2014) who also reported unsatisfactory level of SSIs prevention practices among health workers in two tertiary health institutions in Port Harcourt Nigeria. Factors relating to shortage of supplies in consumables, lack of in-service training and poor monitoring and supervision were highlighted as causes of unsatisfactory practice of SSIs prevention guidelines

Based on the findings of the study, it is concluded that though nurses working in the surgical wards of the teaching hospital investigated demonstrated evidence of good knowledge of SSIs prevention, the level of knowledge did not translate into desired attitude and practices on SSIs prevention. The results of the study also showed that there is positive, moderate and significant association between knowledge and attitude towards SSIs prevention just as the same relationship exists between knowledge and SSIs prevention practices. Again there is high, positive and significant association between attitude and practice of SSIs prevention. It was therefore recommended that there is need for on the job training for nurses to help re-awaken them to the roles expected of them in protecting and preserving life. Also, there is need for close monitoring and supervision of surgical ward nurses to ensure that they strictly adhere to SSIs prevention guidelines. The authorities of hospitals too should provide on regular basis the necessary consumables and supplies to ensure strict adherence to SSIs prevention guidelines. In the same way, the use of education, information and communication materials need to be conspicuously displaced in and around the ward to help keep nurses on their toes on infection prevention. Lastly, there is need for patients' education and empowerment on their rights and the responsibilities and obligations care providers owe them. This is important to enable them realize when their rights are being trampled upon and their safety threatened by the negligence of care providers.

CONFLICT OF INTERESTS

The authors have not declared any conflict of interests.

REFERENCES

Anderson JD, Kaye SK, Chen FI, Schmader EK, Choi Y, Sloan R, Sexton JD (2008). Clinical and Financial Outcomes due to *Methicillin Resistant Staphylococcus aureus* Surgical Site Infection: Amulti-center Matched-Outcomes Study. PloS ONE 4(12):1-8.

Brisibe SFA, Ordinioha B, Gbeneolol PK (2014). Knowledge, Attitude, and Infection Control Practices of two Tertiary Hospitals in Port- Harcourt, Nigeria. Niger. J. Clin. Pract. 17(6):691-695.

Eskander H, Morsy W, Elfeky H (2013). Intensive Care Nurses' Knowledge & Practices regarding Infection Control Standard Precautions at a Selected Egyptian Cancer Hospital. J. Educ. Pract. 4(19):160-174.

Famakinwa TT, Bello BG, Oyeniran YA, Okhiah O, Nwadike RN (2014). Knowledge and Practice of Post-Operative Wound Infection Prevention among Nurses in the Surgical Unit of a Teaching Hospital in Nigeria. Int. J. Basic Appl. Innov. Res. 3(1):23-28.

Humphreys H, Cunney R (2008). Performance Indicators and the Public Reporting of Healthcare-Associated Infection Rates. Clin. Microbiol. Infect. 14(10):892-894.

Lohsiriwat V, Lohsiriwat D (2009). Antibiotic Prophylaxis and Incisinoal Surgical Site Infection Following Colorectal Cancer Surgery: An Analysis of 330 Cases. J. Med. Assoc. Thailand 92:12-16.

Mahmud N, Abdul Sahib S (2011). Assessment of Nurses' Practices toward Infection Control Standardized Precautions in Azady Teaching Hospital in the City of Kirkuk. Iraqi Natl. J. Nurs. Specialties 24(1):52-58.

Mangram AJ, Horan TC, Pearson ML, Silver LC, Jarvis WR (1999). Hospital Infection Control Practices Advisory Committee. Guideline for prevention of surgical site infection, 1999. Am. J. Infect. Control 27(2):97-134.

Weiser TG, Regenbogen SE, Thompson KD, Haynes AB, Lipsitz SR, Berry WR, Gawande AA (2008). An Estimation of the Global Volume of Surgery: A Modelling Strategy Based on Available Data. Lancet 372:139-144.

Wick EC, Gibbs L, Indorf LA, Varma MG, Garcia-Aguilar J (2008). Implementation of Quality Measures to Reduce Surgical Site Infection in Colorectal Patients. Dis. Colon Rectum 51:1004-1009.

18

Determinants of late booking for antenatal care among pregnant women in selected hospitals in South East Nigeria

Ada Carol Nwaneri, Ifeoma Ndubuisi*, Ijeoma Lewechi Okoronkwo, Okwudili Ezike and Umebuani Nkiruka

Nursing Sciences Department, Faculty of Health Sciences and Technology, College of Medicine, University of Nigeria, Enugu Campus, Enugu State, Nigeria.

Late booking for antenatal care is a frequent occurrence among pregnant women in Nigeria unlike in most developed countries. The objective of the study was to determine the maternal, socio-cultural, religious, and institutional/systemic factors that determine late booking for antenatal care among pregnant women in Enugu, Nigeria. Descriptive, cross-sectional questionnaire based method was employed in the study. A proportionate stratified sampling technique was used to select 282 pregnant women from three selected hospitals for the study. A validated structured questionnaire constructed by the researchers was used for collection of data. Findings were analysed using both descriptive and inferential statistics. Respondents revealed that maternal factors such as health status in present pregnancy [205(70.7%)], ignorance of proper gestational age to register for antenatal [125(43.1%)] and experience from previous pregnancies [101(34.8%)] determine timing of booking among pregnant women. Socio-cultural factors such as husband's decision [100(34.5%)] and preference for mother in-law/friends/other women's advice during the early weeks of pregnancy [88(26.9%)] determine timing of booking. Religious factor which mostly determine late booking in the study was preference for prayer and faith healing [157(54.1%)]. Institutional/systemic factors such as long waiting time in hospitals [142(49.0%)] and very frequent antenatal care schedule [129(44.5%)] determine late booking for antenatal care among pregnant women. Health status in present pregnancy, husband's decision, long waiting time at the clinic and frequent number of ante-natal visits are the major determinants of late booking in Enugu. There is need for transitioning from traditional approach of ANC to Focused Antenatal Care (FANC) model recommended by WHO.

Key words: Determinants, Enugu, late ante natal booking.

INTRODUCTION

Each year, approximately one third of a million women worldwide die due to pregnancy related conditions; 99% of these deaths occur in developing countries of Africa and Asia and approximately three quarter of them are

*Corresponding author. E-mail: ifeomaf.ndubuisi@unn.edu.ng.

considered avoidable (WHO, 2014). Preventing problems for mothers and babies depends on an operational continuum of care with accessible high quality care before and during pregnancy, childbirth and the postnatal period, and this also depends on the support available to help pregnant women reach services particularly when complications occur (Lancetto et al., 2010).

An important element of this continuum of care worthy to mention is effective antenatal care. Antenatal care (ANC) can be defined as the care provided by skilled health-care professionals to pregnant women and adolescent girls in order to ensure the best health conditions for both mother and baby during pregnancy (WHO, 2016). The components of ANC according to WHO include: Risk identification, prevention and management of pregnancy-related or concurrent diseases and health education and health promotion. Overtime, this form of care for pregnant women has become an important pillar in reducing maternal mortality rate (Onoh et al., 2013). The goal of antenatal care package is to prepare for birth and parenthood as well as prevent, detect, alleviate or manage the three types of health problems during pregnancy that affect mothers and babies: Complication of pregnancy itself, pre-existing condition that worsen during pregnancy and effects of unhealthy lifestyle (Lancetto et al., 2010). Good antenatal links the woman and her family with formal health system, increases the chance of utilizing a skilled attendant and contributes to good health through the life cycle (Onoh et al., 2013). Inadequate care during this time breaks a critical link in the continuum of care and affects both women and babies (Lancetto et al., 2010).

The first antenatal visit (booking) is a very important component of antenatal care as service providers use the occasion to collect basic medical information that will form the basis of care for the client. Wang et al. (2011) however noted that many women especially in Sub-Saharan Africa tend to wait to start antenatal care until the second or third trimester. Findings of Uganda Demographic and Health Survey (2011) showed that though over 90% pregnant women attended antenatal care at least once, only 48% made four or more antenatal care visits during their entire pregnancy; only 21% of the women made their first antenatal care visit before the fourth month of pregnancy and only 52% of women delivered under the care of skilled birth attendant; the maternal mortality ratio was 438 per 100,000 live birth.

The antenatal policy in Nigeria follows the latest WHO approach to promote safe motherhood. It is worthy to note that despite WHOs' recommendation and antenatal care policy in Nigeria, studies have shown that late booking has become a persistent pathology in the country similar to what is being reported for other developing countries of the world (Ufenne and Utoo, 2013). Ndidi and Oseremen (2010) in their study revealed that vast majority of Nigerian women who utilize modern antenatal care book late which is in sharp contrast with findings in most developed countries. The prevalence of late booking as reported by researchers were as high as 86% in south west and 79% in Niger delta area of Nigeria (Okunlola et al., 2008; Adekanle and Isawumi, 2008).

The researchers in this study through the evaluation of antenatal booking records in selected hospitals found that the prevalence of late booking in South East Nigeria was as high as 75%. The researchers wondered what could be responsible for this late booking of antenatal care and this speculation motivated them to empirically ascertain the determinants of late booking among pregnant women in some selected hospitals in Enugu metropolis. Moreover, this study has not been carried out in South East and the researchers wish to bridge this gap.

The findings from this study will provide information on the factors that determine late booking for antenatal care among pregnant women. The factors identified, especially socio-cultural and organizational/systemic factors will help the policy makers to recognize the need to design new policies and adjust existing ones so as to protect and empower pregnant women as well as improve service delivery in health care setting.

In addition, nurse administrators and managers will be encouraged to enhance nurses' attitude that may deter women from early booking through supervision, seminars, lectures and workshops. Hospital administrators through the findings of this work will provide needed help and changes that may facilitate early booking e.g prompt attention to pregnant women, and reduction in the cost of antenatal services. Finally, the information gotten will provide a solid basis for proper health education with the aim of reducing the prevalence of late booking among pregnant women and consequent high maternal mortality rate.

Objectives of the study

The aim of this study was to assess the determinants of late booking for antenatal care among pregnant women receiving care in some selected hospitals in South East, Nigeria. The specific objectives were to: Assess the maternal factors that predispose to late booking for antenatal care among pregnant women; identify the socio-cultural factors that are associated with late booking for antenatal care among pregnant women; determine the religious factors that contribute to late booking for antenatal care among pregnant women; assess organizational/systemic factors that determine late booking among pregnant women.

RESEARCH METHODOLOGY

This is a descriptive cross sectional study. The study was carried out in three hospitals in Enugu State. The antenatal clinics of ESUT Teaching Hospital, Enugu, Poly Clinic, Asata and Ntasi Obi Hospital

Trans-Ekulu were purposively selected. ESUTTH is a government owned tertiary institution, Poly clinic is a district hospital while Ntasi Obi is a missionary hospital; each located at different areas in Enugu Metropolis. A sample of 310 pregnant women from the three selected hospitals was used for the study. This was drawn from a population of 1061 pregnant women who attend ANC in the selected hospitals using power analysis. Utilizing the sample population for the study (310) and the known population of pregnant women who booked for antenatal in each of the three hospitals (1061) for a six month period, a proportionate stratified sampling method was used to obtain a sample of pregnant women from each hospital. A sample size of 123, 118 and 69 pregnant women constituting 40, 38 and 22%, respectively was obtained from ESUTH, Poly Clinic and Ntasi Obi Hospital, respectively. A researcher developed and pre-tested questionnaire containing 31 questions was used to elicit information from the respondents on their socio-demographic data and factors that determine late booking among pregnant women which include personal, socio-cultural, religious and institutional/systemic factors. Pregnant women who presented for their first ANC visit with a 16 week GA or more were included in the study. Ethical approval was gotten from the research and ethical committee of ESUTH while oral informed consent was gotten from individual respondent before data collection. Data collected was analyzed using descriptive statistics of frequency and percentage. This was done using the statistical tool of IBM statistical package for social sciences (SPSS) version 20.0.

RESULTS

Out of the 310 questionnaire distributed, only 290 were collected and duly filled.

Socio demographic data

The minimum age of the respondents was 17 years while the maximum age was 47 years; the mean age for all the respondents was 29.73 years with a standard deviation of 5.59 years. Out of the 290 respondents 282(97.2%) were married, while 8(2.7%) are single, 86(29.7%) of the respondents are self-employed while 43(14.8%) are civil servants. Most 157(53.3%) of the respondents husbands were self-employed while 72(25.4) are civil servant, 10(3.5%) of the respondents had primary school education, 139(48.1%) of the respondents had secondary education, while 59(20.4%) had OND. Majority 121(43.2%) of the respondent's husbands had secondary education, while only 38(13.6%) had OND (Table 1).

Maternal factors

Health status in present pregnancy (70.7%) and ignorance of timing of registration (43.1%) were the major maternal determinants to late booking. Other minor determinants include poor exposure from past pregnancy (34.8%), poor knowledge of need for early registration (31.4%), lack of money for registration (29.7%), and young maternal age (9.3%) (Table 2).

Socio-cultural factors

The major socio-cultural factors identified by the respondents were husbands' decision (34.5%) and preference of mother in laws (26.9%). Others include lack of adequate information (10.7%), preference for TBA (7.9%) (Table 3).

Religious factors

The respondents identified preference for prayer and faith healing (54.1%) as the religious factor in late booking. Other were engagement with religious activities (16.5%), avoidance of exposure of private parts to male staff (15.8%) and advice from religious leaders/members (14.8%) (Table 4).

System factors

Long waiting time (49%), frequent ANC follow up schedule (44.5%), attitude of nurses and other staff (23.1%), high cost of ANC (25.9%), poor communication by HCP on when to initiate ANC (24.8%) are some of the identified institutional factors that determine late booking (Table 5).

DISCUSSION

Health status in index pregnancy, exposure and knowledge from previous pregnancy, ignorance of the appropriate gestational age to register were very outstanding as maternal factors that determine late booking among the study group. This show that most women book late because of the belief that there are no advantages in booking for antenatal care in the first 4 months of the pregnancy. This may also be due to the fact that antenatal care is viewed primarily as curative among the study population rather than preventive. In this environment, it has been noticed that people visit the hospitals only when they are sick, and that is why wellness clinics do not thrive in this area. This can definitely not be different for pregnant women whose conditions are not seen as sick' but as a natural phenomenon, therefore, there should not be cause for alarm especially if the woman is healthy during this period. Ignorance of time for booking may indicate poor information from health care workers since majority are multigravidas who have attended antenatal in their previous pregnancies. Favorable outcome from previous pregnancy was identified by respondents as a determinant to late booking for ANC. It is pertinent to note that from the demographic history, majority of study respondents were multigravidas and mostly had uncomplicated pregnancy and labour. This further reveals

Table 1. Socio-demographic data of respondents (n=290).

Parameter		Frequency	Percentage
	Mean	29.73	
	SD	5.59	
Age of respondents (Years)	≤ 19	5	1.7
	20-29	150	51.7
	30-39	118	40.7
	40-49	17	5.9
Total		**290**	**100.0**
Religion	Muslim	8	2.8
	Christianity	282	97.2
Total		**290**	**100.0**
Marital status	Single	7	2.4
	Married	282	97.2
	Divorced/separated	1	0.3
Total		**290**	**100.0**
Employment status	Civil servant	43	14.8
	Private employment	48	16.6
	Self-employed	86	29.7
	Unemployed	31	10.7
	House wife	33	11.4
	Student	49	16.9
Total		**290**	**100.0**
Educational status	No formal education	1	0.3
	Primary	10	3.5
	Secondary	139	48.1
	Ordinary National diploma	59	20.4
	Higher National Diploma	40	13.8
	BSc	27	9.3
	PhD	1	0.3
	NCE	12	4.1
Total		**289**	**100.0**
Husband's educational status	Primary	9	3.2
	Secondary	121	43.2
	Ordinary National Diploma	38	13.6
	Higher National Diploma	55	19.6
	BSc	39	13.9
	MSc	15	5.4
	PhD	3	1.1
Total		**280**	**100.0**

the effect of misconception and ignorance that since they are not first timers and have not had problem in any of their previous pregnancy, they need not book early for antenatal care. This further reveals that parity and outcome of previous pregnancy are also maternal factors that influence pregnant women to book late for antenatal and are in keeping with the findings of the studies by Nwagha et al. (2008) and Kisuule et al. (2013), which revealed that parity, ignorance, absence of any problem in current pregnancy are factors that may influence pregnant women's' decision to book late for antenatal care.

Findings from the study revealed that a socio-cultural factor such as husband's decision plays a vital role in

Table 2. Maternal factors in late booking (n = 290).

Parameter	Frequency	Percentage
Health status in present pregnancy	205	70.7
Ignorance of timing of registration	125	43.1
Poor exposure from past pregnancies	101	34.8
Poor knowledge of need for early registration	91	31.4
Lack of money for registration	86	29.7
Tight job schedule	65	22.4
Far distance to the hospitals	44	15.2
Young maternal age	27	9.3

Table 3. Socio-cultural factors in late booking (n = 290).

Response	Frequency	Percentage
ANC depends on husbands decision	100	34.5
Preference of mother-in-law	88	26.9
Lack of adequate media information	47	10.7
ANC is only useful for emergencies	29	10.0
Fear of being attacked by evil powers during early pregnancy	26	8.9
Preference of Traditional birth attendants	23	7.9

Table 4. Religious factors in late booking (n = 290).

Response	Frequency	Percentage
Preference for prayer and faith healing	157	54.1
Engagement with religious activities	48	16.5
Avoidance of exposure of private parts to male staff	46	15.8
Advice from religious leaders/members	43	14.8

Table 5. System factors in late booking (n = 290).

Response	Frequency	Percentage
Long waiting time	142	49.0
Frequent ANC follow up schedule	129	44.5
High cost of ANC	75	25.9
Attitude of nurses and other staff	67	23.1
Long travelling time to health facility	53	18.3
Poor communication by health care providers on when to initiate ANC	29	10.0
Inadequate health facilities	20	6.9

exposing pregnant women to late booking for antenatal care. This may be because in the African culture decisions in the family are male dominant and women are always silent when it comes to deciding on matters that relates to their health due to the cultural inclination of our society and subordinate roles of women. This may also be attributed to the fact that most men in this study are not university graduates. It is believed that the more exposed an individual is the more informed decision they make with regards to their health and that of their family members of which their wives are included. Pregnant women also indicated they booked late due to not receiving enough information from the media. One may reason that this is so because women are too busy these days to seek for information which in turn points to the role reversal as seen in our society today; women are no longer provided for, rather they provide and carry the load of the family and therefore, have no time for their health. In addition, it is usually taken for granted that women are aware of when to book for ante natal care, so it is not usually discussed in media rather topics like complications of pregnancy are given more emphasis. The finding also revealed preference for mother-in-law/older women's advice with reference to booking time.as one of the factors. This might also be due to the outcome of a complex interplay of gendered cultural hierarchies that locate pregnancy related decision making in remote authorities such as older female relatives like mother-in-laws, older female relatives etc. This might be because these women are seen as new members of the family that are not aware of the family tradition therefore, any decision concerning childbirth should be left for older women in the family who understands the tradition and belief of the family. This also showcase the African culture of subordination of younger women's interest with all emphasis on whatever older females whom they believe had gone through the process of pregnancy and childbirth feel about the situation at hand. This is line with the study by Kotecha et al. (2012).

Furthermore, it was shown that fear of being noticed and attacked by evil powers, preference for Traditional Birth Attendants in early weeks of pregnancy were other factors responsible for late booking. This may be so because of the disruptive role of socio-cultural perspective in the use of public health facilities services such as antenatal and perceived threats which are often given socio-cultural interpretation increasing women's anxieties and driving them to seek multiple sources of care. In line with this study, several studies have found a consistent relationship between socio-cultural factors and late booking for antenatal. Study by Dako-Gveke et al. (2013) noted that perceived threats interpreted as socio-cultural increased women's anxiety driving them to seek multiple sources of care from herbalists, traditional birth attendants and spiritualist disrupting the continued use of skilled care providers with resultant increase in prevalence of late booking among pregnant women.

This study revealed the religious factor that has an obvious influence on pregnant women making them to book late for antenatal care was preference for prayer and faith healing. One need not wonder why it is so since there are proliferations of churches and prayer ministries in our societies today. Most Christians attend spiritual/ prayer houses that offer prayers and care during pregnancy as most Christian organizations have spiritual/ prayer houses that offer care to women especially their members that are pregnant. Another, possible explanation could be linked to the belief and fact that pregnancy is surrounded by a lot of uncertainties. Pregnant women always seek shelter from evil by running to these prayer ministries especially during the early months of their pregnancy forgetting or neglecting antenatal care. The study also reveals that advice from religious leaders/ members, engagement with religious activities were some of the religious factors that determine late booking for antenatal. Obviously, due to the trust which people normally have on their religious leaders/ members they tend to heed to their advice even when it is detrimental to their health? They will rather choose to get deeply involved with the religious activities of ministries. This might be the case with this proportion of the study population who booked late due to the advice and engagement in religious activities. This finding implies that mass media should intensify their effort in health education so as to help these religious leaders to understand that while these pregnant women come to them for prayers, they should also advise them to seek orthodox care. A study by Dairo and Owoyokun (2010) on religious factors that affect early booking supports these findings as it revealed that most Christians especially protestants attend spiritual houses for prayer at the expense of antenatal care.

The outcome of the result showed that out of the institutional/systemic factors listed, long waiting time and frequent antenatal care follow-up schedule were most significant factors. In other words, most pregnant women book late for antenatal because they do not want to waste their time or come for antenatal visit frequently. They choose to wait until second or third trimester before booking for antenatal so as to reduce the number of antenatal visits and also reduce the time they will have to wait before being attended to. This finding supports the need for the health institutions to adopt the Focus Antenatal Care approach as was recommended by the WHO in 2002. Under this approach, the WHO recommended only four antenatal visits for normal pregnancy and booking which should occur by 16 weeks gestation. Also implicated under organizational/systemic factors for late booking among pregnant women were attitude of the nurses and other staff and poor communication by healthcare providers on when to initiate antenatal care. This indicates the need for more comprehensive health education on the importance and timing of antenatal care and also the need for attitudinal change among nurses and other health care workers. Owing to the state of Nigeria today, it is obvious from this study that late booking for antenatal care is partly due to harsh economic condition as some of the pregnant women indicated that they booked late due to high cost of antenatal services. In Enugu State, antenatal care services is free in state government hospitals only for civil servants with evidence of tax payment and majority of the respondents and their spouses are not civil servants so they have to pay for the services. The outcomes of this study are in consonance with the findings of a survey by Zegeye et al. (2013) on prevalence and determinants of late antenatal care visit among pregnant women attending antenatal care in Debre, Berhan Health institutions, Central Ethiopia. Their result revealed that poverty, frequent antenatal schedule, long traveling time, long waiting time and inadequate health facilities are factors affecting the timing of antenatal care initiation.

Conclusion

Majority of the respondents booked for antenatal at 5 months gestational age and are multigravidas. Personal/ maternal factors especially health status in present pregnancy, ignorance of the appropriate time (gestational age) to register, exposure (enough knowledge from previous pregnancies) predispose pregnant women to late booking for antenatal care. Husband's decision and preference for mother-in-law/friends/other women's advice during the early weeks of pregnancy are the socio-cultural factors that are mostly responsible for late booking for antenatal. Preference for prayer and faith healings the religious factor that mostly is responsible for late booking among pregnant women. Finally, long waiting time and frequent antenatal care follow-up schedule as institutional/systemic factors are responsible for late booking.

RECOMMENDATIONS

Based on the findings from this study, the researchers made the following recommendations; Health education on the timing and importance of attending antenatal care early should be done in communities where women and other people that influence the pregnant women's decision to attend care live so that they get this information even before they conceive. This can be done through the media, places of worship, schools and community gatherings; Community based health education programs are needed to correct the misconception about antenatal care; The campaign for male involvement in issues of reproductive health such as antenatal care should be sustained so that they will get to know why it is important that their wives should book early for antenatal care; promoting education, public health enlightenment, reduction in poverty and modification of certain cultural practices could be helpful in mitigating hindrances resulting from these factors, thereby contributing towards the improvement in maternal and child health; there is need for transitioning from traditional approach of ANC to Focused Antenatal Care (FANC) model recommended by WHO because some of the pregnant women booked late because of frequent antenatal care follow-up schedule; Efforts should be made to promote maternal education so as to empower women to take care of themselves during pregnancy.

CONFLICT OF INTERESTS

The authors have not declared any conflict of interests.

REFERENCES

Adekanle DA, Isawumi AI (2008). Late Antenatal Care Booking and Its Predictors among Women in South Western Nigeria. Online Journal of Health and Allied Sciences, 7(1):1-6.

Dairo MD, Owoyokun KE (2010). Factors affecting the utilization of antenatal care services in Ibadan, Nigeria. Benin Journal of Postgraduate Medicine, 12(1):3-13.

Dako-Gyeke P, Aikins M, Aryeetey R, Mccough L, Adongo PB (2013). The influence of socio-cultural interpretations of pregnancy threats on health-seeking behavior among pregnant women in urban Accra, Ghana. BMC Pregnancy and Childbirth, 13(1):211.

Kisuule I, Kaye DK, Najjuka F, Ssematimba SK, Arinda A, Nakitende G, Otim L (2013). Timing and reasons for coming late for the first antenatal care visit by pregnant women at Mulago hospital, Kampala Uganda. BMC Pregnancy and Childbirth, 13(1):121.

Kotecha P, Patel S, Shah S, Katara P, Madan G (2012). Health seeking behavior and utilization of health services by pregnant mothers in Vadodara slums. Healthline, 3(1):30-32.

Lincetto O, Mothebesoane-Anoh S, Gomez P, Munjanja S (2010). Antenatal Care: Opportunities for Africa's Newborns. New York: World Health Organization.

Nwagha UI, Ugwu OV, Anyachie US (2008). The influence of parity on the gestational age at booking among pregnant women in Enugu, South East Nigeria. Nigerian Journal of Physiological Sciences, 23(1-2):67-70.

Ndidi EP, Oseremen IG (2010). Reasons given by Pregnant women for late initiation of antenatal care in the Niger Delta, Nigeria. Ghana Medical Journal, 44(1):47-52.

Okunlola MA, Ayinde OA, Omigbodun AO, Owonikoko KM (2008). Factors influencing gestational age at antenatal booking at the University College Hospital, Ibadan. Journal of Obstetrics and Gynaecology, 26(3):195-197.

Ufenne DI, Utoo B (2013). Gestational age at booking for antenatal care in a tertiary health facility in north-central, Nigeria. Nigerian Medical Journal of the Nigeria Medical Association, 53(4):236-239.

Wang W, Alva S, Wang S, Fort A (2011). Levels and Trends in the Use of Maternal Health Services in Developing Countries. DHS Comparative Reports No. 26. Calverton, Maryland, USA: ICF Macro. Available at: https://www.popline.org/node/225045

World Health Organization (WHO) (2002). Antenatal Care Randomized Trial. Manual for the implementation of the new model. Geneva: Department of Reproductive Health and Research. Family and Community Health, World Health Organization. Available at: http://apps.who.int/iris/bitstream/handle/10665/42513/WHO_RHR_01.30.pdf?sequence=1&isAllowed=y

World Health Organization (2014). Maternal mortality fact sheet. Available at: http://apps.who.int/iris/bitstream/handle/10665/112318/WHO_RHR_14.06_eng.pdf;jsession

World Health Organization (WHO) (2016). WHO recommendations on antenatal care for a positive pregnancy experience. World Health Organization. Available at: http://apps.who.int/iris/bitstream/handle/10665/250796/9789241549912-eng.pdf?sequence=1

Zegeye AM, Bitew BD, Koye DN (2013). Prevalence and determinants of early antenatal care visit among pregnant women attending antenatal care in Debre Berhan Health Institutions, Central Ethiopia. African Journal of Reproductive Health, 17(4):130-136.

Unsafe abortion and associated factors among women in reproductive age group in Arsi Zone, Central Ethiopia

Legesse Tadesse Wodajo*, Solomon Tejineh Mengesha and Teresa Kisi Beyen

Department of Public Health, College of Health Sciences, Arsi University, Ethiopia.

Unsafe abortion is one of the major medical and public health problems in developing countries including Ethiopia. Yet, there is no reliable information on induced abortion distribution and its determinant factors in the country. This study assesses the determinants of unsafe abortion among women of reproductive age group in Arsi Zone, Central Ethiopia. Institution based cross-sectional study was conducted in four health facilities in Arsi zone. Client exit interview was conducted on 268 patients using a structured questionnaire and semi-structured guide for in-depth interview with key informants. Bivariate and multivariate logistic regression analyses were performed to identify the factors associated with unsafe abortion. Thematic analysis was done in this study. For variables having association in bivariate logistic regression, multivariate logistic regression test was employed. About 115 (42.9%) underwent unsafe abortion; they were about 15 to 19 years (AOR = 12.5; 95% CI: 3.24, 48.3), 20 to 24 years (AOR= 3.98; 95% CI: 1.27, 12.4) and had no formal education (AOR = 4.3; 95% CI: 1.67, 11.14). The study shows the high level of unsafe abortion to capture the attention of programmers and implementers to prevent unwanted pregnancy and make post abortion care accessible.

Key words: Unsafe abortion, maternal health, Arsi, Ethiopia.

INTRODUCTION

An abortion is said to be unsafe when unintended pregnancy is terminated by unskilled persons and in an environment with no medical standard or both (Singh et al., 2009). Unsafe abortion is an important factor that leads to morbidity and mortality to women of reproductive age group. Globally, 13% of all maternal deaths are attributable to unsafe abortion among which 44% are in Africa. Unsafe abortion endangers the health and life of women from a number of complications (Center for reproductive rights, 1992-2009; IPPF, 2010). Medium and long-term complications range from reproductive tract infections and pelvic inflammatory disease to chronic pain and infertility; delayed complications include increased risk of ectopic pregnancy, miscarriage or premature delivery in later pregnancies.

There are different reasons why women induce abortion. In many situations sexual intercourses are done without thinking and sometimes contraceptives may fail or not be available. Women may not know how to use contraceptives (IPPF, 2010; WHO, 2004). The fact is that, women in different parts of the world especially in developing countries still do not have access to good

*Corresponding author. E-mail: legesset2008@gmail.com.

quality contraceptive services and have no capability to control the circumstances when they become pregnant. Young and poor women may find it difficult to have induced abortion in the hands of skilled persons in an environment with minimum medical hygiene standard. To rise up a child who is born outside wedlock is socially stigmatizing in some communities (Center for reproductive rights, 1992-2009; IPPF, 2010).

In Africa, 25% of all those who underwent unsafe abortion are adolescent girls (Deborah, 2005). In Nigeria about half of the 20,000 women who die from unsafe abortion are adolescents where abortion complications are responsible for 72% of all deaths among teenagers below the age of 19 (Guttmacher Institute, 2006; UKaid, 2010). A study in Uganda showed almost 300,000 induced abortions were done yearly; it resulted in 85,000 abortion related complications as well as 1,200 deaths. These inflict not only morbidity and mortality burden, but also economic cost (Joseph, 2010). In Tanzania 67% of women admitted in hospitals is to due to unsafe abortion that is significantly large in magnitude (Rasch et al., 2014).

In Ethiopia health institutions based study was done on 1075 women who did abortion; one fourth was found to have induced abortion. The mean age of the women who had induced abortion was 22±5; they were younger than the women who had spontaneous abortion (ESOG, 2000). In 2008 in Ethiopia 382,000 abortions were performed of which only 27% were safely induced in health facilities (Singh et al., 2008).

Abortion care report on 2003 mid-year Ethiopian health related indicator shows that 39.7% of national and 37.9% of Oromia State of the year target were given safe abortion services respectively. The 2001 Fiscal Year of Ethiopian Health Related Indicator reported that the number of national and Oromia abortion care given was 66,780 and 25,377 respectively. The reported number of safe abortion shows only slant of the total number of unwanted or unplanned pregnancies. Besides the existence of wide range of unsafe abortion practice, to the investigators' knowledge, no similar study has been done in this area. The output of the study can be done by programmers and implementers of maternal health services.

MATERIALS AND METHODS

Study design and setup

Institutional based cross-sectional quantitative study including qualitative in-depth key-informant interview was conducted in the Gynecology Ward of Asella Hospital, Asella Health Center Maternity Unit, Sagure and Huruta Health Centers, Arsi Zone, Oromia Regional State, located at 175 km South-east of Addis Ababa, from May to September 2012. According to the 2010 population profile Arsi Zone has a total population of over 2.9 million with geographical health coverage of 89%; it has one teaching referral hospital, three district hospitals, 91 health centers and 357 health posts.

Sample size determination

The sample size was calculated by single population proportion formula using 25.6% prevalence of induced abortion from the study conducted by Ethiopia society of Obstetrics and Gynecology (ESOG) from June 1, 2000 to December 31, 2000. It was done in fifteen hospitals of nine of the eleven administrative regions of the country (ESOG, 2000). Considering the 5% non-response rate, the final sample size was 293. From the source population, all the reproductive age (15 to 44) women who visited the selected health facilities during the study period for safe abortion or post abortion, and who can communicate and volunteer were included in the study. Eligible study participants who visited these facilities during the study period were interviewed consecutively after the service was given using an exit interview technique.

Data collection procedure

Asella Teaching Referral Hospital and three Health Centers were taken conveniently taking into consideration the availability of safe abortion and trained staffs. The study sample was divided proportionally among the health institutions after the performance of safe abortion and post abortion care in one year prior to the current study. The performance was taken from the record log books of the selected health facilities. Accordingly from the total 293 study sample, 230 (78.5%) was assigned to Asella Teaching Referral Hospital, 33 (11.26%) to Asella Health Center, 16 (5.46%) to Huruta Health Center and 14 (4.78%) was given to Sagure Health Center. Data were collected from women who intentionally terminated their pregnancies and who visited health institutions for safe abortion or post abortion care. Information was collected on exit from service consecutively until the sample size was reached during the study period from May 1 to September 30, 2012. Questionnaire was prepared in English language and translated to local language by professionals; it was finally re-translated to English language to recheck for possible contextual change. It was pre-tested on 5% of total sample size of clients on other health institutions. Adjustments were made based on the assessment of its appropriateness. The data collectors were trained on how to use data collection tools and techniques. Throughout the data collection supervision was done by supervisors and the principal investigator to keep the quality of the data. To enrich the information obtained by quantitative study, individual key informant in-depth interviews were held between the principal researcher and four nurses/midwives from health centers and hospital gynecology ward.

While the dependent variable was unsafe abortion, the independent variables included important socio-demographic characteristics, number of current alive children, and income of the women or relatives. Response was coded and entered into EPI info 3.5.0. Data were cleaned and then exported to SPSS version 16.0 for windows for analysis. Frequency distributions of dependent and independent variables were worked out; bivariate logistic regression analysis was done to get COR and 95% confidence interval was derived. Then variables which had $p = 0.05$ or less in Bivariate logistic regression were taken to multiple logistic regression module to avoid confusion and show associations between target variables such as; age of respondents, marital status, religion, parity, socio-cultural factors occupational status, educational status etc. Results were reported using adjusted odd ratio and 95% confidence interval. Significance level was declared at p value of 0.05.

Ethical consideration

Ethical approval was secured from the College of Health Sciences of the Adama Science and Technology University, and permission for data collection was obtained from the director office of Assela

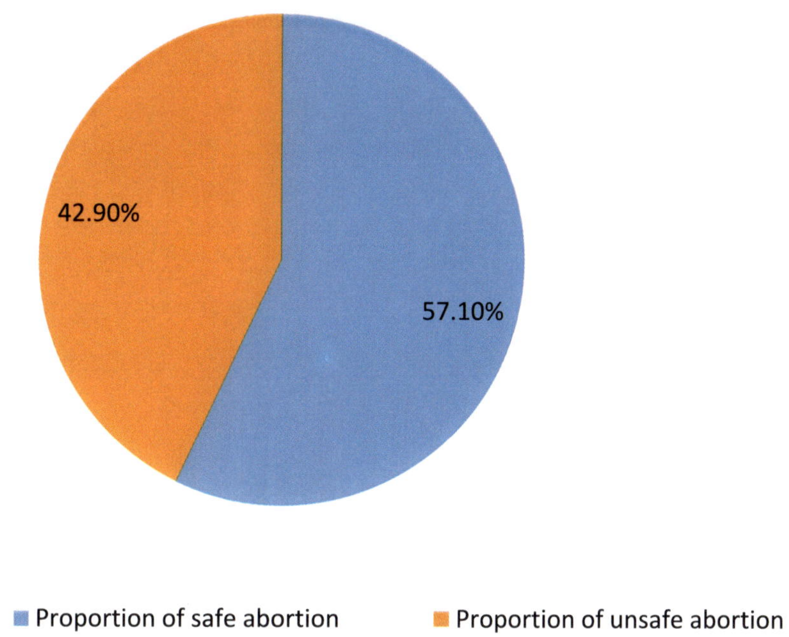

Figure 1. Magnitude of unsafe abortions among the women who intentionally terminated their pregnancies in Arsii zone, Central Region, Ethiopia, in 2012 (n=268).

Teaching Referral Hospital. All issues of ethical consideration, participants' autonomy, privacy, confidentiality, response and non-response, withdrawing at any step were given due attention.

RESULTS

Socio-demographic characteristics of the women who had abortion or post abortion care, Arsi, Oromia, Ethiopia, 2012

Age category distribution shows 46 (17.20%) were age group of 15 to19 years old, 100(37.30%) were 20 to 24 years old age group, 54(20.10%) were 25 to 29 years old age group, and 33(12.30%) were 35 to 44 years old age group. Marital status shows majority 187(69.80%) were currently married, 38(14.20%) were non-married but were either living alone or cohabiting with their partners, 31(11.60%) were single, and 12(4.50%) were divorced or widowed. Educational status shows 120(44.77%) had primary education or at least could read and write, 67(25.00%) were unable to read and write and 81(30.22%) had achieved secondary or above education. Occupational status shows that 107(39.93%) were house- wives, 42(15.70%) were farmers, 41(15.30%) were students, 37(13.80%) were daily laborers, 26(9.70%) were employees of government or other institutions, and 15(5.60%) were merchants. Religion of the study subjects shows that 132(49.30%) were Muslim, 123(45.90%) were orthodox and 13(4.90%) were protestants. For ethnicity, 217(81%) were from Oromo; 44(16.40%) for Amhara and 7(2.60%) for Guragie or Tigrie. The incomes of the women or family as reported by their relatives are as follows: 110(41%) had less than 500 ETB per month; 73(27.20%), 500 to 1000 ETB; 28(10.40%), 1000 to 2000 ETB, while 21(7.80%) had 2001 to 4000 ETB and 36(13.40%) had more than 4000 ETB per month (Table 1). For the women who intentionally terminated their pregnancies, 57.10% underwent unsafe abortion whereas 42.90% undertook safe abortion (Figure 1).

Qualitative results (Key Service providers' interview)

1.30/M

A 30 years old male health professional (Health Officer) in a health center stated that some health service providers trained to do safe abortion including MVA are currently not doing their work due to lack of misoprostol and equipment. Some clients especially students of high school visit health center to know their status of pregnancy when they miss their period. When tested positive for pregnancy, they leave saying they will come back. They appear after some time to recheck their Human chorionic gonadotropin (HCG) or if they have complication from incomplete abortion.

26/F

A female health worker (midwife) explained that when

Table 1. Socio-demographic characteristics of the women who had abortion or post abortion care, Arsi, Central Ethiopia, 2012.

Variable	Age category	Frequency (n)	Proportion (%)
Age of the woman	15-19	46	17.20
	20-24	100	37.30
	25-29	54	20.10
	30-34	35	13.10
	35-44	33	12.30
Marital status of the woman	Currently married	187	69.80
	Cohabiting or none cohabiting partner	38	14.20
	Currently single	31	11.6
	Widowed or divorced	12	4.50
Educational level of the woman	Unable to read and write	67	25.00
	Primary or read and write	120	44.78
	Secondary and above	81	30.22
Occupation of the woman	House wife	107	39.90
	Farmer	42	15.70
	Student	41	15.70
	Daily laborer	37	13.40
	Employee	26	9.70
	Merchant	15	5.60
Religion of the woman	Muslim	132	49.30
	Orthodox or catholic	123	45.90
	Protestant	13	4.90
Ethnicity of the woman	Oromo	217	81.00
	Amhara	44	16.40
	Other (Tigrie or Guragie)	7	2.60
Income category of the woman (ETB)	<500 ETB	110	41.00
	500-1000 ETB	73	27.20
	1001-2000 ETB	28	10.40
	2001-4000 ETB	21	7.80
	>4000 ETB	36	13.4

misoprostol is available at the health center they perform safe abortion for women who conceive after rape or incest at least two to three cases per week. They do not perform dilatation and curette with metal instrument. They interrupt when MVA or medical termination method is unavailable in the health center.

25/M

A male midwife of 25 years old stated that their maternity unit does give abortion care for incomplete abortion. He and another female health officer do not perform safe abortion due to religious reasons. The health center does HCG screening and refers the victim women to other hospitals.

35/F

A 35 years old female nurse in the hospital explained all types of abortion care. Incomplete abortion and safe abortion are performed by trained health service providers and referrals are from all government health institutions and private clinics as well both non-government and non-private associations.

Association of unsafe abortion among women who intentionally terminate their pregnancies with some selected factors, in Arsi Zone, Oromia, Ethiopia, in 2012

Thirty four (83.9%) adolescents of 15 to 19 years and 46 (46%) 20 to 24 years old women underwent unsafe abortion. Among the age group of 25 to 29 years and 30 to 34 years old, 18 (33.3%) and 12 (34.3%) underwent unsafe abortion, respectively. The older group, 34 to 44 years 5(15.2 %) opted for unsafe abortion. Educational status shows that 34(48.4%) women who did not go to school at all, 54(45%) who have primary education or can read and write and 27(33.3%) who have secondary or above education did unsafe abortion. Marital status showed that 55(29 %) of currently married, 33(86.8 %) of those non- married either leaving alone or cohabiting with their partners had unsafe abortion while the singles who have causal sex and are divorced or widowed did unsafe abortion by 19(61.3%) and 8(66.7%), respectively. Occupational status showed that students, merchants and daily laborer did unsafe abortion by 29(70.7%), 10(66.7%), and 22(59.5%), respectively. Sixty two (56.4%) women with income of less than 500 ETB and 12(42.9%) women with monthly income of 1001 to 2000 ETB did unsafe abortion. In a multivariate analysis, adolescents of 15 to 19 years old are more likely (AOR=12.5, 95% CI =3.24, 48.3) to undergo unsafe abortion, while 20 to 24 years old women are also more likely (AOR=3.98, 95% CI =1.27, 12.4) than older (34-44) women to undergo abortion. Education level showed that those illiterate women were more likely (AOR = 4.3, 95 % CI =1.67, 11.14) to undergo unsafe abortion (Table 2).

DISCUSSION

This study is a cross sectional one carried out in selected public health institutions to determine the magnitude and associated factors of unsafe induced abortions in the study area. Age group and educational status were found to have strong association with unsafe abortion. Even though there was an association between unsafe abortion and marital status and occupation in bivariate analysis, these were not statistically significant at the multivariate level.

During the data collection period, a total of 268 reproductive age women were involved making the response rate of 91.47% of the 293 total sample calculated for the study; the proportion of unsafe abortion was 42.91%. The result is almost comparable with Global Report in 2009, which was 48%. However, the result was lower than 55% report for developing countries in the same report (Kebede et al., 2000; Shah and Åhman, 2009). The previous finding in Ethiopia was 25.6% which was lower than the current finding (ESOG, 2000). The discrepancy might be due to small number of facilities with close supervision of data collection and uncovering more cases of unsafe procedures, which otherwise were missed. In Ethiopia the total induced abortion level as seen from facility based studies showed significant decline from 2008 to 2015, from more than 90% (Singh et al., 2008) to 35.6% (Gebeyehu et al., 2015). Though the current result data were generated at the middle of the two findings, the decline is reasonably acceptable due to socio-economic changes happening during the period. But it should be remembered that the methodology for the 2008 country wide estimation for incidence of abortion in Ethiopia was not facility based as in the current study.

Moreover, the interview from the key informants [nurse, midwives, and Health officer] shows that most young pregnant students resort to undergo abortion out of health institutions. After sometime some persons tested negative for pregnancy while some others come with complication from abortion. This is evidence that the cases which come to public health service are only tip of the iceberg of large number undergoing clandestine unsafe abortion. This shows the magnitude of unsafe abortion underestimates the real occurrence similar to other reports (Shah and Åhman, 2009; Singh et al., 2009). It may obviously arise from social, ethical and legal factors that impose difficulty to prevention of unsafe abortion.

Discussion with the health service providers shows that women who conceive out of wedlock do not use health facilities in order to hide their pregnancy from the society. In Uganda, it was found that 23% of women seeking abortion go to traditional practitioners, many of whom employee unsafe techniques and 15% try to do self-induced abortion using highly dangerous methods (Singh et al., 2009).

The mean age of the women who underwent induced abortion was 25.6 while the mean age of the women in the previous study was 22 years (ESOG, 2000). The current study reveals that 86.9% of 15 to 19 years age group and 46% of 20 to 24 years old age group underwent unsafe abortion, which shows the younger age had the highest proportion. There was also a support by multivariate analysis result that the younger groups were more than 12 times likely to undergo unsafe abortion while the 20 to 24 years age groups were nearly four times more likely to undergo unsafe procedure. In Africa the two age groups of 15 to 24 make 60%of women who undergo unsafe abortion; this is comparable to the current finding (Shah and Åhman, 2009).

Among the females involved in the study 17.2% were teenagers. A finding in Pakistan showed that the proportion of adolescents who had unsafe abortion was 11.49%. This shows the significant magnitude of young adolescents trapped in this problem though less than that of the current finding (Rashid, 2017). The current study depicted that women who were not able to read and write were more than four times prone to undergo unsafe

Table 2. Factor associated with unsafe abortion among pregnant women who intentionally terminated their pregnancy in Arsi Zone, Central Ethiopia, 2012 (n=268).

Characteristic	Abortion		COR (95% CI)	AOR (95% CI)	P<0.05
	Safe	Unsafe			
Age group (years)					
15-19	12	34	15.90(4.99.50.46)*	12.50(3.24.48.30)**	0.000
20-24	54	46	4.80 (1.70.13.36)*	3.98(1.27.12.4)**	0.018
25-29	36	18	2.80 (0.93.8.47)	2.90(0.88.9.4)	0.08
30-34	23	12	2.90 (0.89.9.50)	1.96(0.55.7.06)	0.30
35-44	28	5	1.00		
Educational status					
Unable to read and write	33	34	2.06(1.10.4.01)*	4.3(1.67.11.14)**	0.002
Informal education and primary	66	54	1.6(0.91.2.94)	2.1(0.96.4.6)	0.07
Secondary and above	54	27	1.00		
Marital status					
Married	132	55	0.2(0.06.0.72)*		
Non-married cohabiting/ Non-cohabiting partner	5	33	3.3(0.72.15.16)		
Single	12	19	0.8(0.20.3.21)		
Divorced/widowed	4	8	1.00		
Occupation					
Student	12	29	5.4(1.87.0.86)*		
Merchant	5	10	4.5(1.16.0.56)*		
House wife	80	27	0.8(0.3.1.94)		
Daily laborer	15	22	3.3(1.14.0.53)*		
Farmer	23	19	1.9(0.66.5.21)*		
Employee	18	8	1.00		
Woman/family Income					
<500 ETB	48	62	2.6(1.17.5.69)		
501-1000 ETB	50	23	0.9(0.39.2.15)		
1001-2000 ETB	16	12	1.5(0.54.4.16)		
2001-4000 ETB	15	6	0.80(0.25.2.59)		
>4000 ETB	24	12	1.00		

* Has significant association by bivariable logistic regression. **Has significant association by multivariable logistic regression.

abortion than those schooled up to secondary or above level. Among this group of women, 48.4% underwent unsafe abortion and had statistically significant association compared to those who had secondary and above education. This relation is supported by the study in Nigeria in which 84% of women who undergo abortion are illiterate (Guttmacher Institute, 2006).

The study assessed the relation of marital status and occupation to unsafe abortion. Currently, married women were 69.8% of the total study group of which 29.4% undergo unsafe procedure; 86.8% of non-married but either living alone or cohabiting with their sexual partners undergoes similar procedure. The finding is in line with the study in Tanzania that revealed women who conceive from casual sex opt for abortion because they do not want to spoil their chance of getting married again later (WHO, 2004). In Nigeria also 27% of women nationwide who terminated unwanted pregnancy did so because they were not married at the time. Nineteen percent said that they were too young or still in school, 19% said that their partners did not want the child, claiming they were not responsible for the pregnancy, and then left them (Guttmacher Institute, 2006).

More than seventy percent women/girls engaged in schooling resort to terminate their pregnancy in unsafe procedure. The key informant health service providers also indicated that secondary school students practice unsafe abortion more frequently. Several findings support this finding, providing reasons for abortion: fear of dropping out of school, students not wanting to face ridicule from the society and not wanting to bear the burden of single parenthood (Rashid, 2017; Guttmacher Institute, 2006) Similarly, in Philippines 72%of women with unintended pregnancy undergo abortion due to the economic cost of raising children (Singh et al., 2006).

Forty one percent of the women in the current study have lower monthly income of their own; their relatives or families (56.4%) undergo unsafe abortion more than the proportion of women with better income. These women of low income also found in Uganda having clandestine abortions experience health complications more than the better off women (55 versus 38%) (Singh et al., 2009). Similarly, Nigerian study shows women who had abortion and least likely to use contraceptives are poor (80%) (Guttmacher Institute, 2006); especially at personal level, economic issue plays a central role in countries like Philippines (Singh et al., 2006). These indicate that poor women are more exposed to unsafe abortion and its grave consequences.

The qualitative study also showed that lack of safe abortion materials in the facility makes young females turn back to abortion out of health facility. This is in congruent with different findings that adolescents are mostly at high risk of abortion as conception occurs frequently during unplanned and unexpected sexual intercourse and in a number of developing countries where reproductive health family service is not equitably and sustainably provided; where policies and resource assignment are not drawn toward family planning, safe abortion and counseling (Shah and Åhman, 2009; Singh et al., 2009; UN: Center for reproductive rights, 1999; Grimes et al., 2006)

Strengths and limitation

The study used pre- test on 5% similar population at different places to test the consistency of the tools. This cross sectional study cannot explore the temporal relationship.

CONCLUSION AND RECOMMENDATION

The magnitude of the unsafe abortion is greater than that of the National Survey Result in Ethiopia. Uneducated women as well as those between 15 and 24 were more prone to unsafe abortion: the younger the age the more the risk of undergoing unsafe procedure. It would be better if the health systems of the country give more emphasis to the younger uneducated women.

CONFLICT OF INTERESTS

The authors have not declared any conflict of interests.

ACKNOWLEDGMENTS

The authors would like to thank Adama Science and Technology University, Asella College of Health Science for funding the research. The authors would like to extend their special thanks to all data collectors, supervisors and the study participants.

REFERENCES

Center for reproductive rights (1992-2009). In harmed way: The Impact of Kenya's Restrictive abortion Law. Available at: https://www.reproductiverights.org/feature/in-harms-way-the-impact-of-kenyas-restrictive-abortion-law

Deborah M (2005). Unsafe abortion Facts and figures, Washington D.C, USA. Population Reference Bureau. Available at: http://www.prb.org/pdf05/unsafeabortion.pdf

Ethiopian Society of Obstetrics and Gyenacology (ESOG) (2000). Survey of unsafe abortion in selected Health facilities in Ethiopia, Addis Ababa. Available at: esog@ethionet.et

Gebeyehu D, Admassu B, Sinega M, Haile M (2015). Assessment of Prevalence and Reasons for Termination of Pregnancy at Jimma University Teaching Hospital, Ethiopia. Universal J. Public Health 3(6):251-255. Available at: http://www.hrpub.org/download/20151130/UJPH4-17604743.pdf

Grimes DA, Benson J, Singh S, Romero M, Ganatra B, Okonofua FE, Shah IH (2006). Unsafe abortion: the preventable pandemic. Lancet 368(9550):1908-1919.

Guttmacher Institute (2006). Facts on Unwanted Pregnancy and Induced Abortion in Nigeria. Available at: https://www.guttmacher.org/sites/default/files/factsheet/fb_nigeria.pdf

International Planned Parenthood Federation (IPPF) (2010). The health dangerous of unsafe abortion, Addis Ababa, Ethiopia. http://apps.who.int/iris/bitstream/10665/44529/1/9789241501118_eng.pdf

Joseph BB (2010). Economic Impact of Unsafe Induced Abortion in Uganda. University of Washington, USA. Available at: http://poppov.org/Projects/2010/Economic-Impact-of-Unsafe-Induced-Abortion-in-Uganda.aspx

Kebede S, Jira C, Miriam DW (2000). A survey of illegal a abortion, Jimma Hospital, South-western Ethiopia. Ethiop. Med. J. 38(1):35-42.

Rasch V, Sørensen PH, Wang AR, Tibazarwa F, Jäger AK (2014). Unsafe abortion in rural Tanzania–the use of traditional medicine from a patient and a provider perspective. BMC Pregnancy Childbirth 14(1):419.

Rashid M (2017). Unsafe abortion: unnecessary maternal morbidity and mortality. Biomedica 26(2):114-117.

Shah I, Åhman E (2009). Unsafe abortion: global and regional incidence, trends, consequences, and challenges. J. Obstet. Gynaecol. 31(12):1149-1158.

Singh S, Fetters T, Gebreselassie H, Abdella A, Gebrehiwot Y, Kumbi S, Audam S (2008). The incidence of induced abortion in Ethiopia, AA, Volume 36, No 1. Available at: http://aphrc.org/abortionresearch/index.php/other-resources/item/846-the-estimated-incidence-of-induced-abortion-in-ethiopia-2008

Singh S, Juarez F, Cabigon J, Ball H, Hussain R (2006). Unintended pregnancy and induced abortion in the Philippines: causes and consequences. Available at: http://www.popline.org/node/563307

Singh S, Wulf D, Hussain R, Bankole A, Sedgh G (2009). Abortion Worldwide: A decade of uneven progress, New York: Guttmacher Institute. New York, New York, Guttmacher Institute, 2006. 40p. Available at: https://www.guttmacher.org/report/abortion-worldwide-decade-uneven-progress

UKaid Department for International Development (2010). UK's policy position on safe and unsafe abortion in developing countries. https://www.gov.uk/government/publications/safe-and-unsafe-abortion-uks-policy-position-on-safe-and-unsafe-abortion-in-developing-countries

UN: Center for reproductive rights (1999). CIPD+5: Center for reproductive rights; gains for women against opposition, 1999. Available at: https://www.reproductiverights.org/document/icpd-5-gains-for-women-despite-opposition

World Health Organization (WHO) (2004). Unsafe abortion: Global and regional estimates of the incidence of unsafe abortion and associated mortality in 2000: Fourth edition, Geneva. Available at: http://www.who.int/reproductivehealth/publications/unsafe_abortion/9241591803/en/

20

Feto-maternal outcomes in obstructed labor in Suhul General Hospital, North Ethiopia

Gebresilasea Gendisha Ukke[1]*, Temesgen Worku Gudayu[2], Mekdes Kondale Gurara[1], Negash Wakgari Amanta[3] and Mulugeta Shegaze Shimbre[4]

[1]Department of Midwifery, College of Medicine and Health Sciences, Arba Minch University, Arba Minch, Ethiopia.
[2]Department of Midwifery, College of Medicine and Health Sciences, University of Gondar, Gondar, Ethiopia.
[3]School of Nursing and Midwifery, College of Medicine and Health Sciences, Hawassa University, Hawassa, Ethiopia.
[4]Department of Nursing, College of Medicine and Health Sciences, Arba Minch University, Arba Minch, Ethiopia.

Ethiopia is one of the countries with the highest maternal mortality rates, obstructed labor and its complications being the leading causes of maternal deaths in the country. This study was aimed at assessing feto-maternal outcomes in obstructed labor in Suhul General Hospital, North Ethiopia. Institution based cross-sectional study was carried out from May 1 to August 31, 2014 in Suhul General Hospital. All mothers who had given birth in the hospital during the study period were included in the study. Data were collected by using a pre tested structured questionnaire and checklists, entered into Epi Info version 7.1.2.0 and finally transported in to SPSS version 20 software package for analysis. A total of 660 mothers had given birth in the hospital during the study period out of which 44(6.7%) were diagnosed as obstructed labor cases. More than 89% of the mothers with obstructed labor and about 93% of the babies born to them had developed at least one complication. Eighteen (40.9%) of the babies were stillbirths or had died immediately after delivery. Postpartum hemorrhaged and puerperal sepsis 25(56.8%) each and uterine rupture 11(25%) were the main maternal complications among the mothers with obstructed labor. Cesarean birth (68%), hysterectomy (20%), destructive delivery (7%) and repair of the ruptured uterus with bilateral tubal ligation in 5% were interventions done for the mothers with obstructed labor. Inaccessibility of vehicle road and time the women stayed at health centers before they were referred to the hospital have shown association with poor maternal outcomes in Fisher's Exact test. Prevalence of obstructed labor in Suhul general hospital is high with high rate of maternal and fetal complications. Improving vehicle road accessibility and giving training for health centers delivery case teams on when to refer laboring mother to the hospitals is needed in order to decease proportion of Obstructed labor and it sequels.

Key words: Obstructed labor, Ethiopia, low income country, maternal mortality.

INTRODUCTION

Obstructed labor (OL) is defined as the failure of the presenting part to descend in spite of adequate uterine contractions (Dolea and AbouZahr, 2003). The main cause of obstructed labor is cephalo pelvic disproportion which is usually a result of under nutrition during childhood and early childbirth resulting in small pelvis (Dolea and AbouZahr, 2003, Al-Harazi, 2006, Fantu, Segni et al. 2010, Ara 2011, Agrawal et al. 2014).

OL is an important cause of maternal death in low income countries (Dolea and AbouZahr 2003). It is also responsible for a significant short and long term maternal morbidities such as sepsis, uterine rupture, hemorrhage, secondary infertility, obstetric fistulae and other neurologic and skeletal complications (Arrowsmith et al., 1996, Wall, 2012). Moreover, the impact of obstructed labor on the lives of the fetuses is very significant and it is responsible for high proportion of perinatal death. Furthermore, survived children suffer from long-term complications like cerebral palsy and developmental disabilities (Lawn et al., 2005, Fantu et al., 2010; Kabakyenga et al., 2011; Bayou and Berhan, 2012). OL has contributed 8% to the estimated 289,000 maternal death occurred in 2013 globally, 99% of which were in low income countries (Dolea and AbouZahr, 2003; Wall et al., 2005; Gibbons et al., 2010; Khooharo et al., 2013).

Reducing maternal death resulting from obstructed labor is considered as an indication for the improvement of the obstetric care system and socio-economic status of one country (Neilson, Lavender et al., 2003). In Ethiopia, obstructed labor is now the leading cause of maternal death since complications of abortion have reduced. OL now causes 13 to 36% of all maternal deaths in the country (Abdella, 2010, Bayou and Berhan, 2012, EMoH, 2012). Despite the problem, little research has been conducted regarding OL in the country and no research has been conducted in the last decade in the study area. This study was therefore aimed at assessing feto-maternal outcomes in obstructed labor in Suhul General Hospital.

MATERIALS AND METHODS

Institution based cross- sectional study was conducted in Suhul General Hospital from 1st of May to August 31, 2014. Sample size was determined by using a single population proportion formula:

$$n = \frac{(Z\alpha/2)^2 \quad * (p)(1-\mathrm{p})}{\mathrm{w}^2}$$

Where, *n* is sample size required, *p* is estimated proportion of OL among laboring mothers and we took 50% (0.5) to get higher sample size, *w* is maximum tolerable error which is 0.04 and *Z* is value of standard normal distribution (Z-statistic) at 95% confidence level which is1.96.

$$n = \frac{(1.96)^2 \quad *(0.5)(0.5)}{0.04^2} = 600.$$

For possible non response during the data collection time, 10% was added which gave a final sample size of 660.

To get the required minimum sample size all the mothers who had given birth in the hospital from May to August 2014 were included in the study consecutively. The hospital is located in Shire town of Tigray region in north Ethiopia which is about 40 km from Eritrean boarder (14°06'51.03" N 38°18.17" E). The hospital is acting as a referral hospital for the surrounding district hospitals and health centers located in the remote areas of the zone. The proportion of women who give birth at health facilities in the region is 26.7% which relatively higher than the national average which is 16%(CSA, 2014).

Face to face interview was conducted to collect data on socio-demographic status, distance from the hospital, road or ambulance accessibility, diagnosis, maternal and fetal outcomes and interventions done using a pre tested structured questionnaire and checklist.

Three BSc midwives were participated in data collection after getting one day training on how to collect the data. One emergency surgical officer had been supervising the data collectors on a daily bases.

Pretest was conducted on 5% of mothers prior to the actual data collection period. Slight modification was then made to the questionnaire and the checklist. The principal investigator had been reviewing the questionnaires and the checklists every day. Epi info version 7.1.2.0 and SPSS version 20 software package were used for data entry and analysis respectively. Descriptive statistics such as mean and standard deviation were computed and analytic statistical analysis was performed with Fisher exact test.

Ethical clearance was obtained from Ethical Review Board of College of Medicine and Health Sciences, University of Gondar. An official letter of cooperation was written by the University to Suhul General Hospital. The hospital administrator in turn has communicated with the obstetric ward head nurse so that data could be collected in the ward. Informed consent was obtained from each study participants and each study participant was informed about the objective of the study and confidentiality of the information she is giving. The participants were also informed that they have the full right not to participate in the study or to stop participation at any time during the interview.

Operational definitions

Obstructed labor

A labor with the features of obstruction like bandle's ring, excessive fetal head molding or caput, malpresentations, vulvar edema, maternal exhaustion and dehydration in a women either referred form rural health institutions or have been in labor for a long time and diagnosed as obstructed labor by the senior obstetrician of the ward.

Poor maternal outcome

Poor maternal outcomes/complications: Presence of at least one of the undesirable outcomes in the mother like postpartum haemorrhage (PPH), puerperal sepsis, uterine rupture, Vesico-vaginal fistula (VVF), bladder injury, perineal tear, cervical tear and maternal death.

*Corresponding author. E-mail: gebresilasea@yahoo.com.

Table 1. Socio-demographic characteristics of the study participants, Suhul General Hospital, North Ethiopia in August, 2014 (n=660).

Variable	Frequency	Percent
Age (n= 660)		
< 20 years	106	16.1
21 – 34 years	486	73.6
≥ 35 years	68	10.3
Address District (n = 660)		
Indasilassie	279	42.3
Tahtay Koraro	51	7.7
Laylay Adyabo	67	10.2
Tahtay Adyabo	18	2.7
Asgede Tsembla	144	21.8
Medabay Zana	52	7.9
Welqayt/ Tselemt	49	7.4
Occupation (n = 660)		
House wife	542	82.1
Private business	76	11.5
Governmental employee	39	5.9
Others*	3	0.5
Educational status (n = 660)		
Uneducated/unable to read or write	248	37.6
Elementary school (Grade 1 - 4)	108	16.4
Secondary school (Grade 5 - 8)	148	22.4
High school (Grade 9 - 12)	95	14.4
Above high school	61	9.2
Age at first marriage (n = 658)		
< 18 year	379	57.6
18 - 19 years	186	28.3
20 year or above	93	14.1

Others: Daily laborers and housemaids

Poor fetal outcome

Poor fetal outcome/complications: Presence of at least one of the undesirable outcomes in the newborn like birth injury, birth asphyxia, stillbirth, or early neonatal death.

RESULTS

Six hundred sixty mothers had given birth during the study period and participated in this study. The median age of the study participants was 25 year with inter-quartile rage (IQR) of 21 to 29 years. Majority of participants, 606(91.8%) were followers of Orthodox Christianity. More than 98% of them were from *Tigrie* ethnic group. Two hundred ninety eight (45.2%) were rural residents. Six hundred fifty six (99.4%) of the participants were in marital relationship. Concerning the district they came from, most of them, 279(42.3%) were from Indasilassie district followed by *Asgede Tsembla* district, 144(21.8%). Majority (542(82.1%) of the participants economically depend on their husbands.

Nearly three fourth, 248(37.6%) of the study participants had no formal education who cannot read and write while only 61(9.2%) have joined college or university. In case of their husbands, 188(28.7%) were uneducated while 143(21.8%) have educational level above grade 12. Five hundred ten (77.3%) were who grew up in rural area and still living there or had changed their residence to urban area and the rest 150 (22.7) have been urban residents from their childhood. The participants' median age at first marriage was 17 years with interquartile range (IQR) of 16 to 18 years. Concerning the monthly income of their husbands, 146(22.3%) have average monthly income of less than $25 while 324 (49.4%) have a monthly income of above $50 (Table 1).

Thirty two (4.8%) of the mothers had no direct vehicle road access to their home. The maximum distance the participants have travelled to visit the hospital was 140 km. The average time the laboring women had waited for ambulance after calling the focal persons is less than half an hour. The median time the laboring women had

Table 2. Distribution of the study participants in relation to utilization and access to health services, Suhul General Hospital, Shire town, North Ethiopia in August, 2014 (n=660).

Variable	Frequency	Percent
Distance from the hospital (km) (n = 660)		
< 10	313	47.4
10 - 50	284	43.0
> 50	63	9.5
Time to wait after calling ambulance (min) (n=628)		
< 30	598	95.2
30 - 60	22	3.5
> 60	8	1.3
Time to walk on foot to reach vehicle road access (h) (n= 32)		
< 1	9	28.1
1 - 2	14	43.8
> 2	9	28.1
Number of ANC visits (n = 660)		
Less than 4	125	18.9
At least 4	535	81.1
Stay at home before visiting health institutions (h) (n = 589)		
< 1 h	159	27.0
1 - 2	332	56.4
> 2	98	16.6
Stay at health institution before referred to the hospital (h) (n = 327)		
< 8	238	72.8
8 - 12	49	15.0
> 12	40	12.2

stayed at their home after the onset of labor before visiting health institutions was one hour with maximum time of up to 25 h. The average time the mothers who had been referred from other health institutions had stayed at the first health institution was about 4 h with some stayed for more than 70 h (Table 2).

Ten (1.5%) and 115(17.4%) of them have medical and obstetric problems or condition respectively. Post term pregnancy 28(24.3%), hypertensive disorders of pregnancy 24(20.9%), premature rupture of membranes (PROM) 22(19.1%) and ante partum hemorrhage (APH) 14(12.1%) were the main obstetric problems/conditions of the study participants. Forty four out of the 660 (6.7%) study participants were diagnosed as obstructed labor (Table 3).

Most of the participants 445(67.4%) had given birth via vaginal route. The weights of the first babies ranges from 1500 to 5200 g with mean weight of 3117 g (SD = 436.6). Six hundred seventeen (93.5%) of the babies born to the mothers were normal birth weight, 30(4.5%) low birth weight and the rest 13(2.0%) were macrosomic. Caesarean birth was the main intervention done for OL cases (Figure 1). One hundred thirty seven (20.8%) of the babies have at least one problem/complication before they had been discharged from the hospital with birth asphyxia being the main problem encountered in 106(77.3%) of the newborns (Figure 2). Thirty nine out of the 44 mothers with OL (89%) and 41(93.2%) of their babies had developed at least one complication during or after delivery (Figure 3).

Factors associated with poor maternal outcomes

Out of the 44 women with OL, 31(70.4%) had no access to vehicle road from their homes to hospital and absence of access to vehicle road was associated with poor maternal outcomes (p value = 0.02). The second factor which have showed some association with poor maternal outcomes in women with OL is the time the women had stayed at health centers before they were referred to the hospital (p value = 0.05) (Table 4).

DISCUSSION

This study has shown obstructed labor as the main contributor to poor maternal and fetal outcomes. Out of 44 mothers diagnosed with obstructed labor, 39(88.6%) of them have developed at least one complication, PPH and puerperal sepsis being the most common complication each encountered in more than half of the Pakistan where PPH was the main complication of OL

Table 3. Obstetric characteristics of the study participants, Suhul General Hospital, Shire town, North Ethiopia in August, 2014 (n=660).

Variable	Frequency	Percent
Parity (n= 660)		
Primiparous	299	45.3
Multiparous (2- 4)	251	38.0
Grandmultiparous (≥5)	110	16.7
GA at delivery (n = 530)		
Preterm	16	3.0
Term	486	91.7
Post term	28	5.3
Type of the obstetric problem/ condition (n=115)*		
APH	14	12.1
IUFD at admission	3	2.6
Twin pregnancy	18	15.7
Polyhydramnios	1	0.9
Post term pregnancy	28	24.3
Preterm labour	16	13.9
PROM	22	19.1
Hypertensive disorders of pregnancy	24	20.9
Total labour duration (h) (n = 618)		
< 24	567	91.7
≥24	51	8.3
Fetal presentations (n = 660)		
Vertex	573	86.8
Breech	62	9.4
Face	13	2.0
Shoulder	7	1.1
Brow	5	0.8

*One mother can have more than one problems

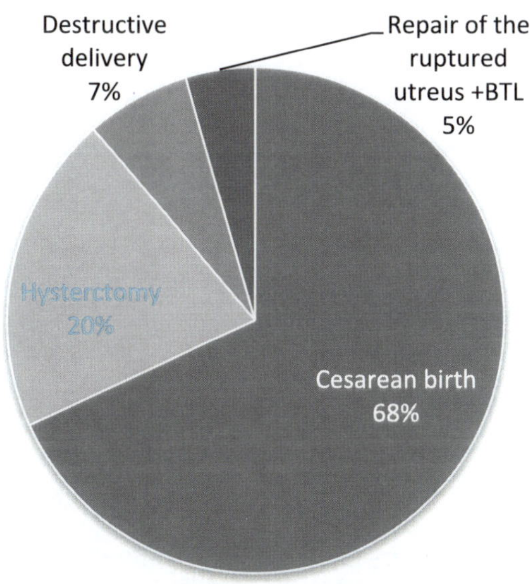

Figure 1. Type of intervention done to manage cases with obstructed labor, Suhul General Hospital, Shire town, North Ethiopia in August, 2014 (n = 44). BTL: Bilateral tubal ligation.

cases followed by puerperal sepsis (Shirin and Nahar 2013). It is also similar with a study done in India where PPH and puerperal sepsis were the main complication among patients with obstructed labour (Omole-Ohonsi and Belga, 2010). This could be due to the fact that women with obstructed labor had been in labor for longer periods after rupture of membrane leading to assessing infection. Manipulations done to manage the cases could also increase the risk of puerperal sepsis. Exhausted uterine muscles fails to contract after prolonged obstructed labor increasing risk of PPH. Rupture of uterus, another complication of OL could have increased rate of PPH in OL cases.

In this study uterine rupture has occurred in 11(25%) of OL cases. This figure is higher than study done in India where only 7.1% of OL cases have developed uterine rupture (Omole-Ohonsi and Belga, 2010). It is however; lower than findings from a study done in Jimma Specialized Hospital in Ethiopia, where uterine rupture has complicated 45.1% of OL cases (Fantu et al., 2010).

This can be attributed to the fact that there is improvement in transportation system in Ethiopia which

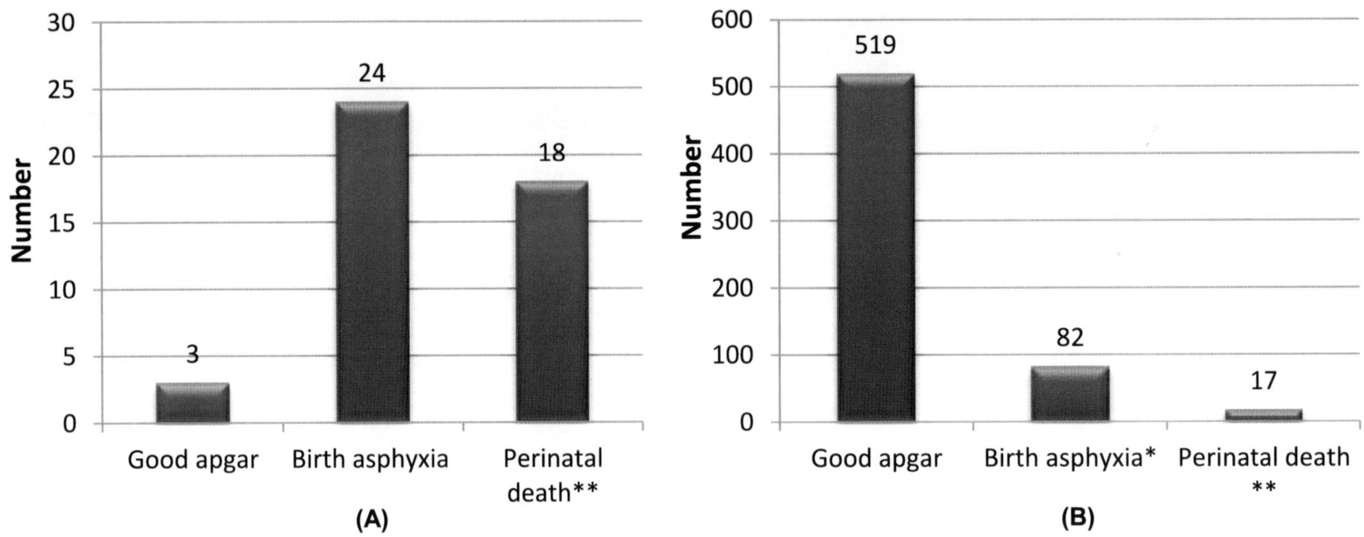

Figure 2. Distribution of birth outcome among the study participants, Suhul General Hospital, Shire town, North Ethiopia in August 2014. (A) OL cases; (B) Non - OL cases. *Two neonates with birth injury included; **Stillbirths + early neonatal deaths that have occurred before discharge from the hospital. One fetus cane have more than one birth outcomes (birth asphyxia and neonatal death.

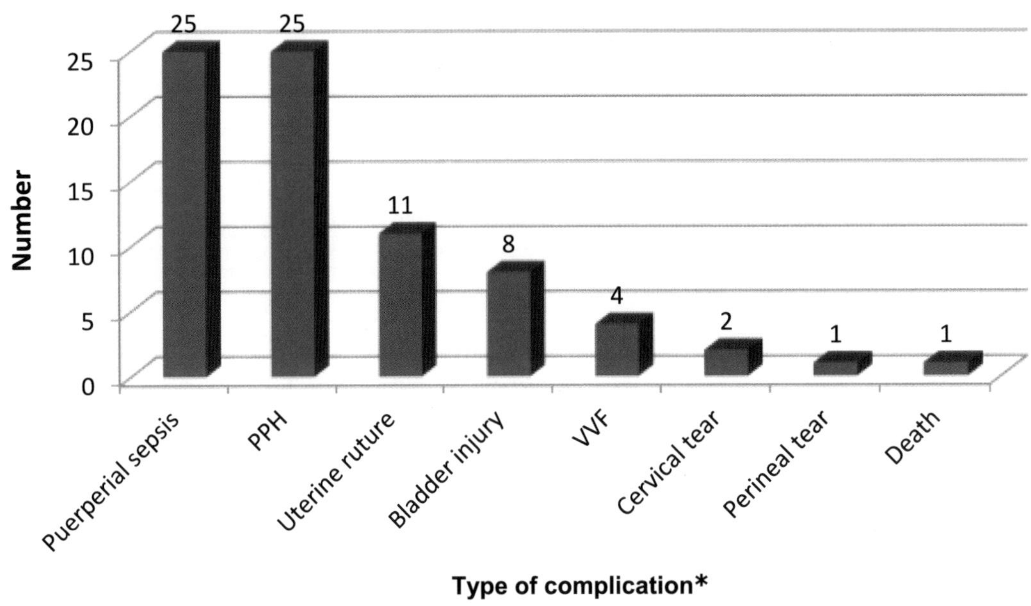

Figure 3. Complications developed by obstructed labor cases at Suhul General Hospital, Shire town, North Ethiopia in August 2014. * One mother can develop more than one complications.

This can be attributed to the fact that there is improvement in transportation system in Ethiopia which could have increased the probability of reaching the hospitals before rupture of the uterus has occurred. The lower figure of Indian study could be due to the difference in the infrastructures from courtly to country.

From this study one mother has died making maternal mortality rate among OL cases to be 2.3%. This is similar to Pakistani study where maternal mortality rate among OL cases was 2% (Shaikh et al., 2013). However; it is slightly higher than Nigerian study and another Pakistani studies where the rate was 1% (Omole-Ohonsi and Belga, 2010; Shazia et al., 2013). This could probably be due to the state at which the patient has admitted to the hospital or availability of drugs and blood products on the day of admission.

Four patients (9.1%) have developed Vesico Vaginal Fistula (VVF) making the rate higher than results from

Table 4. Fisher's exact test analysis of factors associated with poor maternal outcomes among obstructed labor cases, Suhul General Hospital, North Ethiopia in August, 2014.

Variable	Maternal complication/poor outcome		P value
Access to vehicle road	Absent	Present	
Absent	1(3.2%)	30(86.9%)	0.02
Present	4(30.8%)	9(69.2 %)	
Stay at Health centers before referral			
≤ 20 hours	4(25%)	12(75%)	0.05
>20 hours	1(11.4%)	27(88.6%)	

study done in India which was 1.4% and study done in Jimma where the rate was 4.1% (Fantu et al., 2010, Gupta and Porwal, 2012). This could be due to small number of OL cases in this study. It could also be due to difference in time of visiting the hospital after has started as VVF develops about a week after the onset of labor. Out of 44 babies born to women with obstructed labor, 41(93.2%) of the have developed at least one complication. Eighteen (40.9%) of the babies were stillbirths or died immediately after delivery. This is lower than findings from studies done in Nigeria, Pakistan and Jimma Specialized Hospital in Ethiopia where the rate of perinatal loss among OL cases ranged from 50 to 62%(Fantu et al., 2010; Omole-Ohonsi and Belga, 2010; Gupta and Porwal, 2012; Shaikh et al., 2013; Shazia, et al., 2013). However; it is higher than findings from study conducted in six Ugandan hospitals where the rate was 14% (Kabakyenga et al., 2011). This could be due to difference in sample size, differences in availability of equipment to deal with asphyxiated neonates or the status of the fetuses at admission to the hospitals or difference in skill of neonatal resuscitation.

Finding from this study have also revealed that 24(88.9%) of the babies born alive have birth asphyxia (apgar score of less than 7/10 at first minute). This finding is in line with findings from studies done in Pakistan and Jimma Specialized Hospital where 88 to 98% of babies born alive from OL cases have developed birth asphyxia (Fantu et al., 2010, Shazia et al., 2013). However, the rate of birth asphyxia from this study is higher when compared to studies done in Nigeria and India where the rates of birth asphyxia were 37.3 and 35.7%, respectively (Omole-Ohonsi and Belga 2010; Gupta and Porwal, 2012; Shazia et al., 2013). This could be due to difference in skill of assessing apgar score of the neonate's or status of the fetuses at admission or type of intervention done to alleviate the problem.

Conclusions

Prevalence of obstructed labor among mothers who gave birth at Suhul General Hospital is high. Moreover, almost all of the cases with obstructed labor had developed maternal and/or fetal complications. Creating maternity waiting "villages" in a culturally sensitive manner in places where ambulance can access the women so that pregnant women whose homes have no vehicle road access will be admitted to the villages at term is needed. Health professionals working in delivery case teams at health centers need to have training on when to refer/when to send laboring women to the next higher level health institutions. Moreover; strengthening the integrated emergency surgery and clinical midwifery programs to avail emergency obstetric surgeries at health centers in the remote districts of the zone and strengthening universal road access projects including mobilizing men in the community to make each and every house accessed by vehicle is suggested.

Limitations

The first limitation of this study is that it was institution based and therefore did not address the burden of the problem among the women who had given birth at homes where more obstructed labor and its complications including maternal death are expected. Second, the total number of cases with OL is 44 which is a small number to show a reliable association between dependent and independent variables.

CONFLICT OF INTERESTS

The authors have not declared any conflict of interests.

REFERENCES

Abdella A (2010). Maternal mortality trend in Ethiopia. Ethiop. J. Health Dev. 24(1):1.

Agrawal A, Barik S, Mohanta O, Chintamani L, Baru K, Pradhan K, Kuntia P (2014). Fetomaternal outcome in obstructed labour in a tertiary care hospital of Western Odisha. Int. J. Obstet. Gynaecol. 121:135-136.

Al-Harazi AH (2006). Obstructed labor. A real problem in Yemeni s rural areas. Saudi Med. J. 27(9):1435-1436.

Ara A (2011). Outcome of obstructed labour. J. Postgrad. Med. Instit. (Peshawar-Pakistan) 18(3):1-6.

Arrowsmith S, Hamlin EC, Wll LL (1996). Obstructed labor injury complex: obstetric fistula formation and the multifaceted morbidity of maternal birth trauma in the developing world. Obstet. Gynecol.

Surv. 51(9):568-574.
Bayou G, Berhan Y (2012). Perinatal mortality and associated risk factors: a case control study. Ethiop. J. Health Sci. 22(3):153-162.
Central Statistical Agency (CSA) (2014). Mini Demographic and health Survey 2014. Addis Ababa. Available at: https://www.unicef.org/ethiopia/Mini_DHS_2014__Final_Report.pdf
Dolea C, AbouZahr C (2003). Global burden of obstructed labour in the year 2000. World Health Organization (WHO), Geneva, Switzerland. P 17.
EMoH (2012). Maternal Death Surveillance and Response (MDSR) Technical Guideline. Addis Ababa, Ethiopia.
Fantu S, Segni H, Alemseged F (2010). Incidence, causes and outcome of obstructed labor in Jimma University Specialized Hospital. Ethiop. J. Health Sci. 20(3):145-151.
Gibbons L, Belizán JM, Lauer JA, Betrán AP, Merialdi M, Althabe F (2010). The global numbers and costs of additionally needed and unnecessary caesarean sections performed per year: overuse as a barrier to universal coverage. World Health Rep. 30:1-31.
Gupta R, Porwal SK (2012). Obstructed Labour: Incidence, causes and outcome. Int. J. Biol. Med. Res. 3(3):2185-2188.
Kabakyenga JK, Ostergren PO, Turyakira E, Mukasa PK, Pettersson KO (2011). Individual and health facility factors and the risk for obstructed labour and its adverse outcomes in south-western Uganda. BMC Pregnancy Childbirth 11:73.
Khooharo Y, Majeed T, Khawaja MA, Majeed N, Majeed N, Malik MN, Amber A (2013). Even in 21st Century Still Obstructed Labor Remains Life Threatening Condition. Ann. King Edward Med. Univ. 18(3):279.
Lawn J, Shibuya K, Stein C (2005). No cry at birth: global estimates of intrapartum stillbirths and intrapartum-related neonatal deaths. Bull. World Health Organ. 83(6):409-417.
Neilson J, Lavender T, Quenby S, Wray S (2003). Obstructed labour Reducing maternal death and disability during pregnancy. Br. Med. Bull. 67(1):191-204.
Omole-Ohonsi A, Belga F (2010). Outcome of Obstructed Labour in Kano, Nigeria. Nepal J. Obstet. Gynaecol. 5(2):38-42.
Shaikh S, Shaikh A, Shaikh S, Isran B (2013). Frequency of Obstructed Labor in Teenage Pregnancy. Nepal J. Obstet. Gynaecol. 7(1):37-40.
Shazia A, Irum N, Shazia K, Rrafia B (2013). Incidence causes and outcome of obstructed labor in Sheikh Zaid women hospital Larkana-a tertiary care hospital. Med. Channel 19(2):40-43.
Shirin S, Nahar S (2013). Maternal Mortality-A Public Health Problem. Ibrahim Med. College J. 6(2):64-69.
Wall LL (2012). Obstetric fistula is a "neglected tropical disease". PLoS Neglected Trop. Dis. 6(8):e1769.
Wall LL, Arrowsmith SD, Briggs ND, Browning A, Lassey A (2005). The obstetric vesicovaginal fistula in the developing world. Obstet. Gynecol. Surv. 60(7):S3-S51.

The *Igaraçu* fluvial mobile clinic: Lessons learned while implementing an innovative primary care approach in Rural Amazonia, Brazil

Michele Rocha Kadri[1], Debra Rose Wilson[2*], Julio Cesar Schweickardt[3], James G. Linn[4], Lisandra N. Guimarães Farias[5], Adriana Moreira[6] and Rodrigo Tobias Lima[7]

[1]Oswaldo Cruz Foundation - Amazonia, Leonidas e Maria Deane Institute, Rua Terezina, 476 - Adrianópolis, 69057-070, Manaus, Amazonas, Brazil.
[2]Walden University, USA.
[3]Oswaldo Cruz Foundation - Amazonia, Leonidas e Maria Deane Institute, Brazil.
[4]University of Valparaiso, Chile.
[5]Municipal Health Department of Borba, Brazil.
[6]Secretaria Estadual de Saúde do Amazonas, Brazil.
[7]Oswaldo Cruz Foundation - Amazonia, Leonidas e Maria Deane Institute, Brazil.

In Amazonia, which includes regions in eight South American countries (and an enormous area in Northern Brazil) many of the inhabitants live in small communities scattered across a vast territory? Since too often they cannot be accessed by road, health services must be brought to them on specially constructed river barges, which are floating comprehensive primary care clinics. To effectively deliver health services to vulnerable populations living deep in the Amazon Rain Forest, the Municipal Health Authority of Borba, Brazil piloted the innovative technology of the *Igaraçu* Fluvial Mobile Clinic, a boat with full primary care services. The aim of this investigation is to do a case study of the pilot implementation of an innovative technology, *Igaraçu* the fluvial mobile clinic, which delivers primary care services in rural, Amazonas, Brazil. In Borba, the implementation of the *Igaraçu* has increased the number of people receiving primary care by over 10% and improved the quality of primary care provided, in particular, health promotion, maternal and child care, and treatment of chronic disease. Before the *Igaraçu* fewer people used services for the following reasons: (1) Insufficient professional healthcare staff (e. g. medical doctor and advanced practice nurses); (2) Lack of privacy during consultations; (3) Loss of exam samples; and (4) No continuity of care. Implications of this successful healthcare delivery innovation for the importance of coordination between national health authorities and local policy makers are discussed.

Key words: Amazonia, inhabitants, mobile clinic, primary care clinics.

INTRODUCTION

Frequently, the demographic characteristics of a region are associated with poor health outcomes for the local population. This is the case with the Amazonian region of Brazil. Except for a few large cities, the population is dispersed over a vast area in small isolated communities located on riverbanks. This situation is a challenge to the

National Health System, which has a mission of providing universal coverage for 200 million Brazilian citizens wherever they reside. The aim of this investigation is to do a case study of the pilot implementation of an innovative technology (Burns and Grove, 2016), *Igaracu*, the fluvial mobile clinic which delivers primary care services in rural Amazonas, Brazil (Paim et al., 1979).

In this case study, we describe an innovative strategy that has demonstrated the potential for providing comprehensive primary care services for the rural Amazonian population, and we discuss the importance of dialogue between the Ministry of Health (MOH) and the local health authority in the implementation of effective alternative models of care (WHO, 2013). The *Igaraçu* Fluvial Mobile Clinic is a healthcare delivery innovation that was piloted in the rural Amazonian community of Borba, Brazil.

Local setting

Since 1993, Brazil has delivered its primary care program through its Family Health Strategy. The development of the Unified Health System increased access to healthcare for a substantial proportion of the population, but universal coverage has not been realized (Victora et al., 2011). This is particularly the case in Northern Brazil where people in the metropolitan areas have good access to healthcare, but those in rural communities have more limited access to these necessary services (Paim et al., 1979). The rural/urban disparity in healthcare in this region has spurred innovation in the model of health service delivery through a collaborative process involving the MOH and local governmental authorities (Fraxe, 2000).

The municipality of Borba is on the Madeira River, about 208 km from Manaus, the capital of the state of Amazonas. The Madeira is a large tributary of the Amazonas River. Travel from Manaus to Borba by an "express" boat takes 6 h. A small commercial plane carrying 5 passengers takes 50 min to fly between the cities. In Amazonia, it is more accurate to measure distances by time than by kilometers. A river journey's time varies by season and direction (going up or down river). It is less when waters are rising and more when they are receding. In times of flooding water, riverboats can take advantage of "shortcuts" that open up (Fraxe, 2000).

The most recent National census reported that Borba had 34,961 residents (5,931 were self-declared indigenous people) living in a territory that is slightly larger than Switzerland and twice as large as the state of New Jersey in the US. There is a scattered distribution of residents, 60% of whom live in rural areas (Ministério da Saúde, 2013). Population density is low with 0.79 inhab/km^2. GDP per capita is low, around U.S. $800 per year (Instituto Brasileiro de Geografia e Estatística, 2010; Ministério da Saúde, 2013). Also, the HDI is depressed (0.560) which is in the low human development range (Ministério da Saúde, 2015). About 20% of the population above 25 is illiterate.

Residents of rural Amazonas experience the same chronic diseases as other Brazilians (e. g. cardiovascular illnesses, cancer, and diabetes). Children from poorer families often show health conditions (e. g. anemia and stunting related to poor nutrition). However, residents in these tropical areas also suffer from illnesses which are still endemic in the region (e. g. tuberculosis, malaria, and other mosquito borne illnesses, STDS, and leprosy). Individuals who have good access to primary care, and if needed, more complex care, respond well to treatment (Instituto Brasileiro de Geografia e Estatística, 2010). However, many do not and consequently experience high morbidity and mortality from these diseases (Lancet, 2011).

Borba is served by 17 public health units, which are part of the National Health System. These include 12 facilities that are managed by the municipality. Besides that, there are 2 hospitals of medium complexity and 3 federal health units managed by the State of Amazonas and MOH respectively. Nine of the municipal facilities are primary care health centers, including Fluvial Mobile Clinic (United Nations Development Program, 2010).

MATERIALS AND METHODS

This investigation used a case study design (Burns and Grove, 2016). It is an intensive historical exploration of the development and pilot implementation of the *Igaraçu*, the fluvial mobile primary care clinic used in Amazonas Brazil. Following this study design, researchers at the Oswaldo Cruz Foundation-Amazonia: (1) Collected historical information on the policy making relationship between the Brazilian Ministry of Health (MOH) and local health authorities in Amazonas: (2) Studied traditional methods of primary care health service delivery and outcomes in their region; (3) Developed a comprehensive description of the planning, financing, building, supplying and staffing of the fluvial mobile primary care clinic-- *Igaraçu*; and (4) Compiled descriptive information and preliminary outcome data on the pilot implementation of the *Igaraçu*.

All of this information is essential for the case study and is reported in the results section of the manuscript. Therefore, relationships between municipal health authority and the Federal MOH, traditional primary care service delivery, the planning and development of the *Igaraçu*, and the initial outcome data collected on the pilot implementation of the fluvial mobile primary care clinic will be reported.

*Corresponding author. E-mail: debrarosewilson@comcast.net.

RESULTS

Before *Igaraçu,* the healthcare team used a common wooden boat rented by the municipal health authority to deliver primary care services to people living in isolated riverbank communities. Consultations were done in community leaders' houses, churches or schools. There was very little privacy. To complete many exams, such as those for cervical cancer, the nurse had to do home visits and collect their specimens in patients' homes while children and other family members were present. Sometimes the specimens were lost before being analyzed. The mobile health team went to the community every 60 days, six times each year. Rarely a physician accompanied the team.

Dissatisfactions with this model of care delivery resulted in the Borba Health Authority to propose a pilot project to the MOH for the construction of a ship that could provide self-contained full primary care services. In 2012, the MOH responded with additional services and within a year *Igaraçu* Fluvial Mobile Clinic was launched. Currently, *Igaraçu* serves several river bank communities along the Madeira and its affluent. An *Igaraçu* roundtrip in this "liquid" territory takes 20 days. There is an interval of 40 days between trips. The health team includes one nurse unit manager, two nurse assistants, one physician, one dentist, one biomedical technician and twelve community health workers (community based).

In addition, there are six crew members. The community workers have a key role planning the agenda for each *Igaraçu* trip and serve as a communication link between the clinic and the local population. With the nurse supervision, they also develop patient tracking maps with all of the people who must be followed-up with special services such as pregnant women, children and adults with chronic disorders. Patient records are organized according to a therapeutic plan, e.g. maternal and child health, hypertension, diabetes, and geriatric issues (Figure 1).

The mobile health unit is 24 m in length and has two floors. The first deck is devoted to clinical activities, which includes offices for doctor, nurses, dentist and rooms to accommodate a pharmacy, laboratory, immunization and sterilizing suites. The upper deck includes the team's bedrooms, kitchen and administrative space. A typical workday begins at 7:00 a.m. and lasts until the last patient is seen. During the night, *Igaraçu* travels on the river to the next community where it begins seeing patients early in the morning.

Simple tests such as blood, urine, and stool analyses are completed in the *Igaraçu* laboratory while samples from more complex exams are sent to a laboratory in the largest community in Borba or to a clinical laboratory in Manaus. In cases where a patient must be referred for specialized care, sometimes they can be treated in the local hospital in Borba, however, when they require more complex treatment, the municipal health authority assists them, so that they can obtain this needed specialized care in Manaus.

Two constraints on this new model of primary healthcare delivery were identified. First, there had to be an increase in Federal funding (in Brazil, the MOH provides funding for primary care, which is delivered locally). Second, a more effective method of collecting and processing samples and tracking patients had to be developed.

The development and testing of *Igaraçu* was part of a regional program supported by the MOH. Based on Borba's outstanding success, in 2012 the MOH implemented a program to build 64 Fluvial Health Units to be used in the nine Brazilian states of the Amazonian region[1]. Federal funding was also allocated to the local health authorities for the maintenance of these floating clinics. Furthermore, the National Primary Care Policy was updated to address this new model of "Ribeirinha" Population Health. "Ribeirinha" is a riverside population that is deeply influenced by the cycle of waters (floods and droughts), in a type of dependence and symbiosis, traditional beliefs and subsistence family-based agriculture

The cost of providing approximately 3,400 persons with comprehensive primary care including pre-natal, pediatric, chronic disease (especially hypertension and diabetes), infectious disease, immunization, health education and epidemiologic surveillance through the *Igaraçu* is U.S. $26,500 monthly. When this budget is broken down, 65% is for personnel, 23% is for fuel and 12% is for crew food and housing expense. Expenditures for laboratory supplies and pharmaceuticals are not additional because they are no more with the fluvial than the traditional health unit. The overall building cost for one Fluvial Health Unit was US$530,000, which is equal to the cost of constructing four traditional land-based primary care clinics. However, because the population is spread over a vast territory, having 4 additional clinics would not substantially increase the healthcare coverage of the population. In addition, it would cost an estimated U.S.$12,000 more per unit in maintenance expenditure. In Borba, the implementation of the *Igaracu* has increased the number of people receiving primary care by over 10% and improved the quality of primary care provided in particular in the areas of health promotion, maternal and child care and diagnosis and treatment of chronic disease. Before the implementation of the fluvial mobile clinic, fewer people in rural Amazonas used services because of (1) insufficient professional healthcare staff, e. g. advanced practice nurses and medical doctors; (2) lack of privacy during consultations; (3) loss of examined samples; and (4) no continuity of care.

The Ministry of Health of the Federal Government of Brazil had advised that a systematic evaluation of 10 fluvial mobile clinics in the state of Amazonas and Para should be conducted (MOH Communication, January,

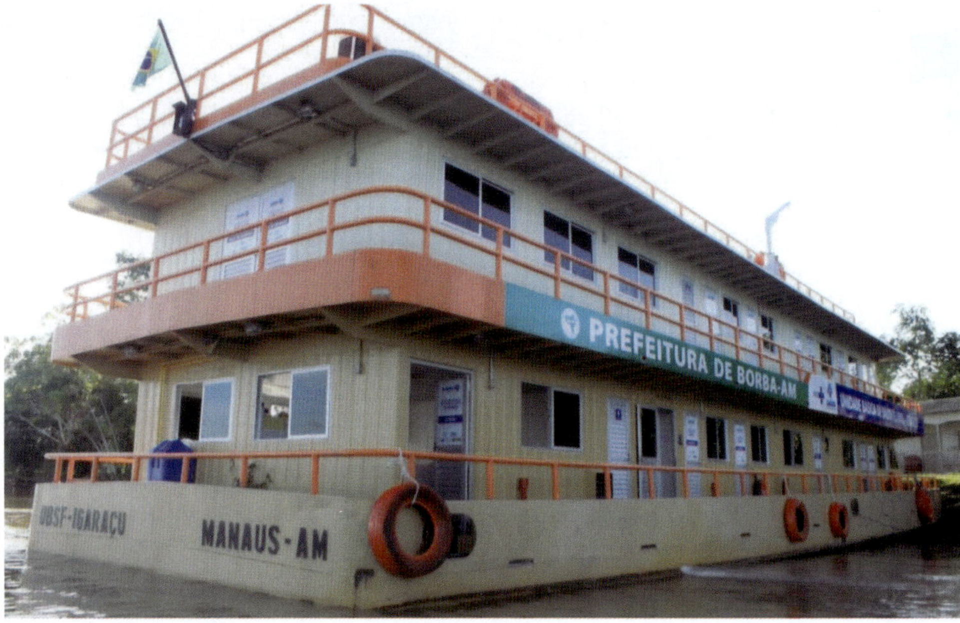

Figure 1. The "Igaraçu" Fluvial Mobile Clinic. A pilot project in Borba, Amazonas, Brazil. Source; Photo from Communication Oswaldo Cruz Foundation (2017).

2017).

DISCUSSION

The Borba pilot project helped the Brazilian MOH to refine and make more effective its Fluvial Mobile Clinic initiative. Key issues that must be addressed for the sustainability of this innovative model of care had been identified. These challenges are assumed to exist in rural areas that have similar characteristics to Amazonia, e.g. vast undeveloped rural regions and widely dispersed populations with low incomes and education levels living along navigable rivers, including other Amazonian countries in South America.

The scheduled predictable and more frequent arrival and functioning of the *Igaraçu* Fluvial Mobile Clinic dispels the community's perception of service unreliability. Families can now return for appointments more regularly because they know they will be assisted by a complete health team, including a medical doctor who have their detailed medical histories, and will be examined and treated as required.

Highly bureaucratic and rigid healthcare delivery models, which often provide fragmented care, must be replaced by more accessible and flexible mobile clinics that have patient oriented highly cohesive clinical staffs (WHO, 2013).

This new model of care requires adjustments in work processes for providing health services (Table 1), and because of crucial differences regarding traditional land-based health units; it is highly desired to keep the same health team and boat crew for no less than two years. This data in the table reflects information collected by the evaluation and monitoring team at the University of the Amazonis.

Conclusions

In countries with vast underdeveloped rural regions and widely dispersed populations with low income and education living on navigable rivers, national health authorities should work with local policy makers to develop innovative models of primary care delivery such as the "Igaraçu" Fluvial mobile clinic. Committed and cohesive teams of primary healthcare workers focused on the family unit, rather than the individual, will more effectively resolve problems of patient tracking, absences, and follow up. The scheduled, predictable, and more frequent arrival and functioning of the "Igaraçu" mobile fluvial clinic dispels the community perception of the unreliability of primary care services.

CONFLICT OF INTERESTS

The authors have not declared any conflict of interests.

FUNDING

The initiative was supported by the Brazilian Ministry of Health.

Table 1. Changes in work process to provide care between a landed based clinic and fluvial mobile clinic.

Parameter	Traditional health clinic	Fluvial mobile clinic
Patient approach	Focuses on individual assistance. Because the service is always available, people usually come to the health center alone or bring one or two family members. The rest of the family stay at home with other children or are doing domestic/agricultural activities	Focuses on familiar assistance. The service is not available full-time, all the family members come for consultation. The quality of care is improved because the clinician knows more about the familiar support, compliance with treatments etc.
Monitoring system	The clinical production can be reported to the national health system databases on a daily basis by internet	There is no internet connection available on board. Data are reported when Igaraçu returns to Borba city. The MOH datacenter has a flexible deadline for the fluvial mobile clinics.
Team	All are health care workers and a community member with basic health training.	In addition to a traditional team, there are the crew members (a captain, navigation assistants, cooker)
Delivering service	Community search for health service. High level of absences and loss follow up.	Health service seeks patients. Patient absences and losses to follow up are reduced.
Cost	About US$ 4.00 per person/month	US$7.80 per person/month
Territory	Land-based. To serve approximately 3.000 people, the unit must cover a large territory, consequently the service is not well accessed	Demographically based. In this "liquid territory" the service is based on the quantity of people, no matter how they are distributed in the territory.

REFERENCES

Burns N, Grove SK (2016). The Practice of Nursing Research: Appraisal, Synthesis, and Generation of Evidence, 8e. Philadelphia, PA: Saunders. pp. 256-257.

Fraxe T (2000). Homens Anfíbios: etnografia de um campesinato das águas. AnaBlume.

Instituto Brasileiro de Geografia e Estatística (2010). Censo Demográfico 2010.

Ministério da Saúde (2012). Unidades Básicas de Saúde Fluviais. Retrieved from http://dab.saude.gov.br/portaldab/biblioteca.php?conteudo=ubs_fluvial

Ministério da Saúde (2013). Financiamento: as necessidades da atenção básica. Rev. Bras. Saúde Fam. 14(35-36):78-81.

Ministério da Saúde (2015). Cadastro Nacional de Estabelecimentos de Saúde 2015. Retrieved from http://datasus.saude.gov.br/cadastro-nacional-de-estabelecimentos-de-saude

Paim J, Travassos C, Almeida C, Bahia L, Macinko J. The Brazilian health system: history, advances, and challenges (2011). Lancet 377(9779):1778-1797.

United Nations Development Program (2010). New Atlas of Human Development in Brazil. Retrieved from http://hdr.undp.org/en/content/new-atlas-human-development-brazil

Victora CG, Barreto ML, do Carmo Leal M, Monteiro CA, Schmidt MI, Paim J, Bastos FI, Almeida C, Bahia L, Travassos C, Reichenheim M, Barros FC I (2011). Health conditions and health-policy innovations in Brazil: the way forward (2011). Lancet 377(9782):2042 2053.

WHO (World Health Organization) (2013). Research for universal health coverage: World health report 2013. Available at: http://apps.who.int/iris/bitstream/10665/85761/2/9789240690837_eng.pdf?ua=1

Pregnancy outcome and early postnatal weights in diabetic and non-diabetic pregnant rats administered ethanolic extract of *Ocimum gratissimum* leaves during pregnancy

Iyare C. O.*, Uzoigwe J., Okorie P. O., Ugwu P. I., Ezeh C. O. and Iyare E. E.

Reproductive and Developmental Programming research Group, Department of Physiology, Faculty of Basic Medical Sciences, University of Nigeria, Enugu Campus, Enugu, Nigeria.

Extract of *Ocimum gratissimum* (OG), also known as scent leaf, is popularly used to treat diabetes mellitus and its hypoglycaemic activity has been confirmed by *in vivo* studies. The aim was to investigate the effect of this extract on placenta development and birth outcome in diabetic pregnancy. Forty two pregnant rats weighing 150-200 g were used. They were divided into control and extract treated diabetic and non-diabetic groups with 6 rats in each subgroup. Extract treated groups were administered 200 and 400 mg/kg of ethanolic extract of OG orally after the induction of diabetes by administration of alloxan monohydrate after an overnight fast. Treatment commenced in the second trimester and lasted till end of pregnancy. On day 18 of pregnancy, 3 rats from each group were sacrificed and placentae harvested and weighed. On the day of delivery, birth weight and other parameters were recorded. Results show that OG administration caused a significant decrease in placental weights, birth weights, litter sizes and placental-birth weight ratio in both diabetic and non-diabetic pregnancy. In conclusion, the observed decrease in placenta-birth weight ratios may suggest a protective beneficial effect of this extract against macrosomia in diabetic pregnancies and increased risk of cardiovascular disease later in life.

Key words: *Ocimum gratissimum*, gestational diabetes, placenta-birth weight ratio, pregnancy outcome, postnatal growth.

INTRODUCTION

There are evidences that diabetic intrauterine milieu is associated with adverse consequences for fetal and postnatal life. Gestational diabetes occurs when pregnant women without a previous history of diabetes develop a high blood glucose level (Casanova et al., 2005) which is characterized by an increased placental transport of

*Corresponding author. E-mail: cordie2age@gmail.com.

glucose and other nutrients from the mother to the fetus, resulting in fetal macrosomia (kamana et al., 2015). However, in severe maternal diabetes complicated by vasculopathy and nephropathy, intra-uterine growth restriction (Dandrea et al., 2001), and in some cases seizures or stillbirth (Dave and Katyare, 2002) can be seen.

Maternal diabetes is also associated with concentration changes of various hormones, cytokines and metabolites in maternal as well as fetal circulation. Hence, these diabetic-associated changes are likely to affect the placenta, because receptors, transporters and enzymes, which are the primary targets of circulating molecules, are expressed often asymmetrically, on both placental surfaces (Desoye and Hauguel-de-Mouzon, 2007). Altered placental function in gestational diabetes may include changes in invasion, ultimately leading to an enhanced risk of early pregnancy loss, growth restriction and pre-eclampsia, as well as a long-term stimulatory effect on placental growth leading to placentomegaly, which is frequently associated with diabetic pregnancies (Emordi et al., 2016).

Gestational diabetes mellitus (GDM) poses a risk to mother and child. The two main risks GDM imposes on the baby are growth abnormalities and chemical imbalances after birth, which may require admission to a neonatal intensive care unit (kamana et al., 2015). Infants born to mothers with GDM are at risk of being both large-for-gestational-age (kamana et al., 2015) in unmanaged GDM, and small-for-gestational-age and intrauterine growth retardation in managed GDM (Godfrey, 2002). In addition, fetal macrosomia in turn increases the risk of instrumentation deliveries or problem during vaginal delivery (shoulder dystocia) (Haavaldsen et al., 2013). Neonates born from women with consistent high blood sugar levels are also at an increased risk of low blood glucose, jaundice, polycythemia, hypokalemia and hypomagnesemia (Irene et al., 2015). GDM also interferes with maturation, making immature babies prone to respiratory distress syndrome due to incomplete lung maturation and impaired surfactant synthesis (Irene et al., 2015).

Treatment of GDM is somehow problematic as care has to be taken to avoid low blood sugar levels due to excessive insulin injections. More injections can result in better control but requires more effort and there is no consensus as to its benefits (Karen et al., 2000; Jones, 2011; Haavaldsen et al., 2013) With the advent of modern obstetric care, the incidence of congenital malformations and neural tube defects have drastically reduced, but macrosomic babies and associated complications remain high (Kaufmann et al., 2003; Kelly et al., 2005).

Studies have shown that extract of OG has been used to treat diabetes mellitus and its hypoglycemic effect has been confirmed *in vivo* (Lee et al., 2005). Unlike most anti diabetic drugs, a study revealed that aqueous extract of OG leaf can significantly reduce postprandial hyperglycaemia in type-2 diabetic model rats, without the risk of hypoglycemia (Lumey, 1998). Most studies on its hyperglycemic effect have been carried out in males using animal subjects (Oguabobi et al., 2012; Shittu et al., 2016). Data on its hyperglycemic effect on diabetic pregnancies is scanty. Secondly, there is high rate of consumption of OG by pregnant women (either as spice or herbal drink) in some rural parts of Nigeria, with speculations that it reduces fetal weight thereby making delivery less laborious. This study was therefore undertaken to investigate whether OG, a confirmed anti-diabetic agent, would have any effect on placentomegaly and fetal macrosomia, which are usual complications of diabetic pregnancy.

MATERIALS AND METHODS

Plant preparation and extraction

Freshly matured leaves were purchased from Ekpoma market in Edo State, mid-west Nigeria and the leaves were identified and authenticated by Mr. Chijioke John Onyeukwu of the Department of Plant Science and Biotechnology, University of Nigeria, Nsukka, where a voucher specimen (UNH Number 360b) was deposited. The leaves were air-dried in a dust-free environment and chopped into pieces using an electric blender. Ethanolic extraction of the leaves was carried out using soxhlet extractor as previously described (Metzger et al., 2008). The extract was then concentrated in a water bath and kept at -4°C until use. Phytochemical analysis of the leaf extract was determined using High Performance Liquid Chromatography method as previously described (Metzger et al., 2008).

Experimental animals

Forty-two matured nulliparous female rats weighing between 150-200 g were used for this study. The rats were housed in special clear-sided cages, with a 12:12 h light-dark cycle and were allowed free access to drinking water and standard rat pellet feed. They were allowed to acclimatize for two weeks.

The estrus cycle was monitored for each rat by daily examination of vaginal smears under the light microscope. At pro-estrus, male rats were introduced into the female cages to allow for mating. Mating was proven successful when spermatozoa were observed in the vaginal smear of the female rats the following morning and this was regarded as the first day of pregnancy.

Experimental design

After pregnancy was confirmed, rats were randomly divided into two broad groups; diabetic and non-diabetic groups. Each group had control and graded doses of extract treated sub-groups. Non-diabetic group consisted of control, 200 mg/kg b.w of extract, and 400 mg/Kg b.w of extract subgroups. Diabetic group consisted of control, 200 mg/Kg b.w of extract, 400 mg/Kg b.w of extract, and 0.5 IU/Kg b.w of insulin subgroups. Each of these seven subgroups had a total of eight rats.

Table 1. Phytochemical analysis of *Ocimum gratissimum* (Qualitative).

Test	Result
Ninhydrin	+
Xantheoprotic	+
Tannin	-
Glycoside	++
Terpernoid	++
Steroid	-
Flavonoid	+
Saponin	++
Resin	++
Alkaloid	++
Anthraqunine	-
Phenol	++

+ = slightly present; ++ = moderately present.

Table 2. Quantitative analysis of OG.

Constituent	% Composition
Alkaloids	2.5
Saponin	3.0
Glycoside	0.0155
Flavonoid	0.5205
Phenol	0.1547

Rats were fasted for 12-h before diabetes was induced on day eight of pregnancy using alloxan monohydrate dissolved in normal saline (Myatt, 2006). The injection site was swabbed using iodine solution. While the rat was held in a dorsal position, the amount of alloxan was injected into the caudal vein at the base of the tail using sterile 1ml syringe.

Blood was taken from the tail vein of all rats, and placed on ACCU-CHEK Active test strips, to check for blood glucose level, before induction of diabetes mellitus, using ACCU-CHEK Active glucometer, Roche Germany. This record was taken as the baseline value for blood glucose. The blood glucose level was subsequently checked 24 h after induction. Animals whose blood glucose exceeded 200 mg/dl were considered diabetic (Nahum et al., 1999).

After confirmation of diabetes, rats in the extract treated groups, both diabetic and non-diabetic, were given graded doses of 200 and 400 mg/kg body weight using oral dosing syringe at the second week of gestation. A subgroup of rats in the diabetic group was given 0.5 international units of soluble insulin per kg body weight and was administered using insulin needle intraperitoneally (Oguabobi et al., 2012). The non-treated control groups received feed and water only. The treatment lasted till parturition.

Body weight (using digital electronic weighing scale), and blood glucose levels were monitored daily, after induction, until delivery. This was to assess the severity of the induced diabetic state.

At day 18 of pregnancy, half the number of rats from each group was sacrificed by cervical dislocation according to Institutional Animal Care and Use Committee (IACUC) guideline on euthanasia (Silverman et al., 2014). The placentae and fetuses were harvested for determination of placental and fetal weights and placental-fetal weight ratio.

On the day of delivery, the litter sizes were noted, birth weight was measured and recorded to the nearest (mg) using an electronic weighing scale, and litters were examined for any anatomical malformations.

Ethical clearance on animal use and handling was obtained from College Of Medicine Research ethics committee, University of Nigeria. A copy of the ethical clearance was attached as an appendix.

Statistical analysis

Results were presented in tables as M±SED and compared using student t-test. Level of significance was taken as $p < 0.05$.

RESULTS

Phytochemical analysis of *O. gratissimum* (qualitative) is shown in Table 1. From the qualitative analysis of O.G, it was observed that saponin, alkaloid, phenol, resin, glycoside, terpernoid and carbohydarate, ninhydrin, xantheoprotic, and flavonoid were present in the extract with alkaloids and saponin relatively higher in concentration as observed in the quantitative analysis result (Table 2).

The result from Table 3 shows that the extract of *O.*

Table 3. Effect of consumption of ethanolic extract of *Ocimum gratissimum* on placental weight (g) at day 18 of pregnancy.

Treatment/Groups	Non-diabetic	Diabetic
Control	0.56±0.04	0.65±0.03
200mg/Kg B.W	0.38±0.01*	0.38±0.03*
400mg/Kg B.W	0.28±0.03*	0.31±0.04*
ITDP 0.5 IU/Kg B.W		0.36±0.01*

Values are expressed as mean ± SEM, n= 6. *Significantly different from the control at $p < 0.05$.

Table 4. Effect of consumption of ethanolic extract of *Ocimum gratissimum* on litter weight at birth.

Treatment/Groups	Non-diabetic	Diabetic
Control	4.44±0.15	5.92±0.27[a]
200mg/Kg B.W	4.75±0.40	4.24±0.40*
400mg/Kg B.W	4.77±0.20	4.48±0.16*
ITDP 0.5 IU/Kg B.W		5.41±0.36

Values are expressed as mean ± SEM, n= 6. *Significantly different from the control in same group at $p < 0.05$. [a]Significantly different between group at $p < 0.05$.

Table 5. Effect of consumption of ethanolic extract of O*cimum gratissimum* on litter size at birth.

Treatment/Groups	Non-diabetic	Diabetic
Control	6.67±0.33	7.00±0.58
200mg/Kg B.W	4.33±0.33*	4.33±0.33*
400mg/Kg B.W	4.67±0.88	6.00±1.00[a]
ITDP 0.5 IU/Kg B.W		5.5±0.50

Values are expressed as mean ± SEM, n= 6. *Significantly different from the control in same group at $p < 0.05$. [a]Significantly different between group at $p < 0.05$.

gratissimum significantly reduced the placental weight in a dose-dependent manner when compared with the control which did not receive the extract. There was no significant difference in the effect of the extract on placental weight between the diabetic and non-diabetic group.

There was no significant reduction in litter weight in the extract treated non-diabetic group compared with the control as shown in Table 4. However, the extract appeared to cause a significant reduction in litter weight in diabetic group when compared with the control and insulin group as shown. In addition, control diabetic group had a significantly higher litter weight when compared to control in non-diabetic group.

The result (Table 5) shows that the 200 mg extract treated group had lesser litter size compared with the control, whereas the 400 mg group was not significantly different from the control and 200 mg group in the non-diabetic group (Table 5). The 200 mg extract treated group had a significantly number of litter size than the 400 mg, ITDP 0.5 IU/kg/bw and control in the diabetic groups. However, litter size was significantly higher in 400 mg/kg/bw in diabetic group when compared to the non-diabetic group as shown in Table 5.

It was observed that the extract reduced the placental-birth weight ratio when compared with the control as shown in Table 6. In the diabetic group, insulin and extract (400 mg/kg/bw) showed a significant decrease in the placental-birth weight ratio when compared with the control. However, on comparison of non-diabetic and diabetic groups, the diabetic groups had significantly greater placental-birth weight ratio as shown below.

The Figure 1 shows a significant increase in weight of the 200 mg extract treated group when compared with the control throughout the three weeks. The 400 mg extract treated group all died two days postpartum.

From Figure 2, there was a steady increase in the weight of the offspring in both the 400 mg treated group

Table 6. Effect of consumption of ethanolic extract of *Ocimum gratissimum* on placental-birth weight ratio.

Treatment/Groups	Non-diabetic	Diabetic
Control	0.09±0.00	0.15±0.01[a]
200mg/Kg B.W	0.06±0.00*	0.08±0.01[a]
400mg/Kg B.W	0.06±0.01*	0.07±0.00*
ITDP 0.5 IU/Kg B.W		0.06±0.01*

Values are expressed as mean ± SEM, n= 6. *Significantly different from the control in same group at $p < 0.05$. [a]Significantly different between group at $p < 0.05$.

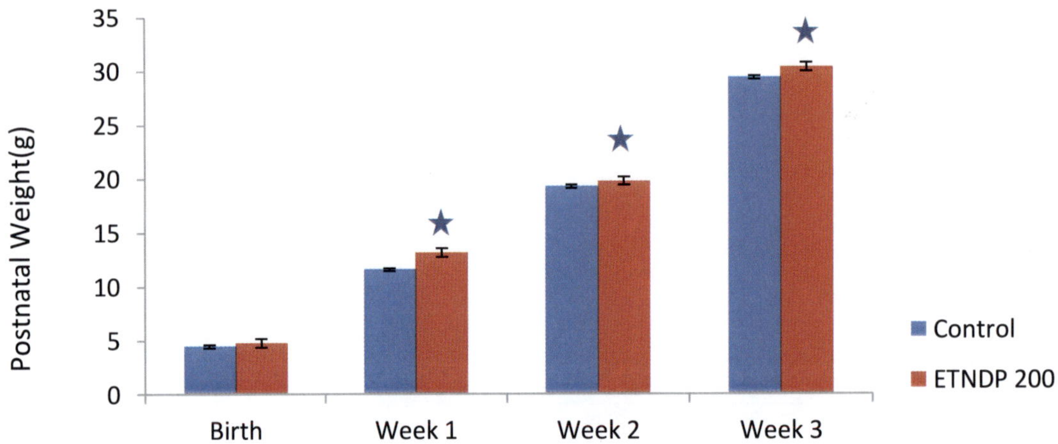

Figure 1. Effect of consumption of ethanolic extract of *Ocimum gratissimum* by non-diabetic pregnant *rats* on postnatal weight of offspring. ETNDP 200 = extract treated non-diabetic pregnant, 200 mg/Kg b. wt; ETNDP 400: all died two days postpartum. N= P<0.05 compared with control.

and the insulin group. The control group and 200 mg treated group all died before the end of the first week postpartum.

DISCUSSION

The observed decrease in placenta weight in both the diabetic and non-diabetic group in the present study, which appeared to be concentration dependent, may be due to the presence of phenol. Phenol was shown to be an active component of the extract (Tables 1 and 2). Omodamiro et al. (2012) has previously reported the presence of phenol in this extract. Lee et al. (2005) showed that phenol decrease placenta weight by significantly reducing levels of placenta lactogen, prolactin-like protein A and C, and decidual prolactin related protein. Placenta lactogen, which is released by a term placenta, affects glucose and insulin metabolism, by decreasing maternal glucose utilization which helps ensure adequate fetal nutrition (Omodamiro et al., 2012). It also decreases maternal insulin sensitivity leading to an increase in maternal blood glucose levels (Rich-Edwards et al., 1997). Consequently, decreasing levels of this anabolic hormone will go a long way in reducing placental weight and by extension, fetal weight. Though prolactin-growth hormones were not quantified in this study, however, the result is in line with previous study by Lee et al. (2005) who reported that bisphenol A, an estrogen-like environmental endocrine disrupter, reduced the secretion of the placental prolactin-growth hormone leading to reduced placental and fetal weight and litter size.

There was a significant increase in the resorption sites following extract administration. This suggests that the extract may have interfered with the normal processes of implantation. This observation may be due at least in part to the presence of alkaloid in the extract (Table 2). Alkaloid administered orally in the second trimester has been reported to cause anti-implantation, anti-gonadotropic, anti-progesteronic, selective estrogenic, embryonic resorption and feto-toxic activities without inducing abortions in animals (Yakubu and Musa, 2012). Ting et al. (2014) reported that Dipsaci Radix (which is

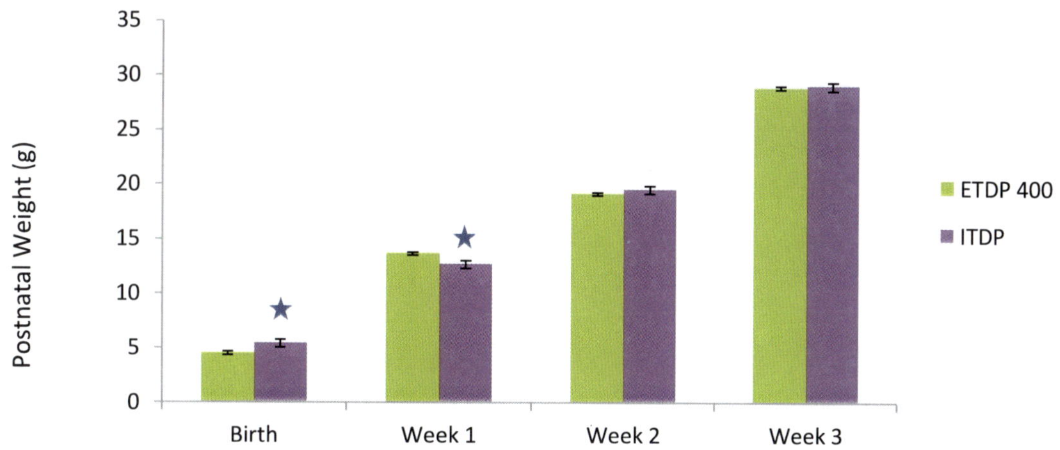

Figure 2. Effect of consumption of ethanolic extract of *Ocimum gratissimum* by diabetic pregnant rats on postnatal weight of offspring. ITDP = Insulin treated diabetic pregnant. ETDP 400 = extract treated diabetic prgnant, 400mg/Kg b. wt; ETDP 200 and Control diabetic: all died within 7 days postpartum; N = P<0.05 compared with control.

high in alkaloid) at a high-dose and long-term administration led to adverse impacts in maternal health and embryo-fetal development in mice and embryonic stem cells. Our results is in support of these previous findings as increased resorption sites may have led to a decrease in the number of viable fetuses that ultimately led to decreased litter size observed in our study.

Adequate placental function is necessary for delivery of nutrients, oxygen, and hormones to the fetus (Setji et al., 2005). The placental-birth weight ratio could be a useful marker for placental efficiency and efficacy (Risnes et al., 2009). Thus, a comparatively large placenta relative to birth weight may be an expression of a relatively inefficient placenta with reduced ability to translate its own growth into fetal growth (Risnes et al., 2009). Studies suggest that a placenta that is large relative to birth weight may be an indicator for reduced nutrient supply to the fetus (Thomas, 2005; Stephanie et al., 2014). In this study, it was observed that extract administration decreased the placental-birth weight ratio possibly in a dose-dependent manner. Both small and large placentae relative to birth weight have been reported to be associated with death in preterm births (Ting et al., 2014). Studies on developmental programming have reported that increased placental-birth weight ratio increases the risk of cardiovascular disease later in life (Van-Assche et al., 1998; Walkinshaw, 2006; WHO, 2014). This observed decrease in the placental-birth weight reported in our study may have been as a result of the extract-induced decrease in the placenta weight reportedly caused by the phenol constituent of the extract.

As shown in Figure 1, it was observed that low dose of OG accelerated early postnatal weight of offspring in non-diabetic pregnancy while Figure 2 shows that high dose extract had similar effect as insulin on early postnatal weight of the offspring in diabetic rat. During the postnatal phase, the litters feed on the breast milk of their mothers. The accelerated growth observed may be from the composition of the breast milk. Since OG is a galactagogue (Yakubu and Musa, 2012), it may have enhanced breast milk production as well as its composition. OG was observed to be toxic at high dose for non-diabetic offspring as there was 100% neonatal mortality. Though low dose extract was not protective against the complications of diabetic pregnancy as both mother and offspring died during the early postnatal period, high dose extract was however protective against the complications of diabetes in the diabetic group.

Limitation to this study

A major limitation to this study is the failure to ascertain the lethal dose of this extract through acute toxicity test. Further studies are recommended to determine the suitable dose of the extract to eliminate fetal resorption associated with the use of this extract as reported in this study.

The research work was done during the raining season between the months of June and July which is usually characterized by low temperature. Failure to maintain a constant room temperature may have contributed to the increase in mortality rate of the offsprings.

Conclusion

In conclusion, these results have shown that ethanolic

extract of *O. gratissimum* has the potentials to reduce placental weight and birth weight, decrease litter size and accelerate early postnatal growth of offspring in both normal and diabetic conditions.

CONFLICT OF INTERESTS

The authors have not declared any conflict of interests.

REFERENCES

Casanova LM, da Silva D, Sola-Penna M, de Magalhaes Camargo LM, de Moura Celestrini D, Tinoco LW (2005). Identification of chocoric acid as a hypoglycaemic agent from Ocimum gratissimum leaf extract in a biomonitoring in vivo study. Fitoterapia 93:132-141.

Dandrea J, Wilson V, Gopalakrishnan G (2001). Maternal nutritional manipulation of placental growth and glucose transporter 1 (GLUT-1) abundance in sheep. Reproduction 122(5):793-800.

Dave KR, Katyare SS (2002). Effect of alloxan-induced diabetes on serum and cardiac butyrylcholinesterases in the rat. J. Endocrinol. 175(1):241-250.

Desoye G, Hauguel-de-Mouzon S (2007). The human placenta in gestational diabetes mellitus: The insulin and cytokine network. Diabetes Care 30(2):120-126.

Emordi JE, Agbaje EO, Oreagba IA, Iribhogbe OI (2016). Antidiabetic and hypolipidemic activities of hydroethanolic root extract of Uvaria chamae in streptozotocin induced diabetic albino rats. BMC Complement. Altern. Med. 16:468.

Godfrey KM (2002). The role of the placenta in fetal programming-a review. Placenta 23:20-27.

Haavaldsen C, Samuelsen SO, Eskild A (2013). Fetal death and placental weight/birth weight ratio: a population study. Acta Obstet. Gynecol. Scand. 92(5):583-590.

Irene L, Eline M, Johan G, Mark JCN, Ricardo DU (2015). Health economic modeling to assess short-term costs of maternal overweight, gestational diabetes, and related macrosomia – a pilot evaluation. Front Pharmacol. 6:103.

Jones CW (2011). Gestational diabetes and its impact on the neonate. Neonatal Netw. 20(6):17-23.

Kamana KC, Shakya S, Zhang H (2015). Gestational diabetes mellitus and macrosomia: a literature review. Ann. Nutr. Metab. 66(2):14-20.

Karen P, George J, Shaish A (2000). Effect of hyperglycemia and hyperlipidemia on artherosclerosis in LDL receptor-deficient mice: establishment of a combined model and association with heat shock protein 65 immunity. Diabetes 49(9):1064-1069.

Kaufmann P, Black S, Huppertz B (2003). Endovascular trophoblast invasion: implications for the pathogenesis of intrauterine growth retardation and preeclampsia. Biol. Reprod. 69(1):1-7.

Kelly L, Evans L, Messenger D (2005). Controversies around gestational diabetes: practical information for family doctors. Can. Fam. Physician 51(5):688-695

Lee CK, Kim SH, Mom DH, Kim JH (2005). Effect of Bisphenol A on the placental function and reproduction in rats. J. Prev. Med. Public Health 38(3):330-336.

Lumey LH (1998). Compensatory placental growth after restricted maternal nutrition in early pregnancy. Placenta 19(1):105-111.

Metzger BE, Lowe LP, Dyer AR, Trimble ER (2008). Hyperglycemia and adverse pregnancy outcomes. N. Engl. J. Med. 358(19):1991-2002.

Myatt L (2006). Placental adaptive responses and fetal programming. J. Physiol. 572(1):25-30.

Nahum Z, Ben-Shlomo I, Weiner E, Shalev E (1999). Twice daily versus four times daily insulin dose regimens for diabetes in pregnancy: randomized controlled- trial. BMJ 319(7219):1223-1227.

Oguabobi NI, Chioli P, Chijioke, Samuel IG (2012). Effects of aqueous leaf extract of Ocimum gratissimum on oral glucose tolerance test in type-2 model diabetic rats. Afr. J. Pharm. Pharmacol. 6(9):630-635.

Omodamiro OD, Ohaeri OC, Nweke IN (2012). Oxytocic effect of aqueous, ethanolic, n-hexane and chloroform extracts of xylopiaaethiopica (Anonaceae) and ocimum gratissimum (Labiate) on guinea pig uterus. Asian J. Plant Sci. Res. 2(1):75-78.

Rich-Edwards JW, Stampfer MJ, Manson JE (1997). Birth weight and risk of cardiovascular disease in a cohort of women followed up since 1976. BMJ 315(7105):396-400.

Risnes KR, Romundstad PR, Nilsen TIL, Eskild A, Vatten LJ (2009). Placental weight relative to birth weight and long term cardiovascular mortality: Findings from a cohort of 31,307 men and women. Am. J. Epidemiol. 170:622-631.

Setji TL, Brown AJ, Feinglos MN (2005). Gestational Diabetes Mellitus. Clin. Diab. 23(1):17-24.

Shittu ST, Oyeyemi WA, Lasisi TJ, Shittu SA, Lawal TT, Olujobi ST (2016). Aqueous leaf extract of Ocimum gratissimum improves hematological parameters in alloxan-induced diabetic rats via its antioxidant properties. Int. J. Appl. Basic Med. Res. 6(2):96.

Silverman J, Suckow MA, Murthy S (2014). The IACUC handbook. CRC Press

Stephanie A, Segovia MH, Vickers CG, Clare MR (2014). Maternal Obesity, Inflammation, and Developmental Programming. Biomed Res. Int. 2014:418975.

Thomas RM (2005). Diabetes Mellitus and pregnancy. Available at: http://revistaamicac.com/dibetesyembarazo.pdf

Ting TX, Min X, Xiao HY, Lam K, Yeuk LC, Zhong ZZ, Kelvin SL, Zhi JY, Xiao YT, Zhi L, Meng YX, Wei X (2014). The evaluation on embryotoxicity of Dipsaci Radix with mice and embryonic stem cells. J. Ethnopharmacol. 151(1):114-122.

Van-Assche FA, Holemans K, Aerts I (1998). Fetal growth and consequences for later life. J. Perinat. Med. 26:337-346.

Walkinshaw SA (2006). Cochrane Database of Systemic Reviews. Available at: http://www.ncbi.nlm.nih.gov/pubmed/17636623

World Health Organization (WHO) (2014). Diabetes fact sheet N° 312. Available at: http://www.who.int/mediacentre/factsheet/fs312/en/

Yakubu MT, Musa IF (2012). Effect of Post-coital Administration of Alkaloids from *Senna alata* (Linn.Roxb) Leaves on some Fetal and Maternal Outcomes of Pregnant Rats. J. Reprod. Infertil. 13(4):211-217.

Italian midwives attitude toward complementary and alternative medicine

Isabella Neri[1*], Maria Cristina Gemmi[2], Alba Ricchi[3] and Elisabetta Romei[2]

[1]Department of Mother-Infant, University of Modena, Italy.
[2]Territorial Service, Reggio Emilia, Italy.
[3]Department of Mother-Infant, University of Modena and Reggio Emilia, Italy

The growing interest in Complementary and Alternative Medicine (CAM) applies also to the field of obstetrics and this encouraged midwives to support the application during pregnancy and delivery. Application of CAM is complete according to the skills and the aims of the midwife's professional profile, representing as it does a safe non pharmacological approach which endorses both the autonomy of women and midwives' professional autonomy. The aim of the present study is to investigate the midwives attitude to CAM application in Emilia-Romagna region located in the North-Italy. This observational study investigated by a written questionnaire 525 midwifes referred to the hospitals and freelancers of Modena, Reggio Emilia, Forlì Rimini and Cesena cities. In such sample, a high involvement of midwives in CAM reaching the 90 to 100% either for hospital/territorial workers or freelancers was observed. Breech presentation and labour management represents the most frequent indication followed by hyperemesis gravidarum. The methods most frequently applied are acupression and moxibustion, homeopathy, relaxation and massage and osteopathy. These midwives were also interviewed about the CAM training expectations: the opportunity to receive teaching during degree is wished by 70% of them, whereas 30% preferred a post-degree training. This represents a preliminary study facing for the first time the attitude toward CAM in Italy, even if the sample size do not allow to reach strong conclusion, some considerations could be drawn: the high compliance showed by midwives should stimulate the increase of CAM offered in public health services and the request also for a qualified training during degree or post-degree studies should promote an enlargement of teaching offer.

Key words: Complementary alternative medicine midwives, training.

INTRODUCTION

The growing interest in Complementary and Alternative Medicine (CAM) applies also to the field of obstetrics. This encouraged midwifes to support the application during pregnancy and delivery. The application of CAM is in complete agreement with the skills and the aims of the midwife's profession, representing as it does a safe non pharmacological approach which endorses both the autonomy of women and midwives' profession (Hall et al.,

*Corresponding author. E-mail: sabella.neri@unimore.it.

2012).

However, the involvement of midwives in the application of CAM raises the question regarding educational training, because non-conventional medications are not included in the teaching program.

The available data in the application of CAM are not consistent and fragmentary. A study performed in South Australia by a postal questionnaire showed that 78% of the 145 midwives interviewed advised women to use CAM during pregnancy and delivery (Gaffney and Smith, 2004). Similar data were found in North-American countries (Hasting-Tolsma and Terada, 2009). Conversely, a study performed in New-Zealand and Canada reported a 40% usage of CAM in a sample of 648, midwives motivated by a lack of interest, religious conflicts and doubts about suitability (Harding and Foureur, 2009). Furthermore, an investigation in Turkey showed that, aside the applications of CAM, 60% of 129 midwives of the family health centers were particularly interested in herbal treatment (Koc et al., 2012).

The aforementioned study reported also that the methods most midwives apply frequently are acupuncture, homeopathy, herbal treatment, and massage (Hall et al., 2012; Gaffney and Smith, 2004; Hasting-Tolsma and Terada, 2009; Harding and Foureur, 2009; Koc et al., 2012). The obstetrics indications requiring CAM application were: fetal malposition, hyperemesis gravidarum, back pain and lactation support (Hall et al., 2012; Gaffney and Smith, 2004; Hasting-Tolsma and Terada, 2009; Harding and Foureur, 2009; Koc et al., 2012). In Turkey report, other indications as common cold, constipation, gastric complaints, insomnia and asthenia are reported (Koc et al., 2012). However, no strong considerations can be drawn considering the relevant heterogeneity of the available studies.

The aim of the present study is to investigate the techniques of the application of CAM by midwives in Emilia-Romagna region located in the Northern Italy. To date, no data about such issue have been published in Italian countries.

MATERIALS AND METHODS

The 525 midwives referred to the hospitals and also freelancers of Modena, Reggio Emilia, Forlì Rimini and Cesena cities were invited to fill questionnaires. The questionnaire included 17 items on CAM techniques. The questionnaires were sent by mail and the answers were requested within 60 days.

A written consent to participate in the study was requested at the end of questionnaire with a specific sentence: "Do you agree that the data obtained by questionnaire be processed and published?"

In details, questionnaire included information as follows (Figure 1):

(1) Demographic data, school degree, previous work experience and actual work position (Group 1-6 items);
(2) Knowledge, motivations and frequency of MNC utilization in the clinical practice (Group 2-7 items);
(3) Most frequent techniques used (Group 3-2 items);
(4) Kind of training received and eventual further training needed to deep the knowledge (Group 4-2 items).

The questionnaire was structured to take into account the interviews reported in the previous studies (1-5). Before commencement of the study, the questionnaire was administered to a sample of 10 midwives who were referred to the Mother-Infant Department, in order to check eventual misunderstanding and difficulties in filling the questions. The results of such evaluation were not included in the final analysis. The e-mail invoice endorsed to reach a large sample of midwives, referred to the whole region. However, such approach caused several methodological biases. Lack of information on the eventual difficulties in filling the questionnaire or misunderstanding causing higher rate of drop-out was more peculiar.

RESULTS

Demographic data

Among the 525 midwives interviewed, only 154 of them filled the questionnaire and the final analysis was performed on 147 cases, because 7 of them were not completely filled. The mean age is about 37.7 (years) and 144 cases were females. The participants' job experience is homogeneously represented: lower than 5 years, 28%; between 5 and 20 years, 35%; and 20 years and above, 37%. All the midwives are graduates and 17% of them have also obtained a post-degree master. The hospital is the most prevalent place of work (71%) followed by territorial service (22%) and Freelancer represent just 7% of the sample.

CAM application

All the midwives interviewed refer to well-known CAM and 75% of them were reported to have conversed with women about the possible use of such methods not just during pregnancy but also in other periods of life like, postmenopausal transition or menstrual disorders.

Also, about 90% of the midwives working at the hospital and all of them at the territorial service (100%) advice women to use CAM. Similarly, the direct involvement is very high. Midwives at the hospital (75%), territorial service (97%), and freelancer midwives (90%) apply CAM during their daily clinical practice with 90% of women's compliance. As far as the midwives motivation to apply CAM is concerned, the most relevant is the safety for both mother and neonate followed by self-resources empowerment (Figure 2).

Breech presentation and labour management represent the most frequent indications to CAM use followed by hyperemesis gravidarum and breastfeeding support. Other indications rarely reported are: low-back pain, neck and arms pain, hemorrhoids, constipation, insomnia, fatigue and common cold.

The commonly applied methods are acupression and moxibustion, homeopathy, relaxation and massage,

How old are you?
What is your gender?
How many years of job experience has you?
What is your place of work?
What is your city of work?
What is your school degree?
GROUP 1

Do you known CAM?
Do you ask to women about their use of CAM during the past or actual pregnancy?
Do you advice the use of CAM during your activity?
Do you use CAM during your activity?
Do you discuss with women before apply CAM?
When you apply CAM? (pregnancy, delivery, puerperium, breastfeeding)
What is the most relevant motivation to use CAM?
(safety, empowerment of self resource, advantage of integration with conventional medicine)
GROUP 2

What are the most frequent techniques advised?
What are the most frequent indications requiring the CAM use?
GROUP 3

How you acquired the training to use CAM?
(University degree, private degree, training organized by the hospital, self…)
What kind of training do you purpose to enlarge the CAM application among midwives?
(University course during degree, after degree, course organized by the hospitals)
GROUP 4

Figure 1. The items of the questionnaire divided into 4 groups accordingly to the issue investigated. Group 1 (6 items): demographic data, school degree, previous work experience and actual work position. Group 2 (7 items): knowledge, motivations and frequency of MNC utilization in the clinical practice. Group 3 (2 items): most frequently techniques used. Group 4 (2 items): kind of training received and also eventual further training needed to deep the knowledge's.

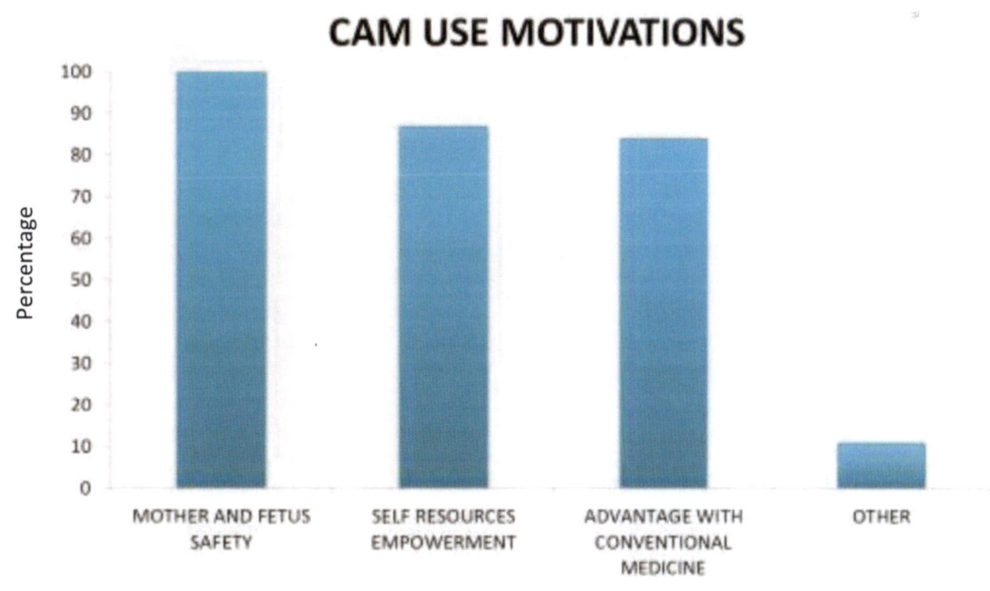

Figure 2. The midwives motivations to apply CAM.

osteopathy and others (Figure 3).

CAM training

The CAM training is performed by private courses (47%), organized by hospital or territorial services (30%) and universities (20%).

The midwives were also interviewed about the importance of CAM training. 70% of them wished for the opportunity to acquire the knowledge during first degree, while 30% preferred a post-degree training. Also, half of

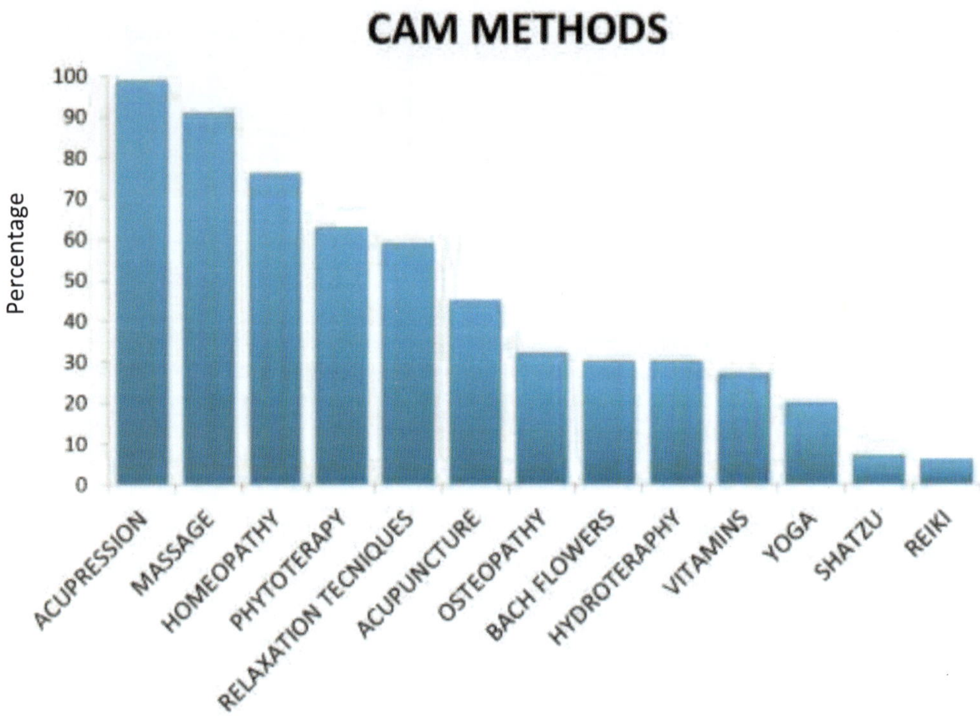

Figure 3. The CAM methods applied.

the midwives look forward to training organized by hospital or territorial services.

DISCUSSION

This study reports a high involvement of midwives in CAM reaching 90 to 100% either for hospital/territorial workers or freelancers. Breech presentation and labor management represents the most frequent indication followed by hyperemesis gravidarum. A further analysis should give more information about the application for labor and delivery which was not particularly be indicated in the questionnaire.

Acupressure and moxibustion are the most frequent methods applied followed by massages, phytotherapy and homeopathy. In Italy, acupuncture application is not allowed by midwives. Five years ago, Emilia Romagna region started with specific moxibustion training for midwives to offer a no pharmacologic approach for breech presentation. This explains the increase in the percentage of midwives who prescribe the use of moxibustion and acupressure.

A plan for acupressure training for labor and delivery has also been organized in order to offer the method to the women considered not eligible or refusing epidural analgesia.

As far as homeopathy and phitotherapy use is concerned, the questionnaire did not investigate the kind or dosage of the substances that are prescribed to the women. Further evaluation should be taken into account, and more details of each method considered.

Midwives stated they would want to be trained by private courses or by hospital and territorial service. In fact, the need to receive a CAM teaching during degree was reported by 70% of them. Such data could be considered by universities institution.

The small sample of questionnaire processed does not allow for strong conclusions about CAM use. Further evaluations should consider different investigation approach in order to avoid the high rate of drop-out experienced at the onset of the present study.

However, considerations that could be drawn from the first study are the high rate of midwives who are looking forward to a qualified training during degree or post-degree studies. Furthermore, their high compliance should stimulate the increase in the application of CAM offered in public health services.

Conflict of Interests

The authors have not declared any conflict of interests.

REFERENCES

Gaffney L, Smith C (2004). Use of complementary therapies in pregnancy: the perceptions of obstetricians and midwives in south Australia. Aust. NZ. Obstet. Gynecol. 44(1):24-29.

Hall H, McKenna L, Griffiths D (2012). Midwives 'support for complementary and alternative medicine: a literature review. Women Birth 25(1):4-12.

Harding D, Foureur M (2009). New Zealand and Canadian midwives' use of complementary and alternative medicine. New Zealand Coll. Midwives J. 40(1):7-12.

Hasting-Tolsma M, Terada M (2009). Complementary medicine use by nurse midwives in the U.S. Complement. Ther. Clin. Pract. 15(4):212-219.

Koc Z, Topatan S, Saglam Z (2012). Use and attitudes toward complementary and alternative medicine among midwives in Turkey. Eur. J. Obstet. Gynecol. Reprod. Biol. 160:131-136.

Perceived socio economic barriers to maternal health seeking behavior among rural women: The case of Raya-Alamata District, Southern Tigray, Ethiopia

Hayelom Abadi Mesele

Department of Sociology, College of Social Sciences and Humanities, Wollo University, Dessie, Ethiopia.

Maternal health care service utilization is one of the components of the reproductive and child health interventions package with the aim of improving both maternal and child health. It is the health of the women during pregnancy, childbirth and postpartum period. Thus, the overall objective of this study is to investigate the perceived socio economic barriers to maternal health seeking behavior of rural women in Raya Alamata District. In doing so, the researcher employed qualitative methods substantiated by the quantitative data. In doing so, a sample of 359 HH units was selected from three 'Tabias' by using simple random sampling techniques. The qualitative data analyzed using thematic analysis whereas the quantitative data analyzed using descriptive statistics. According to the findings of the study, perceived social barriers such as shortage of qualified health workers, ill behavior of health workers, student's internship and poor quality of maternal health services influence the health seeking behavior of the rural women of the study area. On the other hand, the perceived economic barriers such as access to resources, working conditions and cost of transportation and medical treatment also influence maternal health seeking behavior of the women of the study area.

Key words: Antenatal care, delivery care, maternal health, maternal health seeking behavior, postnatal care.

INTRODUCTION

Maternal health care is the health of the women during pregnancy, childbirth and postpartum period which are crucial for the wellbeing of a mother and new born baby (WHO, 2008). It is one of the components of the national package of essential reproductive and child health interventions package focusing on improving quality of life of women and adolescent mothers (Tanzania Ministry of Health and Social Welfare, 2011). Moreover, health seeking behavior is any activity undertaken by individuals and they perceive themselves to have a health problem or to be ill for the purpose of finding an appropriate remedy (Ward et al., 1997). It is situated within the broader concept of health behavior, which encompasses activities undertaken to maintain good health, to prevent ill health, as well as dealing with any departure from a state of good health (WHO., 1995). Besides, health seeking behavior involves identification of pathways to the formal health care system, often commencing with home care and traditional healers and extending to the formal system, pathways differing according to the

E-mail: abadihayelom129@gmail.com.

presenting condition (MacKian, 2003). Along with this, maternal health-seeking behavior is the process and intention of consulting a physician during the prenatal, delivery and postnatal period, especially when disease symptoms are apparent (Caldwell, 1983).

Recent studies show that knowledge about health seeking behavior is essential for the provision of need based health care delivery to any population (Rahman et al., 2011). For example, planning for health care services provision depends on the health needs and health seeking behavior of the population. Thus, determining the health seeking behavior is essential to provide need based health care services to the population (Chauhan et al., 2015). The existing literature on maternal health seeking behavior can be categorized into two; those who studied the issue from an economic point of view and those studied from socio-cultural viewpoints. The first category focuses on economic factors such as income, insurance, cost and availability of medical care (Stekelenburg, 2005).

Besides, lack of money for treatment, costs of transport; formal and informal payments (Ajaegbu, 2013; Reuben Mahiti et al., 2015); and large family size, jobless, unnecessary expenditure on health services; and insecurity, lack of food at home and health facilities, poverty were identified as economic barrier (Lama and Krishna, 2014; Wilunda et al., 2014). These studies showed that poor economic circumstances affect health throughout life (Wilkinson and Marmot, 2003). Therefore, poorest women are generally least likely to use maternal health-care services (WHO, 2009) because of their inability to cover cost of treatment, transport, and other out-of pocket expenses (Yalem, 2013).

On the other hand, the second category focuses on the socio-cultural factors and traditions that affect maternal health seeking behavior. These studies indicate that in the developing countries like Ethiopia, the problem of cultural interference on maternal health has become a catastrophic problem, especially in rural areas (Shole, 2015) and often leads to self-care, home remedies and consultation with traditional healers in rural communities (Nyamongo, 2002). Likewise, Zenebe (2016) found that different cultural malpractices during pregnancy and childbirth affect the maternal health seeking behavior of mothers in Ethiopia.

The issue of maternal health seeking behavior has attracted the interest of some researchers in Ethiopia. Yet the amount of researches and the knowledge obtained from those researches do not suffice to explain the perceived socio economic barriers to maternal health seeking behavior. Furthermore, a critical look at the findings in Ethiopia showed that they mainly concerned with identifying biological aspects that affect maternal health care service utilization. On the other hand, investigating the traditional maternal health beliefs and practices in inclusive manner has been given little emphasis. Moreover, health care seeking behavior as many studies indicate are cultural systems-they are culturally constructed and can only be understood in the context of the wider culture of which they are part.

On top of that, methodologically, the aforementioned studies gave a huge emphasis on quantitative method in the understanding of maternal health care service utilization, for the sake of describing socio-economic and demographic characteristics of study participants' vis-à-vis maternal health. On the contrary, in the present study attempt has been made to incorporate qualitative method intensively due to the fact that perceived socio economic barriers which affect maternal health seeking behavior are more understandable through a detailed and rich data that could be collected by giving more attention to qualitative method.

Hence, it could be said there is a place to conduct a study that assess the issue of maternal health seeking behavior and its socio economic barriers. Thus, the purpose of this study is to identify the major perceived socio economic barriers that affect maternal health utilization and maternal health seeking behavior during pregnancy, labor and delivery in Raya Alamata District. It is also hoped that the results of the study is essential to policy makers to understand the perceived socio economic barriers to maternal health seeking behavior and serve as a groundwork for any possible intervention aimed at improving the low utilization of maternity care services in the study area.

MATERIALS AND METHODS

Description of the study area

Raya Alamata is located at 600 km north of the capital city Addis Ababa and about 180 km south of the capital city of Tigray Regional State, Mekelle. It is the south most administrative district of Tigray Region State bordered in the south with the Amhara Regional State in the east with Afar regional State in the North East with Raya Azeboworeda and in the North with Oflla woreda. Alamataworeda has 15 tabias (peasant associations) and 2 town dwellers associations. The number of agricultural households of the woreda is approximately 17,597. The total population of the woreda was 128,872 in 2003/2004 (IPMS, 2005). Regarding the health infrastructure, the district had one hospital, six health centers and 13 health posts (Rural Raya Alamata district health office, 2004).

Research design

The study is intended to explore the perceived socio economic barriers that affect maternal health seeking behavior among rural women in Raya Alamata District, southern Tigray. In doing so, a cross-sectional study design is employed. Furthermore, the objective of the study requires the integration of both quantitative and qualitative data to best answer questions that cannot be answered by either of the two approaches alone. Therefore, the study employs both data and methodological triangulation.

Study population and sample size determination

The target populations of the study are all women in the

reproductive age group (15-49 years) in Raya Alamata District. Particularly, the study focuses on 5467 households of the study area. Out of this, the researchers selected 359 samples of women from Raya Alamata District based on simple random sampling technique. To do this, Kothari (2004) sample size determination formula would be used as follows:

$$n= \frac{Z2.p.q.N}{e2\,(N-1)+Z2.p.q} n=359$$

Inclusion and exclusion criteria

Inclusion criteria

(1) Women who were mentally and physically capable of being interviewed are included in the study.
(2) Women, who were permanently, reside in the study area.
(3) The elder woman is only selected for the interview (key informant, FGD and in-depth interview) from members of the household.
(4) Women under the age of 15 and above 49 were not included in the survey

Exclusion criteria

(1) Women who are mentally and physically incapable of being interviewed.
(2) Mothers who stayed for less than six month in the study area.
(3) Women, who critically ill, could not talk or listen, were excluded from the study.

Methods of data collection

Four main methods of data collection were employed. These included survey, focus group discussions (FGDs), key informant interviews and in-depth interviews.

Household survey

Survey method is one of the most widely used primary data gathering methods in social research. This method enables researchers to study a given population by relaying only in the portion of that population which is called samples. Thus, it saves time and economy, again access accurate information. Accordingly, in this study the researchers selected 359 samples of women from Raya Alamata district. In order to get a reliable data from respondents, the data collected by using structured questionnaire. The researcher prepared questionnaire in accordance with the research objectives. The entire questionnaire prepared in English for the first time afterward it will be translated in to Tigirigna language in the intention that the majority of the informants are Tigirigna speakers. In addition to, the preparation of the questionnaire, the survey administered by three enumerators for the reason that all women may not read and write. Then, the researcher given one day training for three enumerators to perform their job well and to have clear understanding about the questions put in the schedule. The training includes how the enumerator conducted the survey and the way filling the questions. Besides, it includes further explanation and discussion on the questions to make clear to the enumerators. Finally, the enumerators administered the questionnaires under the supervision of the researcher. Ones the data are gathered from informants, the process of editing, coding, data entry, data cleaning and consistency checking done. The final step was analyzing and interpreting the results.

Focus Group Discussion (FGD)

Focus groups are a form of strategy in qualitative research in which attitudes, opinions or perceptions towards an issue, product, service or programme are explored through a free and open discussion between members of a group and the researcher (Kumar, 2011). It is useful data collection method which helps to generate qualitative data from the discussion by making group interaction between members of the target population. The FGD helps to capture more deeper and comprehensive information from respondents such as model women and males. The researcher conducted three Focus Group Discussions consists of twenty four purposively selected participants. The participants of the FGD were selected from model women, non model women's and husbands/males respectively. The discussion with the participants of the FGD was based on discussion guide that were structured around the key themes by using local Tigrigna language to avoid misunderstandings. Besides, the moderator was sensitive to local norms and customs during discussion. Before the commencement of the discussion, the moderator specified the objective of the focus group discussion and guides the discussion accordingly.

Key informant interview

Key informant interview is used to collect qualitative data from informants that have knowledge and experience on the issue of maternal health. This enabled to get in-depth information from informants. Interview guide with loosely structured conversation is used to collect data. This allows the interviewee to respond flexibly and the interviewer to manage the core issues of the study. In this study, nine model women, six health workers including health extension workers, six religious leaders, three community leaders, were selected purposively and interviewed.

In-depth interview

In-depth interviewing is the most commonly used data collection approach in qualitative research. In-depth interviews are those interviews that are designed to discover underlying motives and desires. Such interviews are held to explore needs, desires and feelings of respondents (Kothari, 2004). This method enabled the researcher to generate highly detailed information and to have better understanding on the perceived socio economic barriers to maternal health seeking behavior. In doing so, in-depth interview is conducted with twelve women with the help of interview guide check lists.

Methods of data analysis

The data obtained from various sources is analyzed using both quantitative and qualitative data analysis methods. The qualitative data was collected from respondent using focus group discussion, key informant and in depth interview. Qualitative data analysis is conducted concurrently with gathering data, making interpretations, and writing reports (Creswell and Creswell, 2017). The researcher listen all audio taped and read the field notes step by step to jot down all the information. After that the audio taped from FGDs, key informant interview and in depth interview it has transcribed verbatim, and translate from Tigrigna to English. Then, the translated data is organized, prepared, and broken up into sections based on their themes. Then a technique of thematic analysis is used to interpret and make sense of the organized data. On the other hand, the quantitative data was processed as an important part of the whole survey operation. It includes editing, coding, data entry, data cleaning and consistency checking. A Statistical Package for Social Sciences (SPSS, version 20) was used to analyze the data. The researcher used descriptive statistical tools to analyze the quantitative data. Descriptive tools such as frequency, percentages, and graphs are employed to present the results. Finally, the quantitative findings are used to substantiate the qualitative findings.

Ethical consideration

In the progress of research, researchers need to respect the participants and the sites for research (Creswell and Creswell, 2017). Thus, due respect was given to the participants during the data collection process. Besides, an informed consent was received from participants before the commencement of the interviews to ensure that participation in research was voluntary. Respondents were informed that they have the right to participate voluntarily and withdraw from the research at any time. Anonymity of respondents and confidentiality of their responses were ensured throughout the research process. Information that was provided by informants would not be transferred to a third party or would not be used for any other purpose.

RESULTS AND DISCUSSION

In this part, the major findings of the study, based on the data obtained through household survey; in-depth and key informant interview and FGD are presented and discussed, in a descriptive rhetoric. Theories relevant to the underlying themes and related literatures are used to interpret the primary data.

Socio-demographic characteristics of respondents

The quantitative data is collected and analyzed on demographic and social characteristics of sample respondents. As indicated in the Table 1, the socio demographic characteristics in this study include age, marital status, ethnic identity, religious affiliation, educational background and income of the respondents.

In this study, a total of 359 rural women aged 15-49 years were included. Out of 359 respondents, the majority 113(31%) of women were found between the age category of 25-34 years. With regard to marital status, the majority of the respondents 314(87.5%) were married followed by divorced consists of 24(6.7%). According to participant's marital status of the respondents has an association with maternal health seeking behavior. Being and becoming divorced and widowed affect maternal health seeking behavior of rural women. Accordingly divorced and widowed women were at risk, lack financial resources, lack emotional, psychological and physical support; and are less likely to receive maternal health care services than the married ones. Moreover, women FGD participants also revealed that most divorced and widowed women were female headed households who have different duties that restrained women from visiting health facilities.

Furthermore, almost all respondents 336(93.6%) belongs to Tigrian ethnic groups followed by 23(6.4%) Amhara ethnic groups. With regard to religious affiliation, the majority of respondents 257(71.6%) are followers of orthodox Christian followed by Muslim 98(27.3%). In relation to educational level of respondents, 218(60.7%) are illiterate, 94(26.18%) are educated up to grade eight, 31(8.63%) are educated up to grade twelve; and the rest 16(4.5%) of the respondents are simply able to read and write. Another important indicator for understanding the socio-economic status is the monthly income of the respondents in the household. Out of 359 respondents, 159(44.7%) of them earn an average monthly income of 501-1000 birr, whereas 132(37.1) of the respondents earn less than 500 birr per month.

Perceived social barriers to maternal health seeking behavior

There are varied perceived social barriers to maternal health seeking behavior in rural areas of Raya Alamata. Among the many perceived social barriers: lack of professional personnel, lack of confidence in the professional competency of health workers, less privacy and confidentiality on health care providers, ill behavior of health workers and poor quality of maternal health services are the major problems of the study area. Each of these perceived social barriers to maternal health seeking behavior has been shown to have strong effects upon the health of rural women of the study area.

Shortage of qualified health workers

As table two showed that more than half 200(55.7%) of the respondent proved the absence of qualified professional personnel in the health institutions whereas the rest 159 (44.3%) of the respondents proved the presence of adequate health professionals. This finding is lower than the findings of study conducted in Southern part of Ethiopia in Duna district in which (62.3%) of women were perceived the availability of health professional personnel as low (Abaychew, 2015). On the other hand, the qualitative data from respondents proved the absence of qualified health workers (physician) in the rural area of the study area. To do this, the quantity of health workers assigned in each health centers and their skill to treat people was taken as a measurement to evaluate their skill. Therefore, in substantiating this idea, A 44 years of old health expert at Raya Alamata District health office described the condition as follows:

There were shortages of skilled and qualified health

Table 1. Demographic and socioeconomic characteristics of respondents (n=359).

Variable	Category	Frequency	Percentage
Age range	15-27	106	30
	25-34	113	31
	35-44	100	28
	45-49	40	11
	Total	359	100
Marital status	Single	14	3.9
	Married	314	87.5
	Widowed	7	1.9
	Divorced	24	6.7
	Total	359	100
Ethnicity	Tigray	336	93.6
	Amhara	23	6.4
	Total	359	100
Religion	Orthodox	257	71.6
	Muslim	98	27.3
	Others	4	1.2
	Total	359	100
Education	Illiterate	218	60.7
	Read and write	16	4.5
	1-8 grades	94	26.2
	9-12 grades	31	8.6
	Total	359	100
Monthly income	Below 500 birr	132	37.1
	501-1000 birr	159	44.7
	1001-1500 birr	43	12.1
	1501-2000 birr	16	4.5
	2001 and above	6	1.7
	Total	356	100

Source: Own survey, 2016.

professionals especially laboratory technician, pharmacy and environmental health expert which are unavailable in the market. Moreover, there are health centers in the district with no laboratory equipments at all. So it is difficult to say we were given adequate maternal health services in the absence of such health personnel's and equipments in the health institutions.

As the narratives of the health worker of the district, indicate that rural women were restrained from getting adequate health personnel particularly laboratory technician, pharmacy and environmental health experts. The health centers are dysfunctional in the absence of those professionals and the necessary equipments. So it is unthinkable to give full fledged maternal health services for rural women like pregnancy checkup, urine test, hemoglobin and blood pressure. It also difficult to give adequate delivery and postnatal care services in the absence of qualified health personnel. The absence of qualified health professional in the rural area compelled women to bypass and travel long distance to get better services. This is one of the causes to delay to get maternal health services and contributes to incur additional cost. Besides, they have compelled to search alternatives medications from traditional healers at home. In support of this, one of the FGD participants noted the shortage of health workers as follows:

There is lack of quick and adequate services given to the clients particularly women due to shortage of health professionals in the health centers. Besides, the health workers assigned to the rural areas were unqualified and

Table 2. Respondents opinion on the availabilities of qualified health workers at health institutions (n=359).

Variable	Alternatives	Frequency	Percentage
	Yes	159	44.3
Availabilities of professional personnel	No	200	55.7
	Total	359	100

Source: Own survey, 2016.

Table 3. Respondents opinion on privacy and trust of health care providers (n=359).

Variable	Alternatives	Frequency	Percentage
	Yes	167	46.5
The presence of privacy and confidentiality	No	192	53.5
	Total	359	100

Source: Own survey, 2016.

they are with inadequate skill to treat severe maternal health problems. They also disclose that most of the rural women often forced to sidestep for further medication in search of better physicians. However, this costs us additional money and which makes us vulnerable to the already burden that we have due to poverty [53 years old participant].

The shortage of skilled health professionals in the health centers has negatively affected the overall health of the community in general and women in particular at the rural areas. It contributes rural women to wait long hours to get maternal health services. Moreover, as a result of shortage of skilled health professionals in the health centers many rural mothers were referring to the district hospital for further medication; and laboratory examination for screening of diseases such as anemia, STIs, Hemoglobin and HIV infection. These conditions restrained rural women of the study area from getting timely treatment and exposes for further complications, pain and extra cost. This condition is very awful for women especially during the period of delivery. Sometimes women delivered before they have reached health facilities. Others died before they have arrived at the district hospital (Table 2).

Lack of privacy and confidentiality

As Table 3 indicates 167(46.5%) of the respondents ensured the presence of privacy and confidentiality while 192(53.5%) of the respondents were not comfortable with privacy and confidentiality. This finding is consistent with the study done in southern Ethiopia among non-user of ANC (55.7%) were proved of the absence of privacy and confidentiality of the service (Abaychew, 2015). Similar studies in Africa also revealed that lack of privacy in health facilities was also mentioned as a contributing factor for home delivery (Mirsho et al., 2007). Another study in Gambia also shows that limited choice for seeking care was one of the reasons for heavy reliance on TBAs, who are considered to be more secretive and friendly than professional healthcare workers (Nyanzi et al., 2007). In line with this, the qualitative data from the majority of the respondents revealed that health workers did not respect their professional ethics why because they were not keeping the privacy of clients. Along this, there are also problems of privacy during the labour and delivery process. According to the statement of the FGD participants, in the district hospital privacy of the birthing woman was not kept. The hospital hosted many apprenticeship students from different colleges and universities of the two adjacent regional states, as a practical attachment fieldwork. The students entered into the delivery room during labour and delivery practice. As a result, birthing women are embarrassed by the crowd for they will be exposed naked in front of them. Some of them refused to deliver at the hospital due to embracement caused by the presence of many individuals in the delivery room. They prefer to deliver at home with the help of elders or TBAs. A 30 year old interviewee from 'Selam Bekalsi' stated that "*I know one woman refuses to deliver and she returns to her home due to this trouble"*. Concomitantly, frequent entry of many health workers to attend the labour woman once at delivery room disrupts the psychology of the birthing woman and raises the issues of privacy. Such incidents erode the confidence of berthing women. Another FGD participant also reported that if you delivered at health facility you would be treated as a doll everyone come and observe the birthing woman. In line with this argument, another 40 years old female key informant reported the condition as follows; "Many rural women do not have interest to deliver at health facilities due to problems related to delivery in the health facilities. During labour the sexual organ (uterus) of the birthing women had

Figure 1. Respondents opinion regarding the behavior of health workers (n=359).
Source: own Survey, 2016.

injured. This bad lived experience of women in the health facilities deter them from delivering at health institution".

Behavior of health workers

As Figure 1 indicates that the majority 219(61%) of the respondents reported that health workers have bad behavior's. This ill behavior of health workers deterred rural women from using modern maternal health services at the earliest time. Similarly, studies showed that the attitude of the health care provider and previous experience of the mothers about the care received influence utilization of maternal health services (Olayinka et al., 2014). Studies in Uganda also revealed that bad staff attitude towards clients was mentioned as a reason for low utilization of health services in general and maternity services in particular (Wilunda et al., 2014). Furthermore, studies in Gondar, north Ethiopia revealed that bad experiences and unwelcome attitude towards health facilities hinder the use of maternal care services (Abebaw et al., 2013). In consistent this, the qualitative data from FGD participants also revealed that health workers have not positive attitude towards rural women. Rural women are being discriminated based on their dressing style and hygiene situations. In strengthening this, one of the FGD participants from 'Tabia' 'Timuga' reported the behavior of health workers as follows:

Some health workers at the district hospital are cruel, impatient and unsympathetic for rural women. The health workers insulting and mistreating women who attend maternal health [A 40 years model woman].

Another FGD participant from 'Tabia' 'Selam Bekalsi' forwarded similar ideas regarding the behavior of health workers as follows:

During labour and delivery rural women entered the health facilities for delivery purpose however, the health workers did not give much attention. They give better attention and follow up for those who have a close acquaintance with the health workers than other patients who are awaiting the health service. Women who do not have someone inside the health facilities do not get the necessary follow up and checkups about the progress of labor. When complication became severe they call them but they abuse us in bad words particularly at night time. They did not like to wake up from their sleep. They were saying wait until the labor is push. This affected our psychology and sometimes we decide not to come again to the health facilities [A 45 year model woman].

As the narratives from FGD participants revealed that the negative attitude and behavior of health workers affect maternal health seeking behavior of rural women. It has discouraged rural women to attend and visit health facilities during pregnancy, delivery and postnatal care services. In addition to this, key informants from Raya Alamata District health office also assured the problems of health workers related to misbehaving and bad working conditions particularly at district hospital. These kind of problems occurred at maternity, OPD and card rooms. The other problem that has taken place at Raya Alamata District hospital is related to discrimination and bias. In substantiating this idea, key informant from 'Tabia' 'Selam Bekalsi' noted that:

Health workers are discriminatory at the district hospital. They are given better services to women who are well dressed and well groomed. On the other hand, those who came from rural areas dressed according to their traditional norms and values were undervalued and mistreated by health workers in the hospital. Moreso, they were treated below the required standard for patients [A 40 years old model woman].

The discriminatory behaviors of health workers inside the hospital affect health seeking behavior of rural women. The health workers provide prompt services for those who have known previously. Besides, those who have relatives in the health facilities get better admiration and care than others specifically at the district hospital. As result of this, rural women preferred to use home based treatment as an alternative of modern health care services. Along with, rural women seek treatment from

Table 4. Respondents opinion on the quality of maternal health services.

Variable	Alternatives	Frequency	Percentage
Quality of maternal health services	Low	201	56.1
	Medium	116	32.4
	High	41	11.5
	Total	358	100

Source: Own survey, 2016.

TBAs, herbalist and other relatives during the time of pregnancy and delivery at Raya Alamata District.

Poor quality of maternal health services

Availability of adequate health facilities determines quality of services provided to a population of a country (Jason, 2005). The quality of health services which has been given for the community also determines maternal health services. However, the quality of maternal health services from the survey indicates that more than half 201(56.1%) of the respondents ranked the quality of maternal health services as low whereas 116(32.4%), 41(11.5%) of respondents ranked it the quality of maternal health services as medium and high respectively.

Quality of care is a major factor for determining the utilization of maternal health services. High quality maternal health services attracted more women. In opposite to that low qualities of maternal health care thrust clients from the health facilities. This low quality of maternal health services causes women to be dissatisfied. Similarly, this finding is consistent with the study done in north Ethiopia which showed that providing incomplete (poor quality) maternal health service had damaging effect on health-seeking behavior of mothers (Abebaw et al., 2013). Besides, there is shortage of drugs and medical supplies, and qualified health professionals in the health facilities. The absence of such facilities in the health centers has negative impacts on the utilization of maternal health utilization as well as maternal health seeking behavior of the rural women of the study area. In view of fact that a key informant from 'Tumuga' health center reported that:

Antenatal care, delivery and postnatal care were given for women. These services were not good enough due to problems related to shortage of manpower and equipment. Now, there were many problems that take place in the health center [A 48 years of old midwife].

In line with this, the health workers stated that the majority rural health centers are not equipped with the necessary equipments, skill personnel and medicines to give quality maternal health services such as antenatal care, delivery and postnatal care services. Except few, the majority health centers do not give quality maternal health services for pregnant women like urine test, hemoglobin, TTC, blood pressure and HIV testing. Additionally, the health centers also could not give quality maternal health services for birthing woman with the necessary and recommended procedures (Table 4).

Perceived economic barriers to maternal health seeking behavior

Perceived economic barriers like less access to resources, bad working conditions and cost of transportation and medical treatment affect maternal health seeking behavior of the rural women of the area under study.

Less access to resources

Women have no decision making power and smaller share of resources and benefits. They have less access to and control over productive resources, land and credit (Kalkidan, 2007). However, the husband/male has the power to own and control every resource. He is the only source of power in the household. On the other hand, women have less access to resources. They do not control and own properties like land, cattle and other products even though this resource are determinants for their health. In the study area women have unequal property right with their husbands. In line with this, a young interviewee from Garjale add that "I have no equal property right with my husband why because I am little girl". According to the view of the informant age gap in marriage is one of the causes to property inequality. This age gap between younger married girls and their spouses creates unequal power relations. The age gap creates favorable condition for the husbands to have a dominant role in the decision-making process of the household; however, it is troubled for the young girl to bargain with her husband and getting timely maternal health services.

Concurrently, another 40 years of old interviewee participant and mother of 6 children noted that:

I knew that the government gave equal property right with my husband but in our culture the husband has the sole

Table 4. Respondents opinion on the quality of maternal health services.

Variable	Alternatives	Frequency	Percentage
Quality of maternal health services	Low	201	56.1
	Medium	116	32.4
	High	41	11.5
	Total	358	100

Source: Own survey, 2016.

power to own and make decision regarding property. Everything was commanded by husband. He has the power to sell and buy any property. I always received money from my husband for purchasing of household consumption and other activities.

The government guaranteed the property rights of women however, some women did not benefit from their constitutional rights. They did not have equal decision making power in the common properties of the household. They lack power to control and own their common properties with their spouse. They are least likely to afford to pay for health service charges. This in turn causes to deter women from getting timely treatment until the husband permit and sold property to the market. The powerlessness of woman to make decisions regarding their communal property causes to suffer from maternal health problems and they are also often at greater risks of vulnerability. Lack of property rights also affects women's ability to make decision on their own health care, contraception use and reproductive health services.

Bad working conditions of women

All rural women were engaged in physical work during their pregnancy. This can be detrimental to their health and damaging for the unborn babies. This also has potential influence on maternal health (Idowu, 2013). Accordingly, the findings from the survey indicates that 282(78.6%) of the respondents have done any work within or outside the home while the rest 77(21.4%) of the respondents were not work within or outside the home. Out of the total women who said, "Yes" regarding the type of work, 179(63.5%) of the respondents executed difficult tasks, 62(22%) carried out moderate works and 41(14.5%) of the respondents carried out easy works. This finding is very low than the findings of study conducted in Bangladesh, 100% of the respondents were engaged in physical work during their pregnancy (Aktar, 2012). In most society's women are the ones who are mostly working at home in the maintenance of the household or very close to home, doing both household activities and small-scale production and trading (Ethiopian societies of population, 2008). Other studies in Gambia by Lowe et al. (2016) shows that women's daily activities were too strenuous and could not get sufficient rest even as they approached their delivery date. In consistent with this, the findings from interviewee, FGD and key informant interview revealed that women are performing different indoor and outdoor activities. Most rural women do routine types of domestic activities from dawn up to the middle night without the assistance of their partner. In substantiate of this idea, a mother of 5 children and participant of the FGD described her lived work experience in the household as follows:

Most of the time, I spent my time doing different household activities. I do different activities like washing clothes, preparing foods, taking care of my children and other household activities. Sometimes, I fetch firewood from the field. Further, I also hauling water and going to the field to reach food to my husband in the farmland. I do not know the time to have rest in my life. My life always come with many ups and downs which enlarge my strain. I do not think so about my health and well being.

The other participant added that most of the rural women had passed difficult time all over their life due to the influence of heavy workload. Womanhood by itself is a problem. Many rural women have accompanied with many life trajectories.

"For instance me, I do a lot of activities until five up to six o'clock at the nighttime; and I do not take rest until I sleep at the mid night". I do not get timely maternal health services because of lack of time. Accordingly, a day has created another day without getting timely medical treatment. This condition affects every rural woman not only me [38 years old Key informant].

In line with the above thought, the following vivid account of the informant will show the role of husbands during pregnancy time: The problem is with our husbands. Because they do not see pregnancy as a thing that needs attention rather they take it as a natural rite of passage that has to be accomplished. That is why during pregnancy my husband gives much attention to his agricultural work, friendship cheers in local alcohol

Table 5. Proportional distribution of respondents according to their working condition and the type of work.

Questions	Alternatives	Frequency	Percentage
Have you done any work within or outside the home? Frequency Percent	Yes	282	78.6
	No	77	21.4
	Total	359	100
What type of work they did?	Difficult	179	63.5
	Moderate	62	21.4
	Easy	41	14.5
	Total	282	100

Source: Own survey, 2016.

houses than me.

If I say something he will lash out to his physical measure that deems his skill to suppress at home. Thus, day in day out I have to silence my voice and pain even during pregnancy [35 years old Key informant].

As the story shows that rural women mostly spent their time in hard physical labour. Such backbreaking working condition in the home created heavy burden on women's' health. Most of the rural women did not get timely treatment particularly maternal health services like ANC. Besides, the majority FGD participants reported that rural women are engaged in physical work during their pregnancy and in the post delivery periods. They participate in pubic work activities like water and soil conservation programs until six months of pregnancy. At this time they were forced to travel more 15 km in one trip every day for about forty days to participate in the public work. It is expected for these women to travel ups and downs in tough geographical area this affect the overall health and wellbeing of the woman. Sometimes rural women has exposed to miscarriage. It has also negatively affected unborn infant (Table 5).

Cost of transportation and medical treatment

Costs of seeking healthcare may include costs for transportation (Gabrysch and Campbell, 2009). However, as Table 6 demonstrated that the majority 232 (64.6%) of the respondents cannot afford the cost of transportation to get maternal health care services while the rest 127 (35.4%) of the respondents can afford the cost of travel to get maternal health services due to different reasons. The quantitative data shows that the majority of the respondents unable to pay their cost of transportation. In substantiating this idea, findings from FGD participants revealed that during the antenatal, delivery and postnatal care rural women traveled by using Bajaj on contract base and it costs up to 150 birr for one trip to reach the nearest health facilities in the absence of ambulances.

Another similar studies by Wilunda et al. (2014) in Uganda showed that the cost of the ambulance were (20,000 Ugandan shillings, about $ 8). These were the most expensive one which is difficult to afford particularly for the poorest rural women. This situation affects rural women treatment seeking behavior. It deters women from utilizing antenatal, delivery and postnatal services. Cost of transportation also causes to delay to get maternal health services. In addition to this, findings from northern part of Ethiopia also showed that inability to cover the costs of transport or service is an important barrier to the utilization of skilled maternal care, especially at the time of complication (Abebaw, 2013).

Correspondingly, lack of money for transportation and other extra costs negatively affected rural women in the study area. This condition deterred rural women from using modern health facilities. It increases delay to diagnosis, put off treatment compliance and it has affected the maternal health seeking behavior of rural woman. The cost of transportation affects the ability of women access to maternal health services. Due to cost of transportation rural women cause to delay to visit health facilities until they get money. They did not go to health institutions at the right time. As the right time was postponed due to lack of money the state of sickness worsens and it affects the overall health of the mother. Besides, the informants argued that women have developed low self esteem and develop feeling of inferiority due to unable to cover the cost of travel. All of these factors affect maternal health seeking behavior of rural women of the study area.

On the contrary to the above narrative, some of the FGD participants and interview schedule respondents said that there was no payment for transportation due to proximity of the health facilities. Thus, they have gone on foot to get maternal health services especially to the health post and health centers. Besides, qualitative data from the majority of FGD participants revealed that rural women were not paid for transportation cost due to convenience of ambulances which were provided by the government during delivery and labour. The ambulance were given free transport services to rural women to ship

Table 6. Proportional distribution of respondents according to the ability to afford the cost of travel (n=359).

Variable	Alternatives	Frequency	Percentage
	Yes	127	35.4
Abilities to afford the cost of transportation	No	232	64.6
	Total	359	100

Source: Own survey, 2016.

women to health institutions. But, there is one problem related to the ambulance services. The ambulances did not come back the birthing woman to her home after delivery this condition forced women to cost extra money for transportation.

Medical costs are expenses for drugs, diagnosis and treatment by the women to get maternal health services. Medical cost for maternal health care services like ANC, delivery and postnatal care become barriers to get timely and appropriate care from health facilities. Due to the presence of medical costs women received delayed treatment which affects the overall health seeking behavior of rural women. In consistent with this, studies in rural Tanzania supports the argument that high direct payments, together with the costs of unofficial payments, are acute barriers to the use of maternal services (Mubyazi et al., 2010) thus contributes to women's inability to access medical services for maternal health care (Lwelamira and Safari, 2012). Another studies in Ethiopia by Abaychew (2015) indicated that cost of medicine and other due costs were the major economic constraints for rural women to get adequate maternal health services.

In order to reduce the problems related to medical costs, the government of Ethiopia provided free maternal health care services for pregnant, delivered and PNC attendants. In line with this, the key informant from district health office said that the federal government of Ethiopia was permitted free medical services for pregnant women from the period of conception to 45 days after delivery. At this phase all pregnant and birthing women were given free medical services at all government health institutions. Then, in our district all the health institution would give free medical services for pregnant women and for birthing women until 45 days of delivery [A 44 year's key informant].

In substantiating to the above idea, one of the FGD participants said that maternal health services are given for free in every public health facilities. What is the problem here is if there is no availability of drugs, the clients referred to private drug stores. Another key informant added that as women went to health institutions there is shortage of medicine; and they did not get adequate medicine in public institutions. The physicians ordered to buy medicine from private clinics which is high in terms of cost and unaffordable especially for the rural poor. The cost of medicine directly or indirectly affects women maternal health seeking behavior. Similar to this, other respondents add that we always expected free medication for mothers in public health institutions but the condition is not found as they expect why because the expose for extra costs urgently (Table 6).

Conclusion

This study has tried to assess the perceived socio economic barriers to maternal health seeking behavior among rural women in the case of Raya Alamata District, southern Tigray, Ethiopia. In doing so, the finding of this study give much emphasis into the perceived socio economic barriers to maternal health seeking behavior among rural women. Accordingly, the shortage of skilled health professionals in the health facilities restrained rural women from getting adequate health services like cheek ups, urine test, hemoglobin and blood pressure. It is also difficult to give adequate delivery and postnatal care services in the absence of qualified health personnel. It causes women to bypass and travel long distance to get better services. They have also compelled to search alternative treatments like traditional healers at home which cause to deter women from getting modern maternal health services. Due to these problems rural women were restrained from getting timely treatment and exposes for further complications, pain and extra cost.

The other problem is related to privacy. Lack of confidence and privacy in health facilities and health care providers were hindered in the use of maternal care services specifically during the labour and delivery process due to the gathering of apparent ship students and frequent entry of many health workers. This bad lived experience of women in the health facilities deter them from delivering at health institution and further debilitate their delivery care seeking behavior. Bad behavior of health workers, lack of respect and mistreatment, abuse and bad staff attitude towards clients are the main reasons for low utilization of maternal health services in the study area. This ill behavior of health workers plus discrimination and bias based on their status negatively affects the maternal health seeking behavior of rural women in the study area. It had discouraged women from seeking them again, discourage other potential users, and possibly affect the degree of compliance with referrals. Availability of adequate health facilities determines the quality services however, the quality of maternal health services were very low in the study area. This low qualities of maternal health care thrust clients from the health facilities. The majority mother's are dissatisfied with maternal health services given in the health facilities due to unavailability of drugs, medical supplies and dearth of qualified health professionals. These poor quality maternal services had damaging effect on health-seeking behavior of mothers.

The study also showed that women have little decision making power and smaller share of resources and benefits. The majority of women in the study area are not capable to control and own property equally with their spouse. They are least likely to afford to pay health service charges; and they do not get timely treatment until the husband permit and sold property to the market. Due to power imbalance between the husband and the woman; women's ability to make decision on their own health care, contraception and reproductive health services were limited.

In addition to this, the indoor and outdoor activities performed by rural women affect their health seeking behavior. These stressed working condition in the home created heavy burden on women health. They did not able to get timely treatment particularly maternal health services such as ANC. The economic costs related to transportation and medical issues were another determinant factor to maternal health utilization. Lack of money for transportation and other extra costs negatively affected rural women in the study area. This condition deterred rural women from using modern maternal health facilities. It could increase delay to diagnosis, put off treatment compliance and it has affected the maternal health seeking behavior of rural woman. Therefore, all concerned government and non government organizations should address these perceived socio economic barriers in order to increase the health seeking behavior of rural women specifically maternal health seeking behavior.

CONFLICT OF INTERESTS

The authors have not declared any conflict of interests.

REFERENCES

Abaychew Z (2015). An assessment of factors affecting the utilization of maternal health care service delivery: The perspective of rural women in the case of DunaWoreda, Hadiya Zone. Addis Ababa, Addis Ababa university (http://etd.aau.edu.et/handle/123456789/6839).

Abebaw G (2013). Determinants of skilled maternal care utilization: A multilevel analysis using mixed method investigation in North Gondar Zone, North West Ethiopia. Addis Ababa, Addis Ababa University.

Abebaw G, Alemayehu W, Mesganaw F (2013). Factors affecting utilization of skilled maternal care in Northwest Ethiopia: a multilevel analysis. BMC International Health and Human Rights 13(1):20.

Ajaegbu OO (2013). Perceived challenges of using maternal healthcare services in Nigeria. Arts and Social Sciences Journal.

Aktar S (2012). Health care seeking behavior for safe motherhood: Findings from rural Bangladesh. Bangladesh e-Journal of sociology 9(2).

Caldwell J (1983). The social component of mortality decline: An investigation is South India employing alternative methodologies. Population studies 37(2):185-205.

Chauhan RM, Anil PJ, Abel S, Zile S (2015). Determinants of health care seeking behavior amongrural population of a coastal area in South India. International Journal of Scientific Reports 1(2):118-122.

Creswell JW, Creswell JD (2017). Research design: Qualitative, quantitative, and mixed methods approaches. Sage publications.

Ethiopian societies of population (2008). Maternal health care seeking behaviour in Ethiopia: Findings from EDHS 2005. Addis Ababa, Ethiopia (https://searchworks.stanford.edu/view/10818112)

Idowu AE (2013). The Socio-Cultural Context of Maternal Health in Lagos State, Nigeria (Doctoral dissertation, Covenant University, Ota, Ogun State).

Improving productivity and market success (IPMS) (2005). Pilot learning site diagnosis and program design: Improving productivity and market success of Ethiopian farmers. Provide a valid link Available at https://cgspace.cgiar.org/bitstream/handle/10568/16756/Alamata.pdf ?sequence=1

Jason OO (2005). Situation analysis on population, reproductive health and gender. Addis Ababa, Ethiopia.

Kalkidan B (2007). Cultural practices that affected the status of women in Benishangul Gumuz Mandura Woreda. Addis Ababa University, Addis Ababa.

Kothari R (2004). Research methodology: Methods and techniques (2nd Ed.). New Delhi, India, New Age International.

Kumar R (2011). Research methodology a step-by-step guide for beginners (3rd ed.). Los Angeles SAGE Publications Ltd.

Lama S, Krishna A (2014). Barriers in utilization of maternal health care services: Perceptions of Rural women in Eastern Nepal. University Medical Journal 48(4):253-258.

Lowe M, Chen DR, Huang SL (2016). Social and cultural factors affecting maternal health in rural Gambia: An exploratory qualitative study. PloS one 11(9):e0163653.

Lwelamira J, Safari J (2012). Choice of place for child birth: prevalence and determinants of health facility delivery among women in Bahi district, Central Tanzania. Asian Journal of Medical Sciences 4(3):105 112.

MacKian S (2003). A review of health seeking behaviour: Problems and prospects. Health Systems Development Programme.

Mrisho M, Schellenberg JA, Mushi AK, Obrist B, Mshinda H, Tanner M, Schellenberg D (2007). Factors affecting home delivery in rural Tanzania. Tropical Medicine and International Health 12(7):862-872.

Mubyazi GM, Bloch P, Magnussen P, Olsen OE, Byskov J, Hansen KS (2010). Women's experiences and views about costs of seeking malaria chemoprevention and other antenatal services: a qualitative study from two districts in rural Tanzania. Malaria Journal 9(1):54.

Nyamongo IK (2002). Health care switching behavior of malaria patients in a Kenyan rural community. Social Science and Medicine 54(3):377-386.

Nyanzi S, Manneh H, Walraven G (2007). Traditional birth attendants in rural Gambia: Beyond health to social cohesion. African Journal of Reproductive Health 11(1):43-56.

Olayinka A, Achi T, Amos O, Chiedu M (2014). Awareness and barriers to utilization of maternal health care services among reproductive women in Amassoma community, Bayelsa State. International Journal of Nursing and Midwifery 6(1):10-15.

Rahman M, Islam M, Islam MR, Sadhy G, Latif MA (2011). Disease pattern and health seeking behavior in rural Bangladesh. Faridpur Medical College Journal 6(1):32-37.

Reuben M, Dickson AM, Angwara DK, Columba KM, Anna-Karin H, Isabel G (2015). Women's perceptions of antenatal, delivery, and postpartum services in rural Tanzania Glob Health Action 8(1):28567 http://dx.doi.org/10.3402/gha.v8.28567

Rural Raya Alamata district health office (2004). Annual report.

Shole (2015). An impact of socio-cultural practices on maternal mortality in Masasi District, Tanzania. Malaysian Journal of Medical and

Biological Research 2(3):45-78.

Stekelenburg J (2005). Health care seeking behavior and utilization of health services in Kalabo District, Zambia. Vrije University.

Tanzania Ministry of Health and Social Welfare (2011). A performance audit on the monitoring, evaluations and budget allocation for maternal health care activities in Tanzania, National Audit Office of Tanzania.

Ward H, Thierry M, Carol T (1997). Health seeking behaviour and the control of the sexually transmitted disease. Health Policy and Planning 12(1):19-28.

Wilkinson R, Marmot M (2003). Social determinants of health: the solid facts. Copenhagen: World Health Organization.

Wilunda C, Gianluca Q, Giovanni P, Peter L, Giovanni D, Fabio M, Andrea A, Rose ML, Risa T, Aline M, Koyejo O (2014). A qualitative study on barriers to utilization of institutional delivery services in Moroto and Napak districts, Uganda: Implications for programming. BMC Pregnancy and Childbirth 14(1):259.

Zenebe K, Alem H, Merga A, Abate G, Taha H (2016). Prevalence of cultural malpractice and associated factors among women attending MCH Clinic at Debretabor Governmental Health Institutions South Gondar, Amhara Region, North West Ethiopia, 2015. Gynecol Obstet (Sunnyvale) 6: 371. doi:10.4172/2161-0932.1000371

World Health Organization (WHO) (1995). A rapid assessment of health seeking behavior in relation to sexually transmitted disease: Draft Protocol.

World Health Organization (WHO) (2008). Maternal Health. Available at http://www.who.int/topics/maternal_health/en/

World Health Organization (WHO) (2009). Women and Health: Today's Evidence Tomorrow Agenda. Geneva, Switzerland.

Yalem T (2013). Determinants of antenatal care, institutional delivery and skilled birth attendant utilization in Samre Saharti District, Tigray, Ethiopia. Umeå University, Sweden.

25

Premenstrual symptoms in young students and in their mothers at their ages

Miwa Fukuoka[1*], Yuna Hamada[2], Mari Fujikawa[3], Sayuri Hatanaka[4] and Toshiyuki Yasui[1]

[1]Department of Reproductive and Menopausal Medicine, Graduate School of Biomedical Sciences, Tokushima University, Tokushima, Japan.
[2]Tokushima Red Cross Hospital, Irinokuchi-103 Komatsushimacho, Komatsushima, Tokushima Prefecture 773-8502, Japan.
[3]Takamatsu Public Health Center, Kagawa Prefecture, Shikoku, Japan.
[4]Kitano Hospital, 2 Chome-4-20 Ogimachi, Kita Ward, Osaka, Osaka Prefecture 530-8480, Japan.

Premenstrual symptoms are gradually becoming recognized socially and measures taken to cope with premenstrual symptoms are changing. The purpose of this study was to determine the differences in degree of recognition, in physical and emotional symptoms and in means for coping with premenstrual symptoms between nursing students and their mothers at the ages of the nursing students. This study was conducted between July and November, 2016. 272 nursing students and 272 mothers of the students were recruited. This study was approved by the Ethics Committee of Tokushima University Hospital. A self-administered questionnaire that took about 15 min to complete was designed. The proportion of students who recognized premenstrual symptoms was 98% and the proportion of mothers who recognized premenstrual symptoms at the same age as the students was 76%. The proportions of students who had moderate to severe physical and emotional symptoms were higher than those of the mothers. The items with the highest percentages of students and mothers who answered moderate to severe physical and emotional symptoms were desire for sweets and irritability, respectively. The proportion of students who took measures to cope with premenstrual symptoms was higher than that of the mothers. Physical symptoms in the students were significantly correlated with those in their mothers. The degrees of physical and emotional symptoms in the students were greater than those in the mothers at the same age as the students and measures taken for coping with these symptoms were diversified. The increasing availability of information on premenstrual symptoms and changes in lifestyle may contribute to the increase in prevalence of premenstrual symptoms.

Key words: Premenstrual symptoms, coping, nursing students, mothers.

INTRODUCTION

Many women of reproductive age experience physical or emotional symptoms associated with the menstrual cycle. Premenstrual syndrome (PMS) is a cluster of mood, behavioral and physical symptoms occurring during the

*Corresponding author. E-mail: fukuoka@medsci.tokushima-u.ac.jp

late luteal phase of the menstrual cycle that interfere with daily activities and are relieved by the onset of menstruation (Yonkers et al., 2008). It has been reported that the frequency of premenstrual symptoms is quite high (80-90%) (Angst et al., 2001) and that about 5% of women have severe symptoms that interfere with personal or social relationships or work and may require pharmacological management (Dimmock et al., 2000). In Japan, it has been reported that 95% of women aged 20 to 49 years suffered from premenstrual symptoms (Takeda et al., 2006) and that 64.8% of high school students suffered from premenstrual symptoms (Takeda et al., 2010).

The etiology of PMS has remained unknown, although hormonal changes and serotonin dysregulation have been suggested (Grady-Weliky, 2003). Lifestyle factors such as diet, exercise and sleep are considered to be involved. A potential role of dietary fat in premenstrual symptoms in Japanese women has been proposed (Nagata et al., 2004). Relationships of PMS with calcium intake, caffeine-containing beverages and chocolate or sweets containing refined sugar have also been reported (Tadakawa et al., 2016). Tadakawa et al. (2016) reported that a preference for salty food and a lack of regular exercise were identified in girls aged 15 to 19 years with physical premenstrual symptoms as risk factors for school absenteeism. It has been reported that exercise could be used as treatment for premenstrual disorders, suggesting that there is an association between PMS and lack of exercise (Daley, 2009). Skipping breakfast, insufficient sleeping and insufficient exercise were suggested to be exacerbation factors of PMS (Ogata and Daitou, 2013; Mori et al., 2004). Sakuma et al. (2008) reported that no feeling of fatigue when getting up, sufficient sleeping and appropriate exercise were associated with mild degrees of premenstrual symptoms. Considering the current lifestyles of young women, the prevalence of PMS may gradually increase.

Premenstrual symptoms and PMS had not been recognized as health concerns in Japan. However, premenstrual symptoms have gradually become recognized due to the availability of information regarding premenstrual symptoms. Lifestyle modifications including regular exercise, avoidance of stressful events, adjustment of sleeping habits, cognitive behavior therapy and dietary supplementation as well as pharmacological treatments have been proposed for coping with premenstrual symptoms (Ryu and Kim, 2015). However, the means of coping with premenstrual symptoms may have changed with times. The degree of recognition of symptoms, the physical and emotional symptoms, and coping strategies may be different for young women at present and their mothers at young ages because of differences in life style, background knowledge of symptoms and means for coping.

Premenstrual syndrome experienced by premenopausal women greatly interferes with the quality of life (Rapkin and Winer, 2009). Bertone-Johnson et al. (2015) showed in a prospective study that women who experienced moderate to severe PMS had a 40% higher risk of developing hypertension than did women who experienced few premenstrual symptoms. Symptoms such as hypersomnia and general fatigue in the daytime may increase since it has been reported that the quality of night sleeping deteriorated before menstruation (Baker and Driver, 2004). It has been reported that restriction of sleeping hours and disturbance of deep sleep induce insulin resistance (Tasali et al., 2008), suggesting that sleeping disorder due to premenstrual symptoms may be involved in the occurrence of diabetes mellitus.

The purpose of this study was to determine the differences in degree of recognition in physical and emotional symptoms and in the means for coping with premenstrual symptoms between nursing students and their mothers at the ages of the nursing students.

SUBJECTS AND METHODS

This study was conducted between July and November in 2016. 272 nursing students (66 first grade, 67 second grade, 71 third grade and 68 fourth grade students) and 272 mothers of the nursing students were recruited. The nursing students for whom agreement could be obtained were asked to complete a questionnaire after explanation of the study at the end of a lecture, and questionnaires were collected on the same day. Subsequently, invitation letters and questionnaires were mailed to their mothers through the nursing students for whom agreement had been obtained. The participants were informed of the purposes and procedure of the study in the invitation letter. It was stated in the invitation letter that cooperation in the questionnaire survey is based on free will and that there is no advantage for the subjects who do not cooperate. Agreement for participation in this study was obtained by having the questionnaire form returned by mail. The same connection numbers on the questionnaire forms we used for a nursing student and her mother. Each nursing student was asked to send her mother an envelope containing a questionnaire form with the same connection number as that on the nursing student's questionnaire form. The questionnaire forms from the students and their mothers were anonymous, and questionnaire forms from the mother and her daughter could be identified by same connection numbers. Sufficient considerations were given to private information. This study was approved by the Ethics Committee of Tokushima University Hospital (2625).

A self-administered questionnaire that took about 15 min to complete was designed. The first part of the questionnaire consisted of questions on age, body height and weight, past history of hypertension, menstrual status including age of menarche, menstrual regularity and menstrual cycle, and degree of dysmenorrhea assessed by using a visual analogue scale (VAS). The second part of the questionnaire consisted of questions on recognition of premenstrual symptoms including PMS and physical symptoms beginning within 5 days before menstruation, including abdominal tension and pain, bloating, breast swelling and tenderness, headache, low back pain, hot flashes, rough skin, fatigue or lack of energy, overeating, food cravings/desire for sweets, hypersomnia, insomnia, constipation and diarrhea, and psychological symptoms including irritability, anger, anxiety, depressed mood, decreased interest in social relationships, and confusion/out of control. Items were rated as "not at all", "mild", "moderate", or "severe". The third part of the questionnaire

Table 1. Background characteristics of the students and their mothers.

Parameter		Students	Mothers	p values
Age at menarche (years)		12.2 ± 1.45	12.5 ± 1.31	0.008
Menstrual cycle (days)	≤24	14(5.5)	4(2.4)	0.073
	25-38	209(83.2)	146(89.5)	
	≥39	28(11.1)	13(7.9)	
Menstrual pain	No	50(19.8)	42(25.7)	0.156
	Yes	202(80.1)	121(74.2)	
Use of medicines for pain	No	87(44.6)	81(67.5)	<0.001
	Yes	108(55.3)	39(32.5)	
VAS		5.6 ± 2.3	4.7 ± 2.3	0.001

VAS, Visual analogue scale. Age at menarche and VAS are shown as means ± standard deviation.

consisted of questions on coping with premenstrual symptoms: lying down, warming the lower back and lower abdomen, having a massage, visiting a gynecologist, taking medicines, consulting somebody, appropriate exercise, sufficient sleeping, doing something to take one's mind off the symptoms, refraining from favorite food and caffeine, restricting intake of water and salt, and telling somebody that one is now before menstruation. The mothers were asked to answer the questions based on their memory at the same age as their daughters.

Statistical analysis

Statistical analyses for data evaluation were carried out using SPSS version 20 for Windows. All p values are two-tailed and those less than 0.05 were considered to be statistically significant. The significance of differences in the degree of premenstrual symptoms between the students and their mothers was evaluated by the Wilcoxon rank sum test. Physical and emotional symptoms were scored according to the degree of symptoms (severe: 4 points; moderate such as having an impact on daily life: 3 points; a little: 2 points, and no symptom: 1 point) and total points of 14 physical symptoms and 6 emotional symptoms were calculated. Spearman's correlation test was used for the correlation between the students and their mothers in physical and emotional symptoms. Scores of physical and emotional symptoms in the mothers with and those without hypertension were assessed by using the Mann-Whitney U test.

RESULTS

The response rates of the questionnaire were 93.0% (253 /272) in the students and 59.9% (163/272) in their mothers. Mean (± standard deviation: SD) ages of the students and their mothers were 20.1 ± 1.8 and 49.8 ± 4.1 years old, respectively. Mean body heights, body weights and body mass indices (BMIs) were 157.5 ± 4.9 cm, 50.9 ± 5.9 kg and 20.5 ± 2.1, respectively, in the students and 157.9 ± 4.9 cm, 53.7 ± 7.5 kg and 21.5 ± 2.7, respectively, in their mothers.

As is shown in Table 1, age of menarche in the students was significantly younger than that in their mothers. The proportion of students with an irregular menstrual cycle tended to be larger than the proportion of mothers with an irregular menstrual cycle at the same age as the students. The proportion of students who had menstrual pain was significantly larger than that of the mothers who had menstrual pain at the same age as the students. The mean score of VAS in the students was significantly higher than that in their mothers.

Four students had a past history of hypertension. Twenty-five mothers had a past history of hypertension and 15 mothers had taken anti-hypertensive drugs. Scores of physical symptoms and emotional symptoms were not significantly different in the mothers with and those without hypertension (p=0.575 and p=0.876, respectively).

Proportion of women who recognize premenstrual symptoms

The proportion of students who recognize premenstrual symptoms was 98%. The proportion of mothers who had recognized premenstrual symptoms at the same age as the students was 76%, and the proportion of mothers who now recognize premenstrual symptoms was 98%.

Physical and emotional symptoms in the students and the mothers at the same age as the students

The mean (± SD) numbers of moderate to severe physical symptoms and emotional symptoms in the students were 2.6 ± 2.4 and 1.7 ± 1.0, respectively. The mean (± SD) numbers of moderate to severe physical symptoms and emotional symptoms in the mothers at the same age as the students were 1.4 ± 0.85 and 0.75 ± 0.25, respectively. Both the number of physical symptoms and the number of emotional symptoms in the students were significantly larger than those in the mothers at the same age as the students (p<0.001).

As shown in Table 2, the item with the highest

Table 2. Physical symptoms before menstruation in the students and their mothers (Students: n=253; Mothers: n=163)

Physical symptom		Degree of symptom				p values
		Not at all	Mild	Moderate	Severe	
Abdominal pain and distension	Students	74(29.2)	156(61.7)	16(6.3)	7(2.8)	0.170
	Mothers	34(21.0)	115(71.0)	10(6.1)	3(1.9)	
Bloating of the face, hands and feet	Students	138(0)	105(91.3)	6(5.2)	4(3.5)	<0.001
	Mothers	126(77.8)	36(22.2)	0(0)	0(0)	
Breast pain and distension	Students	80(31.6)	150(59.3)	17(6.7)	6(2.4)	0.094
	Mothers	31(19.1)	124(76.5)	5(3.1)	2(1.2)	
Headache	Students	158(62.5)	65(25.7)	26(10.3)	4(1.6)	0.088
	Mothers	112(69.1)	41(25.3)	9(5.6)	0(0)	
Low back pain	Students	123(48.6)	102(40.3)	22(8.7)	6(2.4)	0.750
	Mothers	71(43.8)	81(50.0)	9(5.6)	1(0.6)	
Hot flashes	Students	187(73.9)	56(22.1)	4(1.6)	6(2.4)	0.002
	Mothers	140(86.4)	21(13.0)	0(0)	1(0.6)	
Rough skin	Students	85(33.6)	136(53.8)	19(7.5)	13(5.1)	<0.001
	Mothers	82(50.6)	72(44.4)	6(3.7)	2(1.2)	
General fatigue/lack of energy	Students	51(20.2)	134(53.2)	55(21.8)	12(4.8)	<0.001
	Mothers	63(38.9)	92(56.8)	7(4.3)	0(0)	
Hypersomnia	Students	65(25.7)	112(44.3)	53(20.9)	23(9.1)	<0.001
	Mothers	80(49.4)	73(45.1)	9(5.6)	0(0.0)	
Insomnia	Students	215(85.0)	32(12.6)	5(2.0)	1(0.4)	0.119
	Mothers	146(90.1)	15(9.3)	1(0.6)	0(0)	
Constipation	Students	121(47.8)	95(37.5)	28(11.1)	9(3.6)	0.410
	Mothers	79(48.8)	70(43.2)	11(6.8)	2(1.2)	
Diarrhea	Students	152(60.3)	77(30.6)	20(7.9)	3(1.2)	0.105
	Mothers	106(65.4)	55(34.0)	1(0.6)	0(0)	
Overeating	Students	63(24.9)	68(26.9)	85(33.6)	37(14.6)	<0.001
	Mothers	88(55.0)	41(25.6)	17(10.6)	14(8.8)	
Desire for sweets	Students	61(24.8)	55(22.4)	87(35.4)	43(17.5)	<0.001
	Mothers	66(50.8)	35(26.9)	20(15.4)	9(6.9)	

Table 3. Psychological symptoms before menstruation in the students and their mothers (Students: n=253; Mothers: n=163).

Psychological symptom		Degree of symptom				p values
		Not at all	Mild	Moderate	Severe	
Irritability	Students	60(23.8)	113(44.8)	50(19.8)	29(11.5)	0.002
	Mothers	43(26.4)	100(61.3)	15(9.2)	5(3.1)	
Anger	Students	137(54.4)	82(32.5)	22(8.7)	11(4.4)	0.450
	Mothers	88(54.7)	64(39.8)	9(5.6)	0(0)	
Anxiety	Students	102(40.5)	100(39.7)	30(11.9)	20(7.9)	<0.001
	Mothers	115(70.6)	42(25.8)	6(3.7)	0(0)	
Depression	Students	82(32.5)	116(46.0)	31(12.3)	23(9.1)	<0.001
	Mothers	77(47.2)	82(50.3)	4(2.5)	0(0)	
Decreased interest in social relationships	Students	135(53.6)	86(34.1)	18(7.1)	13(5.2)	0.020
	Mothers	123(75.9)	38(23.5)	1(0.6)	0(0)	
Confusion/out of control	Students	213(84.5)	29(11.5)	7(2.8)	3(1.2)	0.020
	Mothers	149(92.0)	13(8.0)	0(0)	0(0)	

percentage of students who answered moderate to severe in physical symptoms was desire for sweets, followed by overeating and hypersomnia. The item with the highest percentage of mothers who answered moderate to severe symptoms was desire for sweets, followed by overeating. The degrees of physical symptoms including bloating, hot flashes, rough skin, general fatigue, hypersomnia, overeating and desire for sweets in the students were significantly greater than those in the mothers at the same age as the students.

As shown in Table 3, the item with the highest percentage of students who answered moderate to severe in emotional symptoms was irritability, followed by depression and anxiety. The item with the highest percentage of mothers who answered moderate to severe in emotional symptoms was irritability. The degrees of emotional symptoms including irritability, anxiety, depression, decreased interest in social relationships and confusion in the students were significantly greater than those in the mothers at the same age as the students.

Correlations between premenstrual symptoms between students and their mothers

Physical symptoms in the students were significantly correlated with those in the mothers at the same age as the students ($r=0.199$, $p=0.012$), but emotional symptoms in the students were not correlated with those in their mothers ($r=0.093$, $p=0.240$).

Coping with premenstrual symptoms

The proportion of the students who took measures to cope with premenstrual symptoms (54%) was higher than that of the mothers (29%). The measures taken to cope with premenstrual symptoms are shown in Table 4. The measures taken to cope with premenstrual symptoms were diversified in the students. The proportions of both students and mothers who answered "taking medicine" and "lying down" were high. The proportions of students who answered "consulting somebody" and "telling somebody that I am now before menstruation" were high. All of the 22 mothers who had taken medicine had used analgesic agents. Seventy-two students had used medicine, and 65 (90%) of the 72 students had taken analgesic agents as medicine. The students also used Japanese herbal medicines (8%), oral contraceptives (6%) and supplements (3%).

DISCUSSION

In the present study, it was shown that the

Table 4. Coping with premenstrual symptoms.

Coping measure	Students (n=118)	Mothers (n=44)
Lying down	58	18
Warming lower back and lower abdomen	33	14
Massage	25	5
Visiting a gynecologist	1	0
Taking medicine	72	22
Consulting somebody	17	0
Appropriate exercise	8	2
Sufficient sleep	40	8
Diversion to change mood	41	6
Refraining from favorite food	3	0
Refraining from caffeine	9	0
Restricting intake of water and salt	1	1
Telling somebody that you are now before menstruation	31	4

Multiple answers were allowed.

proportions of students who had moderate to severe physical symptoms and emotional symptoms were higher than those of the mothers at the same age as the students and that the degrees of the symptoms in the students were significantly greater than those in the mothers at the same age as the students. Physical symptoms in the students were significantly correlated with those in the mothers at the same age as the students. The proportion of students who took measures to cope with premenstrual symptoms was higher than that of the mothers at the same age as the students.

It was confirmed that the rate of recognition of premenstrual symptoms including PMS was extremely high (98%). Ogata and Daitou (2013) reported that the proportion of nursing students who recognized PMS was only 18.6% in the first grade but increase with advance of grade and reached 69.6% in nursing students in the fourth grade. Recognition of PMS by a high proportion of nursing students might be due to a high level of awareness of health care. Sakuma et al. (2008) reported that not only knowledge of menstrual disorders including premenstrual symptoms but also knowledge of health care was insufficient in non-medical vocational school students. Possible reasons for the relatively high rate of recognition in the nursing students' mothers are that the mothers obtained medical information through their daughters as nursing students and that the proportion of mothers working as medical staff was high.

It was shown that the proportions of nursing students with bloating, general fatigue, desire for sweets, overeating and hypersomnia in physical symptoms and with irritability and depression in emotional symptoms were high. In Iranian university students, the most common symptoms were tiredness, depression and anxiety in emotional symptoms and backache and bloating in physical symptoms (Bakhshani et al., 2009). Another study showed that mood lability, anger and sadness were the most frequent emotional symptoms and that acne was the most frequent physical symptom (Lajoie and Desindes, 2002). The most frequent symptoms in Turkish medical students were bloating, irritability and breast tenderness (Goker et al., 2015). The frequencies of physical symptoms in the present study were rather low compared to those in a previous study (Czajkowska et al., 2015). The differences in physical symptoms may be due to differences in race and lifestyle.

Compared to the results of a previous study for Japanese high school students, the frequencies of overeating, irritability, depression and decreased interest in social relationships were high in the present study (Takeda et al., 2010). In addition, compared to the results of a previous study for Japanese women whose mean age was 36 years, the frequencies of overeating, depression, decreased interest in social relationships, fatigue and hypersomnia were high in the present study (Takeda et al., 2006). The symptoms may change with advance in age.

The symptoms with significant differences between the students and mothers at the same age as the students were bloating, hot flashes, rough skin, general fatigue, hypersomnia, overeating and desire for sweets in physical symptoms and irritability, anxiety, depression, decreased interest in social relationships and confusion in emotional symptoms. The reasons for the differences are an increase in the general recognition of symptoms and availability of information on premenstrual symptoms. Students nowadays freely talk about premenstrual symptoms with their friends. However, their mothers about 30 years ago did not have opportunities to talk about menstrual disorders with their friends because of a lack of understanding of the symptoms. About 30 years ago Japanese women might have suppressed verbal expression of premenstrual symptoms in order to promote maintenance of social harmony.

According to the National Health and Nutrition Examination survey in 2014, the proportion of women aged 20 to 29 years who skipped breakfast was 23%, which was highest among all age groups, and the proportion of women aged 20 to 29 years who regularly did exercise was 10.1%, which was lowest among all age groups. Otsuka et al. (2015) reported that irregular sleeping was a risk factor for deterioration of premenopausal symptoms. Also, the proportion of women aged 20 to 29 years, whose sleeping time was less than 6 h was 45.1% in 2015, which was higher than the proportion in 2007, and the proportion of women aged 20 to 29 years who could not get adequate rest due to sleep disturbance was 24.5% in 2014, which was higher than that in 2012 (Ministry of Health, Labour and Welfare. National Health and Nutrition Examination survey, 2014). Thus, lifestyle has become irregular compared with that in the past. In addition, the proportion of women in whom psychological stress in daily life affected premenopausal symptoms was significantly higher for women being treated for PMS, suggesting that psychological stress as well as an irregular lifestyle were involved in the occurrence of PMS (Koda et al., 2012). According to the comprehensive survey of living conditions, the proportion of women who were suffering from stress (43.2%) in 1995 increased to 52.2% in 2013 (MHLW, 2013), and the proportion of women aged 20 to 29 years who were suffering from stress was 54.4%. The irregular lifestyle and increase in psychological stress may be involved in the intergenerational differences in degrees and types of premenstrual symptoms between the students and their mothers.

It was shown that measures taken to cope with premenstrual symptoms were diversified. Women can easily obtain information on coping with premenstrual symptoms through the internet. Also, various pharmacological treatments for PMS including treatments with oral contraceptives, selective serotonin reuptake inhibitors and gonadotropin-releasing hormone analogues have become available (Ryu and Kim, 2015). Students can get information on treatments for premenstrual symptoms through the internet, but they might easily believe the information without evidence. Selection of appropriate information regarding health care is needed. Communication with family and friends may also be needed. Exercise may improve emotional and physical premenstrual symptoms by increasing physical well-being (Delara et al., 2012). A previous study revealed beneficial effects of exercise on physical symptoms including breast tenderness and bloating (Daley, 2009). However, it was pointed out in that report that evidence-based recommendation regarding the effectiveness of exercise is needed because of the small sample size and low methodological quality in the study (Daley, 2009).

In the present study, a weak correlation was found between physical symptoms, but not between emotional symptoms, in the students and their mothers. Further study on predisposition of physical symptoms is needed. Ogata and Daitou (2013) reported that lifestyle-related factors such as no exercise habit, skipping breakfast, no mood change and short sleeping time were significantly associated with emotional symptoms. The fact that emotional symptoms are affected by individual lifestyle might be the reason for no correlation being found between emotional symptoms in the students and their mothers.

Derman et al. (2004) reported that there was an association between dysmenorrhea and PMS in adolescent girls aged 10 to 17 years and that 71% of the girls with dysmenorrhea had PMS. Kitamura et al. (2012) also reported that the prevalence rate of moderate to severe PMS increased with increase in the severity of dysmenorrhea. The reason for the correlation between PMS and dysmenorrhea has not been clarified. Prostaglandin (PG) may have a role in the biochemical etiologies in both PMS and dysmenorrhea. It has been reported that PGE2 and its receptor mediated elevated anxiety and social avoidance induced by repeated social defeat through attenuating a stress-coping action of the meso-prefrontal dopaminergic pathway (Tanaka et al., 2012). Haack et al. (2009) reported that increase in PGE2 metabolite levels in response to sleep loss was associated with the degree to which participants in their study reported spontaneous pain complaints. Lifestyle-related factors may influence both PMS and dysmenorrhea. It has been reported that the proportions of women with dysmenorrhea who skipped lunch and had a short sleeping time were significantly higher than those in women without dysmenorrhea (Yuasa et al., 2013). In the present study, the proportion of students with dysmenorrhea was higher than that of the mothers who had dysmenorrhea at the same age as the students, and the degree of pain in the students was higher than that in their mothers. Unfortunately, in the study questions regarding lifestyle were not asked so the association of lifestyle with dysmenorrhea could not be clarified.

This study has several limitations. A self-administered questionnaire was used to assess premenstrual symptoms. Therefore, the reliability of answers could not be verified. The recall bias of the mothers is of a serious nature. Retrospective recall regarding premenstrual symptoms at the time when mothers were about 20 years old is a limitation of this study. Since the contexts of behavior during menstruation may be changed by large time gaps, comparison between the nursing students and their mothers may not be valid. The subjects in this study were nursing students, who have basic medical knowledge. Therefore, further study in non-medical students is needed. The reasons for the drop-out were not known for there was no response on that since this study was a questionnaire survey. The results for the mothers who did not return the questionnaire form might be significant.

Conclusion

The degrees of physical symptoms and emotional symptoms in the students were greater than those in the mothers at the same age as the students, and measures taken to cope with these symptoms were diversified. The increasing availability of information on premenstrual symptoms and changes in lifestyle may contribute to the increase in prevalence of premenstrual symptoms.

CONFLICT OF INTERESTS

The authors have not declared any conflict of interests.

ACKNOWLEDGEMENT

The author extends their thanks to the nursing students and their mothers who made this study possible.

REFERENCES

Angst J, Sellaro R, Stolar M, Merikangas KR, Endicott J (2001). The epidemiology of perimenstrual psychological symptoms. Acta Psychiatr. Scand. 104:110-116.

Baker FC, Driver HS (2004). Self-reported sleep across the menstrual cycle in young, healthy women. J. Psychosom. Res. 56:239-243.

Bakhshani NM, Mousavi MN, Khodabandeh G (2009). Prevalence and severity of premenstrual symptoms among Iranian female university students. J. Pak. Med. Assoc. 59:205-208.

Bertone-Johnson EB, Whitcomb BW, Rich-Edwards JW, Hankinson SE, Manson JE (2015). Premenstrual syndrome and subsequent risk of hypertension in a prospective study. Am. J. Epidemiol. 182:1000-1009.

Czajkowska M, Drosdzol-Cop A, Galazka I, Naworska B, Skrzypulec-Plinta V (2015). Menstrual cycle and the prevalence of premenstrual syndrome/premenstrual dysphoric disorder in adolescent athletes. J. Pediatr. Adolesc. Gynecol. 28:492-498.

Daley A (2009). Exercise and premenstrual symptomatology: a comprehensive review. J. Womens Health 18:895-899.

Delara M, Ghofranipour F, Azadfallah P, Tavafian SS, Kazemnejad A, Montazeri A (2012). Health related quality of life among adolescents with premenstrual disorders: a cross sectional study. Health Qual. Life Outcomes 10(1):1.

Derman O, Kanbur NO, Tokur TE, Kutluk T (2004). Premenstrual syndrome and associated symptoms in adolescent girls. Eur. J. Obstet. Gynecol. Reprod. Biol. 116(2):201-206.

Dimmock PW, Wyatt KM, Jones PW, O'Brien PM (2000). Efficacy of selective serotonin-reuptake inhibitors in premenstrual syndrome: a systematic review. Lancet 356:1131-1136.

Goker A, Artunc-Ulkumen B, Aktenk F, Ikiz N (2015). Premenstrual syndrome in Turkish medical students and their quality of life. J. Obstet. Gynaecol. 35:275-278.

Grady-Weliky TA (2003). Clinical practice. Premenstrual dysphoric disorder. N. Engl. J. Med. 348:433-438.

Haack M, Lee E, Cohen D, Mullington JM (2009). Activation of the prostaglandin system in response to sleep loss in healthy humans: Potential mediator of increased spontaneous pain. Pain 145:136-141.

Kitamura M, Takeda T, Koga S, Nagase S, Yaegashi N (2012). Relationship between premenstrual symptoms and dysmenorrhea in Japanese high school students. Arch. Womens Ment. Health 15:131-133.

Koda C, Takahashi M, Koda K, Sadamoto K (2012). Differences in premenstrual symptoms and life styles between healthy women and patients diagnosed with premenstrual syndrome. J. Jpn. Soc. Psychosom Obstet. Gynecol. 17:112-120.

Lajoie F, Desindes S (2002). Improving treatment for premenstrual syndrome. Can. J. CME 14(8):81-94.

Ministry of Health, Labour and Welfare (MHLW) (2013). Comprehensive survey of living conditions, 2013. Available at:http://www1.mhlw.go.jp/toukei/ksk/htm/ksk016.html

Ministry of Health, Labour and Welfare. National Health and Nutrition Examination survey (2014). http://www.mhlw.go.jp/file/04-Houdouhappyou-10904750-KenkoukyokuGantaisakukenkouzoushinka/0000117311.pdf

Mori K, Kawase K, Yoshizaki A, Wada M, Matsumoto S (2004). A study of premenstrual syndrome in mature Japanese women and their life-styles. J. Jpn. Soc. Psychosom. Obstet. Gynecol. 9:134-145.

Nagata C, Hirokawa K, Shimizu N, Shimizu H (2004). Soy, fat and other dietary factors in relation to premenstrual symptoms in Japanese women. BJOG 111:594-599.

Ogata T, Daitou M (2013). The study on the actual situation of female college student's premenstrual syndrome and their personal lifestyle and self-care. J. Kyushu Univ. Nurs. Soc. Welfare 13(1):57-65.

Otsuka Y, Takahara M, Sakuragi S (2015). Risk Factors Related to the Onset and Aggravation of Premenstrual Syndrome. Bull. Aichi Univ. Educ. 64:27-31.

Rapkin AJ, Winer SA (2009). Premenstrual syndrome and premenstrual dysphoric disorder: quality of life and burden of illness. Expert Rev. Pharmacoecon Outcomes Res. 9(2):157-70.

Ryu A, Kim TH (2015). Premenstrual syndrome: A mini review. Maturitas 82:436-440.

Sakuma Y, Kanoya Y, Ishimitsu F, Hosona M, Mochizuki Y, Sato C (2008). The Factors Affecting Premenstrual and Menstrual Symptoms Among Young Women-Comparison of the Lifestyle/Health Behavior in Nursing Students and Non-medical Vocational School Student. J. Jpn. Soc. Nurs. Res. 31(2):25-36.

Tadakawa M, Takeda T, Monma Y, Koga S, Yaegashi N (2016). The prevalence and risk factors of school absenteeism due to premenstrual disorders in Japanese high school students –a school-based cross sectional study. Biol. Psychol. Soc. Med. 10:13.

Takeda T, Koga S, Yaegashi N (2010). Prevalence of premenstrual syndrome and premenstrual dysphoric disorder in Japanese high school students. Arch. Womens Ment. Health 13:535-537.

Takeda T, Tasaka K, Sakata M, Murata Y (2006). Prevalence of premenstrual syndrome and premenstrual dysphoric disorder in Japanese women. Arch. Womens Ment. Health 9:209-212.

Tanaka K, Furuyashiki T, Kitaoka S, Senzai Y, Imoto Y, Segi-Nishida E, Deguchi Y, Breyer RM, Breyer MD, Narumiya S (2012). Prostaglandin E2-mediated attenuation of mesocortical dopaminergic pathway is critical for susceptibility to repeated social defeat stress in mice. J. Neurosci. 32:4319-4329.

Tasali E, Leproult R, Ehrmann DA, Van Cauter E (2008). Slow-wave sleep and the risk of type 2 diabetes in humans. Proc. Natl. Acad. Sci. USA 105:1044-1049.

Yonkers KA, O'Brien PMS, Eriksson E (2008). Premenstrual syndrome. Lancet 371:1200-1210.

Yuasa Y, Kobayashi Y, Niibori T, Hatsushika S, Akedo Y (2013). Examination of the lifestyle-related factors affecting on menstrual symptoms. Int. J. Hum. Cult. Stud. 23:282-286.

Disparities in adverse pregnancy outcomes between advanced maternal age and younger age in Ethiopia

Mekiya Ediris[1*], Tefera Belachew[2], Fekadu Yadassa[3] and Kidest Getu[3]

[1]Department of Midwifery, College of Health Sciences and Medicine, Wolaita Sodo University, Wolaita Sodo, Ethiopia.
[2]Department of Population and Family Health, College of Health Sciences, Jimma University, Jimma, Ethiopia.
[3]Department of Nursing and Midwifery, College of Health Sciences, Jimma University Jimma, Ethiopia.

Women older than 35 years are known to beat "advanced maternal age" and considered to be at risk of adverse pregnancy outcome. Data on adverse birth outcomes and the risk factors are still scarce in developing countries including Ethiopia. The aim of this study was to examine the obstetrical outcomes among primiparous and multiparous women of advanced age (35 and above) when compared to the younger age group (20 to 34) and identify its predictors among women delivering at public health facilities of Shashemene Town, Ethiopia. Institution based comparative cross sectional study were conducted from March to April, 2016. A consecutive sampling technique was employed to select 306 study participants. Data were collected using pretested structured questionnaires through face to face interview and checklist. Data were entered into Epi-data version 3.1 and analyzed using SPSS version 20.0. Logistic regression analyses were used to identify associated factors. A total of 306 mothers were involved in this study with response rate of 100%. Advanced maternal age, antenatal follow up, mode of current delivery and previous caesarian section were factors associated with adverse pregnancy outcome.

Key words: Adverse pregnancy outcome, advanced maternal age, participants.

INTRODUCTION

Globally, women and children are among the most vulnerable in terms of unfavorable influences in the environment including insufficient nutrition, inadequate health care and poor education. In addition, pregnancy brings those factors as high risk for women. Worldwide, it is estimated that more than 50 million women suffer from poor reproductive health and serious pregnancy related complications (Tesfay et al., 2015).

Mothers age 35 and above at estimated date of delivery is known to be old maternal age (Yogev et al., 2010). Older age is risk factor for decreasing fertility and increasing miscarriage. For women who succeed in

*Corresponding author. E-mail: mekediris@gmail.com.

conception at higher age, the risk of complication during pregnancy and delivery is high (Almhfooth et al., 2013). Older pregnant mothers have an increased risk of pregnancy, labour complications and adverse fetal outcome. Medical complications like hypertensive disorders, gestational diabetes and preterm birth and labour related complications like induction of labour, prolonged labour and hemorrhage are the most common ones. This aged group mothers mostly delivered with caesarean section and their children will have a higher risk of congenital anomalies and will face fetal and neonatal mortality (Tromp et al., 2010). Even if the issue is essential and its effect is bad to the mother and fetus, studies on this area lack adequate data. Therefore this study aimed to compare pregnancy outcomes between advanced maternal age and younger age and identify predicting factors among women delivering at public health facilities of Shashemene Town.

MATERIALS AND METHODS

Study setting and study period

Shashemene town is situated in West Arsi Zone in Oromia Regional State, Ethiopia ("CSA-Ethiopia", 2012). The city lies on the trans-African highway 4 of Cairo-Cape town, about 150 miles (240 km) from Addis Ababa. Based on the 2007 population Census, the population size of Shashemene were 102,062 of which 51,477(50.4%) are males and 50,585 (49.6%) are females. According to the Central Statistical Agency of 2005, females 35.2% (16,288.5) were in reproductive age group (15 to 49), the total fertility rate was 4.2. The population expected for 2013 using the census data in 2007, was 129,084, of which 65,091 were men and 63,993 were women.

Study design and population

A comparative cross sectional study was conducted on pregnancy outcomes among women aged 20 to 34 years and 35^{+} delivering at public health facilities in Shashemene town. All pregnant mothers who gave birth at public health facilities of Shashemene town, Ethiopia, from March to April, 2016 were taken as source population and selected mothers who gave birth during the study period at public health facilities of Shashemene town, Ethiopia taken as study population. All mothers 20 years and above who gave birth at public health facilities of Shashemene town, Ethiopia during data collection period were included and women who were seriously ill and unable to respond were not included in the study.

Ethical consideration

Ethical clearance was obtained from the Institutional Review Board (IRB) of Jimma University College of Health Sciences to shashemene town health facility authorities. Permission letters were obtained from Shashemene Referral Hospital and Melkaoda Hospital Administration, after the objectives of the study were explained, consent was obtained from head of maternal and child health unit. Written and verbal consent were taken from selected participant to validate willingness to participate in the study before the interview. Privacy and confidentiality were ensured by using coding.

Sampling technique

A comparative cross sectional study was conducted among women aged 20 to 34 years and 35^{+} delivering at public health facilities in the town.

Data collection tools

Data were collected using pretested and structured questionnaire and through chart review. Questionnaire contained socio demographic, obstetrics, medical history and other characteristics.

Data analysis and quality control

Collected data were entered into Epi data version 3.1 and exported to SPSS version 20.0 for analysis. After cleaning data for inconsistencies and missing value in SPSS, binary logistic regressions with p value < 0.25 were transferred to multivariable logistic regression. Variables with p value < 0.05 were considered significant variable. Training for data collectors, pretest and supervision were undertaken to control data quality.

RESULTS

Socio demographic characteristics of the respondent

Three hundred and six study participants participated with a response rate of 100%. The mean age of women (20 to 34) was 24.39 (SD ± 3.865). Regarding residence in the age group 20 to 34, 88 (50.3%) were living in urban. Married women between age 20 to 34 was 151. Those mothers who can read and write were 49(32.02) and 31(20.2) in both age group, respectively. Oromo was the dominant ethnicity is the study area with 110 (71.89%) and 102 (66.69%). Majority of participants in both age group were housewives in their occupation 116 (48.7%), 112(79.7%) and their Income ranged from 1801 to 3000 48.3 (31.37%) (Table 1).

Obstetric characteristics of participants

Majority of normal reproductive age group participants are multigravida which accounts for 92(41.3) and 131(58.7) in advance reproductive age group. Moreover, multiparas were 86(41.1%) and 123(58.9%). Those mothers with 1 to 3 antenatal visits were 89(50.9%) and 86(49.1%), respectively. Mothers who took iron/folic acid during antenatal care visit were 98(44.1%) and 124(55.9%). For mothers in both age group, their current mode of delivery of SVD was 112(73.2%) and 106(26.8). Current labour with no complication in advanced age group was 129(84.3%) (Table 2).

Medical related complications of the respondents

Advanced reproductive age group mothers who do not

Table 1. Sociodemographic characteristics of participants in women attending public health facilities of Shashemene Town, Ethiopia, 2016 (N =153).

Variable	Normal reproductive age group (20-34) N (%)	Advanced reproductive age group (35-49) N (%)
Residence		
Rural	65(49.6%)	66(43.1%)
Urban	88(50.3%)	87(56.86%)
Marital status		
Married	151(98.69)	152(99.34)
Others[1]	2(1.31%)	1(0.65%)
Educational status		
Can't read and write	35(22.87)	39(25.49)
Can read and write only	49(32.03)	31(20.26)
Elementary	38(24.8)	47(30.72)
Secondary	14(9.1)	25(16.34)
College and above	17(11.11)	11(7.19)
Ethnicity		
Oromo	110(71.89)	102(66.66)
Amhara	26(16.99)	28(18.3)
Silte	11(7.19)	15(9.8)
Gurage	5(3.28)	9(5.88)
Others [2]	1(0.65)	9(5.88)
Occupation		
Housewife	116(48.7)	122(79.74)
Merchant	17(51.5)	16(10.46)
Others[3]	20(13.07)	15(9.8)
Income		
300-1000	44(28.76)	46(30.06)
1001-1800	43(28.1)	27(17.64)
18001-3000	48(31.37)	48(31.37)
>3000	18(11.76)	32(20.9)

Others[1]- Single, widowed
Others[2]- Wolayita, Hadiya, Tigire, Kambata
Others[3]- farmer, daily labour

report medical illness before pregnancy was 136(88.88). Whereas in both age group from those who reported previous medical illness 22(14.37) and 17(11.11) anemia is commonly mentioned one 17(11.11) and 6(3.92) respectively (Table 3).

Frequency of maternal adverse pregnancy outcomes of the respondent

While comparing the prevalence of adverse maternal pregnancy outcomes among women aged 20 to 34 and 35^{+}, the risks were high among advanced maternal age (Table 4).

Frequency of fetal adverse pregnancy outcomes of the respondent

Adverse pregnancy outcome at normal reproductive age group was 45(29.41%) and in advanced age group it was 62(40.5%). Adverse fetal outcomes were more at advanced maternal age in comparison with normal reproductive age group except still birth which was the

Table 2. Obstetric characteristics of participants in women attending public health facilities of Shashemene Town, Ethiopia, 2016 (N= 153).

Variable	Normal reproductive age group (20-34) N (%)	Advanced reproductive age group (35-49) N (%)
Gravidity		
Primigravida	61(73.5)	22(26.5)
Multigravida	92(41.3)	131(58.7)
Parity		
Multipara	86(41.1%)	123(58.9)
Primiparous	67(69.1%)	30(30.9)
Number of visit		
1-3	89(50.9)	86(49.1)
>=4	31(38.3)	50(61.7)
Take Iron /folic acid during ANC		
Yes	98(44.1)	124(55.9)
No	55(65.5)	29(34.5)
Mode of current delivery		
SVD	112(73.2)	106(26.8)
Caesarian section	41(46.6)	47(53.4)
Current labor have any problem or complication		
Yes	26(16.99)	24(15.69)
No	127(83)	129(84.3)
Type of complication		
Prolonged labor	13(8.49)	8(5.23)
Mal position or mal presentation	8(5.23)	11(7.19)
Obstructed labor	2(1.31)	4(2.61)
Others	4(2.61)	2(1.31)

[2]Obstructed labour, Failure of VBAC, uterine rupture, Postterm, APH.

same frequency among the two age group (Table 5). In binary multiple logistic regression age, education, ethnicity, occupation, outcome of last delivery, previous caesarian section and antenatal follow up showed association with p value < 0.2, these variables transferred to multivariate logistic regression then age, antenatal follow up, previous caesarian section and mode of current labour showed significant association with p value < 0.05 (Table 6).

DISCUSSION

The study revealed that the prevalence of adverse pregnancy outcomes was 45(29.41%) and 62(40.5%) among mothers aged 20 to 34 and 35^{+}, respectively. This study showed that adverse pregnancy outcomes were highly prevalent in advanced maternal age when compared to younger age group. The study done in Norway from 2004 to 2007 ruled out that the prevalence of adverse pregnancy outcomes among advanced maternal age was 33.4% (Laopaiboon et al., 2014). Another study conducted in Taiwan found that the prevalence is from 11.4 to 19.1% (Jahromi and Husseini, 2008). A large, population-based cohort study in the UK showed an 18.2% prevalence of adverse pregnancy outcome among maternal ages of 35 years or older (Kenny et al., 2013).

The prevalence of hypertensive disorder of pregnancy in advanced maternal age was higher when compared to their younger counterparts. This study was similar to the study conducted in Nigeria (Liou et al., 2010). This might

Table 3. Medical related complications of women attending public health facilities of Shashemene Town, Ethiopia, 2016. N =153.

Variable	Age	
	Normal reproductive age group (20-34)	Advanced reproductive age group (35-49)
	N (%)	N (%)
Medical illness before pregnancy		
Yes	22(14.37)	17(11.11)
No	131(85.6)	136(88.88)
Type of medical illness		
Anemia	17(11.11)	6(3.92)
Malaria	0(0.0)	3(1.96)
Upper urinary tract infection	4(2.61)	2(1.31)
Chronic hypertension	1(0.65)	2(1.31)
Diabetes mellitus	0(0.0)	4(2.61)
On treatment		
Yes	17(11.11)	13(8.49)
No	136(88.88)	140(91.5)

be due to the reason that old age is one of a risk factor for pregnancy induced hypertensive disorder.

The prevalence of postpartum hemorrhage in advanced maternal age was higher when compared to their younger counter parts. This study was supported by the study done in Israel (Tesfay et al., 2015). Also according to Laopaiboon et al. (2014), the prevalence of caesarian delivery was 6 times higher among advanced maternal age when compared to younger mother. Study done in Nigeria supports this result; advanced age has higher incidence of cesarean delivery than their counterparts (Bako et al., 2013). These two findings can be based on the reason that advanced age women are more likely to be grand multi-para and this may lead them to face postpartum hemorrhage due to uterine atony. Obstructed labour, prolonged labour, mal presentation and related fetal complications which is more common in advanced maternal age may lead them to caesarean section than their counter part.

Adverse fetal outcome like low birth weight, preterm birth, Apgar score 5 min < 7, congenital anomaly, admission to neonatal intensive care unit (NICU) and fetal death are highly related with advanced age group. This result is similar with a study conducted in Turkey which ruled out that advanced maternal age were significantly associated with fetal complication and Apgar score 5 min < 7 (Lamminpää, 2015). Similarly, study conducted in Flemish found that advanced maternal age were associated with very preterm and low birth weight (Delbaere et al., 2007).

Advanced maternal age (35^{+}) was 2 times risky of wide range of adverse pregnancy out come when compared to mothers in normal reproductive age group (20 to 34). The result is in line with a case control study conducted in Iran, which revealed that advanced maternal age of 40 and above were more complicated by maternal and neonatal complication (Khalil et al., 2013). A retrospective study done in Spain supports this result (Jahromi and Husseini, 2008). In this study antenatal care follow up was significantly associated with adverse pregnancy outcome. Studies done in Gondar University Hospital, Northwest Ethiopia rule out that lack of ANC follow up were associated with adverse pregnancy outcome like still birth (Adane et al., 2014).

A prospective study done at University Hospital UZ Brussels proved that lack of antenatal follow up was associated with adverse pregnancy outcome like preterm (Beeckman et al., 2012). Mode of current labour is significantly associated with adverse pregnancy outcome. Most mothers who came to this hospital were referred from health center with complication that leads to caesarian section. Mothers who deliver by caesarian section were more risky to develop adverse pregnancy outcome than those who delivered by spontaneous vaginal delivery. Caesarian section is a major operation which can be associated with significant maternal and fetal, morbidity and mortality. This can be due to the fact that bleeding in caesarian section is higher than vaginal delivery, this can lead mother to risk of death (Arulkumaran, 2016).

Conclusion

In this study, adverse pregnancy outcome is high in advanced maternal age. Postpartum hemorrhage and Hypertensive disorders are mostly observed adverse outcomes in advanced maternal age. Age, antenatal

Table 4. Frequency of maternal adverse pregnancy outcomes of women attending public health facilities of Shashemene Town, Ethiopia, 2016.

Variable	Age	
	Normal reproductive age group (20-34) N (%)	Advanced reproductive age group (35^+) N (%)
Pregnancy induced hypertension		
Yes	18(46.2)	21(53.8)
No	135(50.6)	132(49.4)
Type of pregnancy induced hypertension		
Gestational Hypertension	9(42.9)	2(57.1)
Preeclampsia	7(50)	7(50)
Eclampsia	2(50)	2(50)
Ante partum hemorrhage		
Yes	19(57.6)	14(42.4)
No	134(49.3)	139(50.7)
Post-partum hemorrhage		
Yes	23(48.9)	24(51.1)
No	130(50.2)	129(49.8)
Instrumental delivery		
Forceps	3(2%)	2(1.3)
Induction		
Yes	150(98)	151(98.7)
No	25(59.5)	17(40.5)
Cesarean section		
Yes	126(48.5)	136(51.5)
No	41(46.6)	47(53.4)
Indication for cesarean section		
Previous cesarean section	12(46.2)	14(53.8)
Fetal distress	20(43.5)	26(56.5)
Others[2]	7(58.3	5(41.7)

[2]Obstructed labour, Failure of VBAC, uterine rupture, Postterm, APH

Table 5. Frequency of fetal adverse pregnancy outcomes among women at public health facilities of Shashemene Town, Ethiopia 2016.

Variable	Age	
	Normal reproductive age group (20-34) N (%)	Advanced reproductive age group (35 and above) N (%)
Neonatal condition		
Live birth	143(93.5)	143(50)
Still birth	10(0)	10(50)

Table 5. Cont'd.

Gestational age		
Term	146(50.7)	142(49.3)
Preterm	5(45.5)	6(54.5)
Post term	2(28.6)	5(71.4)
Current pregnancy condition		
Single	152(50.3)	150(49.7)
Others	1(33.3)	2(66.7)
Twins	0(0)	1(100)
Birth weight (g)		
<1500	1(14.3)	6(85.7)
1500-2500	4 (28.6)	10(71.4)
2500-4000	145(52.5)	131(47.5)
≥4000	3(33.3)	6(66.7)
5 minute APGAR score <7		
Yes	13(27.7)	34(72.3)
No	140(54.1)	119(45.9)
Congenital anomaly		
Yes	7(33.3)	14(66.7)
No	146(51.2)	139(48.8)
Death	2(28.6)	5(77.4)

Table 6. Multivariable logistic regression Analysis of Adverse pregnancy outcome among women age 20-34 and 35$^+$ delivering at public health facilities of Shashemene Town, Ethiopia 2016.

Predictor		P value	AOR	95% C.I. for EXP(B)	
				Lower	Upper
Age	20-34 35$^+$	0.026	1.00 1.883	1.078	3.288
Antenatal follow up	Yes No	0.004	1.00 3.902	1.529	9.960
Previous caesarian section	No Yes	0.000	1.00 0.094	0.027	0.321
Mode of current labour	SVD Caesarian section	0.002	1.00 3.381	1.581	7.234

follow up, mode of current delivery and previous caesarian section are risk factors for adverse pregnancy outcome.

CONFLICT OF INTERESTS

The authors have not declared any conflict of interests.

REFERENCES

Adane AA, Ayele TA, Ararsa LG, Bitew BD, Zeleke BM (2014). Adverse birth outcomes among deliveries at Gondar University hospital, Northwest Ethiopia. BMC Pregnancy Childbirth 14(1):90.

Almhfooth WF, Cabog D, Dahos MB (2013). Advance Maternal Age and Pregnancy Outcome. Karbala J. Med. 6(1):1531-1538.

Arulkumaran S (2016). Best practice in labour and delivery: Cambridge University Press.

Bako B, Umaru I, Geidam AD, Garba MA (2013). Pregnancy outcome in elderly primigravidae at the University of Maiduguri Teaching Hospital, Maiduguri, Nigeria. International Journal of Medicine and Medical 3(7):476-480.

Beeckman K, Louckx F, Downe S, Putman K (2012). The relationship between antenatal care and preterm birth: the importance of content of care. European Journal of Public Health 23(3):366-371.

Delbaere I, Verstraelen H, Goetgeluk S, Martens G, De Backer G, Temmerman M (2007). Pregnancy outcome in primiparae of advanced maternal age. European Journal of Obstetrics andGynecology and Reproductive Biology 135(1):41-46.

Jahromi BN, Husseini Z (2008). Pregnancy outcome at maternal age 40 and older. Taiwanese Journal of Obstetrics and Gynecology 47(3):318-321.

Kenny LC, Lavender T, McNamee R, O'Neill SM, Mills T, Khashan AS (2013). Advanced maternal age and adverse pregnancy outcome: evidence from a large contemporary cohort. PloS one 8(2):e56583.

Khalil A, Syngelaki A, Maiz N, Zinevich Y, Nicolaides KH (2013). Maternal age and adverse pregnancy outcome: a cohort study. Ultrasound in Obstetrics and Gynecology 42(6):634-643.

Lamminpää R (2015). Advanced maternal age, pregnancy and birth. PhD. University of Eastern Finland.

Laopaiboon M, Lumbiganon P, Intarut N, Mori R, Ganchimeg T, Vogel JP, Souza JP, Gülmezoglu AM (2014). Advanced maternal age and pregnancy outcomes: A multicountry assessment. International Journal of Obstetrics and Gynaecology 121(s1):49-56.

Liou JD, Hsu JJ, Lo LM, Chen SF, Hung TH (2010). Advanced maternal age and adverse perinatal outcomes in an Asian population. European Journal of Obstetrics and Gynecology and Reproductive Biology 148(1):21-26.

Tesfay K, Gebrehiwot H, Bruh G, Fantahun A (2015). Health promotion practice and its associated factors among pregnant mothers attending ANC services in public health institution of Mekelle City. Tigray Ethiopia 4:18-25.

Tromp M, Ravelli A, Reitsma J, Bonsel G, Mol B (2010). Increasing maternal age at first pregnancy planning: health outcomes and associated costs. Journal of Epidemiology and Community Health 2010:095422.

Yogev Y, Melamed N, Bardin R, Tenenbaum-Gavish K, Ben-Shitrit G, Ben-Haroush A (2010). Pregnancy outcome at extremely advanced maternal age. American Journal of Obstetrics and Gynecology 203(6):558.e1-7.

The effect of the health-based supportive plan on primiparous mothers' performance in neonatal care

Sima Kermanshahi

Department of Nursing, Tarbiat Modarres University, Tehran, Iran.

Infancy is the most vulnerable period of life often faced with mortality and morbidity. Appropriate care is important for maintaining and improving the health of newborns. Therefore, this study was designed to determine the effect of health-based supportive plan on the performance of primiparous mothers in the care of infants. This is a quazi-experimental study with two groups of intervention (30) and control (33) selected by census. Data were collected by a demographic information questionnaire designed to assess the primaparous mothers'knowledge and practice of infant care. The designed plan for the intervention group consisted of three stages (recognition, support and evaluation). The results were analyzed and compared with the control group by the SPSS software (ver. 16). Chi-square test demonstrated that the two groups were identical in terms of the demographic variables of age, job, education level and being a housewife. The knowledge level of performance in the two groups before intervention was not significant ($p>0.05$).The independant T-test and Chi-square showed significant differences between the maternal action and fetal complications in both groups after the intervention ($p<0.05$). The results showed that the designed plan was effective in maternal performance of infant care suggesting that the support program is an effective method for improving maternal and neonatal health.

Key words: Health-based supportive plan, primiparous mothers, neonatal care.

INTRODUCTION

In all societies, improvement in individual health and wellbeing of both society and persons is crucial for maximum social and economic capacity.Infants' health determines the future of the country and is of special importance, indicating the health and welfare of the future of society (Mirgafoorvand and Mohammad Alizadeh, 2000). Childhood consists of several phases with the newborn period identified as the most vulnerable period needs to be recognized as a critical phase of development for physiological accommodation for the out of uterus life and for potential congenital illness and other issues that threaten life and normal development. These occur more frequently in this period, as well as deaths and accidents when compared to other phases of life (Nelson Textbook of Pediatrics, 2006).The World Health Organization (WHO, 2012) has declared that annually approximately 40% of all deaths below the age of 5 occur foundation of infants'health (Beake et al., 2010).This

E-mail: kerkerman_s@modares.ac.ir.

among newborn infants that 3.4 of them die in the first week and more than 1.4 in the first 24 h after birth (Jehan et al., 2009; Boskabadi et al., 2010; Lawn et al., 2009). According to WHO, in the Islamic Republic of Iran, the rate of newborn death in 2006 was equal to 13.3 out of 1000 births (World Health Organization (WHO), 2008). Based on the statistics of the Ministry of Health in Iran, 13 to 15 newborns die per 24 h. In other words, about 20,000 newborns die before the age of one month annually (Ministry of Health, 2008). The mortality index in Tehran has been 23.8 since 1990. Despite the fact that newborn mortality has been increasingly declining in recent decades, it still accounts for 65% of deaths below the one year (Ghorat et al., 2016).

According to the WHO's "Hygiene for Everyone Program", the Third Millennium Development Goal, all countries in the world are committed to improve infants' health (World Health Organization, 2001), and infant mortality should be decreased by 2.3% up to 2015. To achieve this goal, mortality rate among newborns should decrease to less than 8 cases in 1000 births by 2015. Despite numerous activities during the two recent decades, the death index of newborns has not significantly decreased and has not met the Third Millennium Goal based on the WHO recommendations and international commitments. Effective interventions should be implemented with the aim of lessening newborn mortality (Kiasari et al., 2009). Previous studies show that newborn mortality can be prevented by up to 70% by improving conditions (Titaley et al., 2008). Reduction in newborn mortality rates has been noted with the implementation of special prenatal care (Ballard, 2000; Curley and Halliday, 2001; Eichenwald and Stark, 1999). Efforts must be made to prepare for protecting and promotion of a high level health in newborns as a vulnerable group requiring special attention in health care (Dadipoor et al., 2014). Inaccessibility of care in human violates the rights of the newborn. Care requires prioritizing hygiene and prevention as well as efficient treatment and training of persons in health care (Chiabi et al., 2014).

Therefore, mothers' health awareness and health care before and after childbirth affects mother's and infants'health, and is the most important factor in preventing undesirable health problem of the mother and newborn (Chiabi et al., 2014; Boskabadi et al., 2010). Many multiparous mothers are not neccesarily ready for becoming a mother and need family, friends and assistance with hygiene (Cronin and McCarthy, 2003). Klein (1998) also belived that mothers usually feel weak after delivery and need more information for taking care of themselves and their children (Kline et al., 1998). In new postnatal situations, mothers are faced with responsibilities and new problems, creating the need for new knowledge (Mohseni et al., 2009). As primiparous mothers are inexperienced and may be unaware of what is needed, their level of readiness and awareness has an important effect on the newborns' health. Thus it is necessary to pay more attention to mother and newborn health improvement programs. An evidence-based program to improve the mothers'performance of newborn care was designed with the aim of determining the effect of the health-based supportive plan on the performance of primiparous mothers in newborn care.

MATERIALS AND METHODS

This study is a quazi-experimental intervention design that was conducted with the participation of 70 primiparous mothers in 2013 to 2014. Sampling was done by census method. Data collection tools consisted of a demographic questionnaire, knowledge assessment tool, and a mothers'performance checklist in the field of prevention and care of jaundice, colic, respiratory aspiration and diaper dermatitis. The validity of the data collection tools was established by the method of content validity and by 10 members of the faculty of the Department of Nursing and Midwifery of Medical Faculty of Shiraz and TarbiatModares University.The reliability of knowledge assessment tool was calculated as 0.84 through renewed examination with test -retest, and the reliability of performance tool through simultaneous examination between the two groups was 0.87.

The designed program consisted of three stages (recognition, support and evaluation) before and after childbirth. After entering the center, a list of all mothers that had inclusion criteria (being primiparous, singleton pregnancy, and mothers who were not physically or mentally impaired at pregnancy), was prepared. Their phone number was obtained, and next referral to the center was recorded. About the control group, the researcher referred to the center and talked with the mothers face to face about the program, and all of participants signed written informed consent prior to their participation.The demographic information questionnaire and educational need assessment were collected.After completing and delivering these questionnaires, a survey checklist of mothers' performance after childbirth was left with them, and how and when to complete it was explained. In the test group, explanations about the goals'study method and intervention time duration (from 7 to 8 months before delivery to one month after childbirth) were given to them.This was explained via phone, and questions were answered clearly to dissolve ambiguity.

They were then invited to the first session of the class. In the first session, the data of demographic information and the assessment questionnaire (related to jaundice, aspiration, colic and diaper dermatitis) were gathered to determine the educational needs of mothers and to compare the knowledge level of the two groups before beginning the intervention. The knowledge level of the two groups was compared with no significant difference. After the mothers' educational needs were identified, the intervention program in second stage (physical, educational and emotional support) started. Mothers who were 7 to 8 months pregnant were in the training class. The class period was 1 to 1.5 h. The elements of educational support for the intervention group included mothers' role and self-care in the recent months of pregnancy (proper breastfeeding, activity, etc.), type of delivery and benefits and problems, and postpartum self care (breast care,suture care, personal hygiene, and nutrition), as well as care of newborn (umbilical cord care, bathing, restraint of neonate, etc.). The program also delivered education on the mothers' role, the most relevant newborn problems (jaundice, infantile colic, dermatitis caused by clothing and aspiration), their causes and treatment, and the role of participating fathers to deliver emotional and physical support to the mother and newborn after childbirth. The classes were both theoretical and practical. The first 15 min of every

Table 1. Relative and absolute frequencies distribution of maternal in terms of demographic characteristics between the two groups.

Demographic data		Test	Control	χ square
Age	30 years<	26 (87)	27 (82)	0.59
	> 30 years	4 (13)	6 (18)	
	Total	30 (100)	33 (100)	
Literacy	< Diploma	5 (17)	6(18)	0.65
	Diploma	12 (40)	17(52)	
	>Bachelor	13 (43)	10(30)	
	Total	100	100	
Mothers' job	Housewife	28(93)	26(79)	0.16
	Employed	2(7)	7(21)	
	Total	100	100	
Delivery type	Normal delivery	9(30)	5(15)	0.22
	Elective caesarean	4(13)	9(27)	
	Emergency cesarean	17(57)	19(58)	
	Total	30 (100)	33 (100)	

session was allocated to review the information of the previous session, answer the mothers'questions, and correcting mothers'false beliefs.The learning level of the participants was evaluated by asking the mothers some specific questions. In these classes, the mothers talked about their anxieties related to childbirth and the expectations of health workers. At the end of each session, there was time for questions and discussion, and the time of the next session was determined with the mothers' agreement. Individual counsult, in person or by phone, was possible after class. At the last session, the mothers were instructed on how to use a performance checklist on newborn care. During the interval between finishing the classes and childbirth, there were contact with the mothers and they were asked their physical and mental health status; their anxiety and stress was decrease by talking with them and encouraging the fathers' to engage in the mothers' care. The mothers had given the nurse's phone number to one of their support persons who were instructed to call her whenever the mother's labor pain began. If it was possible and the authorities cooperated, the nurse visited the mothers in the maternity ward, tried to reduce their anxiety, and immediately after delivery, accompanied them to the ward.

The mother was asked to give an educational pamphlet to her husband in order to increase his knowledge.At least one postpartum home visit was made to all the women. Future visits depended on the nurses' discretion and if there were problems, the numbers of visits were increased. During the home visit, the mothers'total health and the newborns' health were assessed, and a record of the mothers'appetite, sleep and bowel status was taken. For the newborns, skin condition and signs of colic, mothers' capability to calm her neonate and bathing were assessed by the nurse on an observation form. During the home visit, the nurse assessed the maternal and neonatal complications and devised a care plan. If the problem did not clear up, the nurse then made a referral to the mother's need.This care continued to the end of the neonatal period.During the neonatal period, the mothers filled out the assessment performance checklist. The nurses phoned the mothers once a week to assess the relationship of mother and neonate, recall the mothers'essensial caring points,and record her knowledge.The control group did not receive any of these interventions but their check lists were filled out independently and they were only called once after childbirth.

RESULTS

Most of the participants in the test (87%) and control (82%) groups had less than 30 years, had diploma (test group 40% and control group 52%), and were housewives (test group 93% and control group 79%). Most of the partipcants in the test group (57%) and in control group (58%) have had emergency cesarean delivery, and the Chi-square test results showed no significant differences between the two groups in terms of delivery (p=0.22). But the rate of normal delivery in the test group (30%) was more than in the control group (15%).The rate of elective cesarean in the test group (13%) was less than in the control group (27%). Also the rate of natural childbirth in the test group was twice the control group, and only 13% of the test group mothers' preferable childbirth has been cesarean, while in the control group, cesarean has been twice (Table 1).

Before intervention, 23.1% of the mothers in the test group and 18.6% of the mothers in the control group had good knowledge about neonatal care. Chi-square test showed there was no significant difference between the two groups before intervention in this regard (p=0.754).That both groups had almost equal awareness level. After intervention, 87% of the mothers in the test group and 18% of the mothers in the control group had good knowledge about neonatal care. 73% of the mothers in the test group and 10% of the mothers in the control group had good performance about neonatal care. Chi-square test showed there was a significant difference in knowledge and performance between the two groups (p=0.001) (Tables 2 and 3). Acccording to the results, the mothers'performance in preventing and treatment of colic (p=0.22) and jaundice (P=0.04) was significantly different in the two groups (Table 4). The rate

Table 2. The relative and absolute frequency in terms of mothers' knowledge in infants' care in two groups before and after intervention.

Knowledge level	Group			
	After intervention		Before intervention	
	Test	Control	Test	Control
Poor	6(20)	9(28)	0(0)	7(21)
Moderate	17(57)	18(54)	4(13)	20(61)
Good	7(23)	6(18)	26(87)	6(18)
Total	30(100)	33(100)	30(100)	33(100)
χ square	P=0.754		P=0.001	

Table 3. The relative and absolute frequency in terms of mothers' performance in infants' care in two groups after intervention.

Performance level	Group	
	After intervention	
	Test	Control
Poor	0(0)	22(66)
Moderate	8(27)	8(24)
Good	22(73)	3(10)
Total	30(100)	33(100)
χ square	P=0.001	

Table 4. The relative and absolute frequency in terms of mothers' Performance in "the colic and jaundice of infants" in two groups

Performance		Group				Chi-square test
		Test		Control		
		Absolute frequency	Relative frequency	Absolute frequency	Relative frequency	
Performance in colic	Desirable	3	67	2	17	
	Undesirable	1	33	22	83	(p=0.22)
	Total	4	100	24	100	
Performance in jaundice	Desirable	7	70	6	30	
	Undesirable	3	30	14	70	P=0.04
	Total	10	100	20	100	

of inffection to respiratory aspiration in the control group was twice that of the test group. Regarding the mothers' performance in putting the head higher than the body and putting the pacifier in the neonate's mouth, there was significant relation (p=0.001) (Table 5). Acccording to the results, the mothers'performance in preventing skin infection (diaper dermatitis) in infants was significantly different in the two groups (p<0.05) (Table 6).

DISCUSSION

In this study, the effect of a health-based supportive plan on primiparous mothers'performance in prevention of colic, aspiration, skin problems and care in jaundice was investigated. Mojalli et al. (2010) demonstrated that with increasing age and higher levels of education, mothers exhibit better performance. Therefore, by eliminating the effect of these variables on our results; the two groups were equal in all demographic variables and Chi-square test showed no significant relationship between the two groups. There was a significant statistical diffrence (p=0.04) in the test group with more mothers employing correct strategies in care. This demonstrates the effect of the protective health improvment program on mothers'recognition of jaundice and its management and

Table 5. Absolute and relative frequency in terms of mothers' performance in infants' aspiration in the two groups.

Measurement in aspiration	Group				Chi-square test
	Test		Control		
	Yes	No	Yes	No	
Getting neonate to burp	30 (100)	0 (0)	33 (100)	0 (0)	P= 0/001
Putting a pacifier in to baby's mouth	7 (23)	23 (77)	25 (76)	8 (24)	P= 0/001
Positioning the child	26 (87)	4 (13)	11 (23)	22 (67)	P= 0/001

Table 6. Relative and absolute frequency distribution by mothers' performance in preventing skin infection (diaper dermatitis) in infants.

Mothers' performance in skin problems	Group				Chi-square test
	Test		Control		
	Yes	No	Yes	No	
Repetitively changing	30 (100)	0 (0)	30 (91)	3 (9)	P= 0/09
Use allergen detergents	5 (17)	25 (83)	19 (58)	14 (42)	P= 0/02
Washing after each bowel movement	30 (100)	0 (0)	25 (76)	8 (24)	P= 0/004
Putting in air	17 (57)	13(43)	9(27)	24(73)	P= 0/01

how this is reflected in their performance in newborn care. According to Hosseinzade et al. (2012), only 42% of mothers knew about neonatal jaundice (Hosseinzade et al., 2012). In addition, the findings of Saravi Ghaffari (2006) showed that 302 mothers (75.5%) had little, 93 (23.3%) had moderate and only 5 mothers had good awareness about neonatal jaundice (Ghafari et al., 2007). Hosseini and Nikbakht (2011) also reported that the measure of awareness and information about the nature of jaundice in the newborn period is minimal (Hosseini and Nikbakht, 2011).

This is during a time when the health of the newborns that have jaundice is critical and dependent on early diagnosis and treatment (Pang and Ling, 2000). Avasady et al. (2006) noted that traditional curing is an important factor in delaying going to the hygiene and cure stations in India (Awasthi et al., 2006). Pang and Ling (2000) and Chap Jambo (2008) showed that the traditional cure using medical plants has a significant relationship with severe neonatal jaundice (Pang and Ling, 2000; Chappjumbo and Ohanenye, 2008). In the present study, regarding not giving medical plants to newborns resulted in significant difference between the two groups. Results in the control group, were two times higher than in the test group (test group 30% and control group 63/3%). The increases in the control group were attributed to mothers not being aware, being impressible and accepting traditional beliefs. The results demonstrated that the rate of pulmonary aspiration in the control group was twice that of the test group, a clinically important finding. The Chi-square results comfirmed the performance in aspiration prevention (p=0.001). There was no difference between the two groups in making the newborn burp after feeding, and the reason is that breastfeeding classes were attended in all centers. The mothers' performance in preventing respiratory aspiration had a positive effect on neonatal respiratory health. More mothers showed appropriate performance for preventing respiratory aspiration at home in the test group.Appropriate performance demonstrated in the test group included burping newborns after feeding and positioning the infant, The pacifier was given in 23.3% of the cases, while the desired mothers' performance in the control group was making the newborn burp after breast feeding.The Chi-square test results regarding the rate of skin infection demonstrated a significant difference between the two groups (p=0.02), being three times more in the control group.

A significant difference was noted in the mothers' performance of washing the buttocks after every defecation of baby, allowing the genital area to air and not using allergen cleaning materials that cause skin problems.Decreasing skin infection in newborns occurred due to the correct performance of the mothers in the test group. This shows the effect of supportive teaching during the intervention. Caring points to mothers, investigating newborn skin position at home, performing primary care program when the primary sign was observed, and correcting mothers behavior prevented the occurance of dermatitis diaper, and if any problem occured, corrected primary care were employed, and simultaneously the nurse aids were used. Emdadi and Bazmazmun, (2005) emphasized teaching the mothers about infant hygiene to prevent dermatitis diaper (Emdadi and Bazmazmun, 2005). Renjinidevi (2005) investigated the effect of teaching mothers to prevent newborn infections and concluded that mothers' knowledge about dermatitis before and after the intervention had a significant difference. In the present study, 3 infants in the test group and in the control group 12 infants had colic.According to these results, mother' performance in preventing and curing colic was significantly different (p=0/02). 3 mothers in the test group preformed the correct performance, however, one infant was referred to a physician and two other infants were cured with appropriate performance at home. In the control group, only 2 mothers used the appropriate performance, 10 mothers had undesired performance.The results showed that health based supportive plan before and after delivery and following the mother and baby at home help mothers' learn about the best performances. Also there was a significant difference between the two groups' regarding the behaviours of calming in the home atmosphere, not responding to the newborn's cries, putting the baby on its abdomen and going to the physician for curing colic. Both groups adhered to not eating flatulent foods and making the baby burp. The present knowledge indicates that curing behaviors, as well as consultive and trusted supports to parents are the most effective of all options. Furthermore, teaching the mothers about colic symptoms, and using health preventive correct behavior were considered. Also, the results showed that the average grade of mothers desired performance in taking care of a newborn in the test group was 18.1, and in the control group, it was 12/4. The independent t-test results showed a significant relationship between the two groups in this regard (p=0.001). Most of the mothers in the test group (66.1%) had well performance while most of them others in the control group (64%) showed weak performance in taking care of the baby. In total, the results of the present research confirm the effect of health-based supportive plan in preventing the specific problems in infants and this is while prevention is prior to treatment.There was no limitation in this study.

Conclusions

Teaching emotional and consultive support in the pregnancy period, continuing supports after childbirth and during home visiting after childbirth and following how mothers perform are effective in taking care of newborn. That is why the number of desired performance among the mothers in the test group is more than in the control group. Also supporting mothers in all dimensions is effective in helping them in taking care of themselves and their children and promoting quality of life. It is necessary to encourage nurses as a part of the medicine team to continually support mothers in this critical period after childbirth. This significantly helps mothers and newborns towards higher level of health improvement, increasing the quality of life, decreasing the possible side effects of childbirth and consequently, decreasing the mothers' and new borns' mortality. Impoverment in the performance of the mothers' in the present study as a result of health-based supportive plan implies that supporting mothers before childbirth and continuing these supports after birth,visiting newborn at home, and following, this program can be used in improving both mother and newborns' health and promoting their quality of life.

CONFLICT OF INTERESTS

The author has not declared any conflict of interests.

Ethics and consent

The study was conducted in accordance with the guidelines of the Declaration of Helsinki and was approved by the Institutional Review Board (IRB) of Tarbiat Modares University (Approval number:IR. TMU.REC. 1067779). All pertinent study information was explained to the patient about the nature, scope and objectives of the study and they were informed that rejection or withdrawal from the study will not affect any medical service provided. A summarized study information sheet was shown to all cases before obtaining their verbal agreement. Finally, an informed verbal consent was obtained and witnessed by the attending nurse. The IRB waived the requirement for taking a written consent as the research had minimal risk of harm to subjects and involved no risky procedures for which written consent is required.

ACKNOWLEDGEMENTS

The authors are grateful to all midwives and nurses who conducted the plan, and to all the mothers who agreed to participate in this study. Research was supported by the Fund of the Tarbiat Modares University.

REFRENCES

Awasthi S, Verma T, Agrawal M (2006). Danger signs of neonatal illnesses: Perception of caregivers and health workers in Northern India. Bull. World Health Organ. 84(10):819-825.

Ballard PL (2000). Scientific rationale for the use of antenatal glucocorticoids to promote fetal development. Pediatr. Rev. 1(5):E83-90.

Beake S, Val R, Debra B, Weavers A, Wray J (2010). A qualitative study of the experiences and expectations of women receiving in-patient postnatal care in one English maternity unit. BMC Pregnancy Childbirth 2010:1-9.

Boskabadi H, Maamouri G, Sadeghian MH, Ghayour-Mobarhan M, Heidarzade M, Shakeri MT, Ferns G (2010). Early diagnosis of perinatal asphyxia by nucleated red blood cell count: A case-control study. Arch. Iran Med. 13(4):275-281.

Chappjumbo AUN, Ohanenye C (2008). Awareness of neonatal jaundice among women seen at an immunization clinic in Aba. J. Med. Investig. Pract. 7:66-70.

Chiabi A, Takou V, Mah E, Nguefack S, Siyou H, Takou V, Tchokoteu PF, Mbonda E (2014). Risk factors for neonatal mortality at the

Yaounde Gynaeco-Obstetric and Pediatric Hospital, Cameroon. Iran J. Pediatr. 24(4):393-400.

Cronin C, McCarthy G (2003). First-time mothers- identifying their needs, perceptions and experiences. J. Clin. Nurs. 12(2):260-267.

Curley AE, Halliday HL (2001). The present status of exogenous surfactant for the newborn. Early Hum. Dev. 61(2):67-83.

Dadipoor S, Rajaei M, Naderi S, Ghanbarnejad A, Safari Moradabadi A (2014). Investigating causes of infant mortality in hospital of children during 2010-2011 in Bandar Abbas. Iranian J. Neonatol. 5(1):12-18.

Eichenwald EC, Stark AR (1999). High-frequency ventilation: Current status. Pediatr. Rev. 20(12):e127-33.

Ekhtiyari A, Emami P (2009). The success rate of mothers' breast feeding in vaginal delivery and cesarean section in Tehran. Med. Sci. J. Islamic Azad. Univ. 18(1):51-54.

Emdadi M, Bazmazmun H (2005). Prevalence of dermatitis in children under 2 years old in Hamedan nurseries. Res. Paper. J. Hamadan Univ. Med. Sci. 11(1):44-46.

Ghafari V, Vahidshahi K, Alitaleshi B (2007). Knowledge and attitudes of mothers about neonatal jaundice in neonates in Sari Hospitals. J. Mazandaran Univ. Med. Sci. 16(52):92-97.

Ghorat F, Ghafarzadeh R, Jafarzadeh Esfehani R (2016). Perinatal Mortality and Its Associated Risk Factors: A Study in the North-East of Iran. Iranian J. Neonatol. 7(1):47-51.

Hosseini L, Nikbakht NA (2011). The experience of mothers with newborn jaundice: A qualitative study. Nurs. Res. 5(18):66-72.

Hosseinzade M, Ezataghajari P, Hashtrudizade M (2012). Comparison of mothers' knowledge of neonatal care, in maternal health centers - Health care homes in rural and urban Maraghe. Congress on Clinical Audit and Quality Improvement, Tabriz. Univ. Med .Sci. 2012; 4436 (poster).

Jehan I, Harris H, Salat S, Zeb A, Mobeen N, Pasha O, McClure EM, Moore J, Wright LL, Goldenberg RL (2009). Neonatal mortality, risk factors and causes: A prospective population-based cohort study in urban Pakistan. Bull. World Health Organ. 87(2):130-138.

Kiasari AZ, Kabirzadeh A, Saravi BM, Rezazadeh E, Khademlou M, Biazar T (2009). Rate and causes of perinatal mortality in Imam Hospital, Sari 2007. Iranian J. Obstet. Gynecol. Infertil. 12(2):23-30.

Kline CR, Martin DP, Deyo RA (1998). Health consequences of pregnancy and childbirth as perceived by women and clinicians. Obstet. Gynecol. 92(5):842-848.

Lawn JE, Kerber K, Enweronu-Laryea C, Massee Bateman O (2009). Newborn survival in low resource settings-are we delivering? Br. J. Obstet. Gynaecol. 116(11):49-59.

Ministry of Health (2008). Neonatal status of Iran and providing solution to reduce neonates' mortality. Tehran: Ministry of Health.

Mirgafoorvand M, Mohammad alizadeh SC (2000). Infant care knowledge of primiparous urban mothers in hospitals of Tabriz. Med. Sci. J. Islamic Urmia. Univ. 11(4):234-242.

Mohseni M, Bahadoran P, Abedi H (2009). The quality of postpartum care from mothers' viewpoint. Hakim Res. J. 12(1):27-34.

Mojalli M, Basiri Moghadam M, Shamshiri M (2010). Effectiveness of Instructional Environment and Related Factors on Breast feeding Function of Mothers. Horizon Med. Sci. 16(1):59-64.

Nelson Textbook of Pediatrics (2006). (Trans: Kavehmanesh Z), 18th ed.Part 11, Philadelphia: WB Saunders company. 2006.

Pang MF, Ling SG (2000). Factors affecting severity of neonatal jaundice in patients presenting from home. JUMMEC 1:24-27.

Renjinidevi S (2005). Effectiveness of planned teaching programme on prevention of neonatal infections for primigravidae in a selected hospital at Mangalore. Dissertation submitted to the Rajiv Gandhi University of Health Science, Karnataka, and Bangalore.

Titaley CH, Dibley M, Agho A, Roberts CH, Hall J (2008). Determinants of neonatal mortality in Indonesia. BMC Public Health 8:232.

World Health Organization (WHO) (2008). Representative Office in Iran. Statistical indicators of health. Available at: http://www.whoiran.org/index-farsi.htm

World Heath Organization (WHO) (2001). Millennium development goals and challenges under five year-child mortality rate: 1. 2001.

28

Evaluation of the quality of postnatal care and mothers' satisfaction at the university college hospital Ibadan, Nigeria

Rose Ekama Ilesanmi and Janet Atinuke Akinmeye*

Department of Nursing, College of Medicine, University of Ibadan, Ibadan, Oyo State, Nigeria.

Globally, postpartum care is a neglected part of maternal health, even though 50% of maternal deaths occur in the first weeks after childbirth. Literature is sparse on the quality and content of postnatal care provided in Nigeria. This study aimed to assess the quality of Postnatal Care (PNC) for mothers using the World Health Organization (WHO) practice guideline of postnatal care. An exploratory cross-sectional design was employed among 57 purposively selected mothers in postnatal clinic and wards. Data were collected in two phases using three checklists to examine facility resources and quality of postnatal care provided; and one questionnaire to evaluate mothers' satisfaction in both the clinic and the wards. Data were analyzed using descriptive statistics. The facility assessment showed an inadequate infrastructure and human resources. Only 47.9% of the recommended routine postnatal care was provided on the postnatal wards and 42.3% in the postnatal clinic. Level of satisfaction was found to be poor among 63.2% of the women on the wards, and good among 82.5% of the women in the clinic. Findings suggest that inadequate resources for PNC. Organizations need to strengthen PNC services by providing recommended resources and a standard guideline that will serve as a framework for provision of quality postnatal care services.

Key words: Postnatal care, postnatal care guideline, quality care, maternal satisfaction.

INTRODUCTION

The postnatal period is the first six weeks after birth, which is critical to the health and survival of the mother and her newborn. The most vulnerable time for both is during the hours and days after birth (WHO, 2014). Despite this long-standing definition, the postpartum period frequently lasts for several months and it is documented as a neglected aspect of modern maternity care. Accordingly, Pallangyo et al. (2017), reported that the global picture confirms that postpartum care is a neglected part of maternal and neonatal health, yet 50% of maternal deaths occur in the first weeks after childbirth. It is therefore not surprising that literature is sparse on the puerperium and where it exists; it deals primarily with abnormal involution and pathology (Kearns et al., 2016). The WHO has highlighted widespread and persistent health problems, including death experienced

*Corresponding author. E-mail: atinukeedache@gmail.com.

by women after childbirth, many of which are unreported by women and not identified by healthcare professionals (WHO, 2014). Furthermore, WHO (2014) reports that of the 289,000 maternal deaths that occur each year, worldwide and 50 to 71% occur within the postnatal period. Unfortunately, 99% of these maternal deaths occur in low and middle income countries including Nigeria (Blencowe et al., 2012).

Despite the more than 20 years fight against maternal deaths, Nigeria still documents one of the worst maternal mortality statistics in the world. With a maternal mortality ratio of 576 per 100,000 live births, Nigeria is second only to India in the global estimates of maternal mortality.

Consequently, Nigeria loses about 153 women of childbearing age every day and a woman's chance of dying from pregnancy and childbirth in Nigeria is 1 in 13 (NDHS, 2013). Specifically, over 40,000 maternal deaths occur in Nigeria yearly (APHRC, 2017). Reports from other low income countries such as Uganda also suggest poor Postnatal Care (PNC) services. There is no document to suggest an adapted standard for PNC services in Nigeria. However, effort is geared towards achieving the recommended standard specified by the WHO.

Khanal et al. (2014), reported that the postnatal care indicated that standards were infrequently met as only 2 in 5 women in their study were reported to have received a postnatal check-up within one hour of delivery. In another study in Pakistan, Munawar et al. (2017) revealed verbalization of the low quality of maternity care by most of the participants.

In Nigeria an extensive review of the literature suggests a dearth of researches on the content and quality of postnatal care, even though care is routinely provided for women. However, several important indicators such as mortality indices reported from recent studies raise concern about its quality and effectiveness, consequently the question of quality and coverage.

Accordingly, Kinney et al. (2010) reiterates that the burden of maternal death can effectively be reduced when efforts are geared towards overcoming both the coverage and quality gaps in postnatal care. This is also consistent with other reports. For example, Carvajal-Aguirre et al. (2017) in an audit review of the content of ANC and PNC services concluded that the gap between coverage and content as a measure of quality of care is tremendously wide in all countries.

Therefore, in order to accelerate maternal and newborn survival, the authors suggested an urgent need for increased efforts targeted at improving both the coverage and actual contents of maternal and newborn health interventions.

In response to the morbidity and mortality indices, the WHO in 2014 established guidelines of postnatal care, to promote quality and ensure effectiveness. Again in 2016 the organization indorsed the availability and the use of all recommended resources to achieve optimal health care outcomes and improve the use and satisfaction of individuals, families and communities with maternal health services.

Implicitly, a first step towards achieving the goals for maternal health in the Sustainable Development Goals (SDGs 3): ensuring healthy lives and promoting the well-being of all at all ages. For women this would mean to routinely monitor quality along the continuum of care in terms of structure, process and outcome, within the context of Donabedian model of quality care. The aim of this study was to assess the available resources (Structure) used in the provision of postnatal care in the facility, evaluate routine postnatal practices on the postnatal wards and clinic in accordance with WHO guidelines (Process), and to examine women's level of satisfaction (Outcome) with the care they received in the study setting. The Donabedian model of quality care was used as the framework to evaluate the extent of implementation of WHO guideline for quality postnatal care. The three dimensions of quality care identified in the model namely; structure, process and outcome dimensions served as the basis for assessment in this study.

MATERIALS AND METHODS

This study was an exploratory cross-sectional survey. It employed a mixed method of data collection, which consists an initial phase of qualitative data collection followed by a second phase of quantitative data collection. The observation was the dominant method and it was employed in order to examine the actual care being provided by the care providers. On the other hand, the structured interview with questionnaire was used to assess the level of satisfaction among mothers.

The sample size of 57 mothers was determined using the formula $n = N / [1 + N (e)^2]$ Where; N = estimated population, e = level of error of tolerance (5%). A purposive sampling method was used in the selection of the mothers who gave consent to participate and affirmed that they would return to postnatal checkup. Purposive sampling method was used because only few of the mothers who had normal delivery confirmed they would return for postnatal follow-up in the facility. Mothers with still borne, postpartum hemorrhage or instrumental deliveries and caesarean section were excluded. Four data collection instruments were designed to achieve the objectives of the study, which included three checklists and one questionnaire. The checklists were adapted from WHO (2014) guideline for postnatal care to assess the structure (human resources, material resources and infrastructure), the process dimension (care provided) on the postnatal wards and postnatal clinic. A structured questionnaire was administered to the mothers to determine their level of satisfaction with postnatal care on the postnatal wards and postnatal clinic.

Ethical approval to conduct the study was issued after review by the University of Ibadan/University College Hospital Ethical Committee (NHREC/05/01/2008a). The respondents' participation in the study was voluntary and consent was obtained after giving an explanation of the study. The respondents were assured of the absence of risk by their participation and confidentiality.

The qualitative data was collected first through non-participant observation using the prepared checklists to record relevant information on the available resources in the facility and on the postnatal care provided to the women. The duration of the

Table 1. Facility Assessment.

Items	Available	Not available
facility readiness	√	
24 h availability	√	
Emergency preparedness	√	
Equipment		
Weighing scale	√	
Sphygmomanometer	√	
Stethoscope	√	
Thermometer	√	
Sterilizer	√	
Instruments	√	
Medicine		
Analgesics	√	
Antibiotics	√	
Haematinics	√	
Supplies	√	
Infection Prevention Measures	√	
Infrastructure	**Adequate**	**Not adequate**
Functional Ambulance	√	
Backup Source of Electricity?	√	√
Comfortable Beds		
Toilet and Bathroom facilities		
Regular water supply		√
Regular electricity supply		√
Staffing		√
General Medical Doctors	√	
Specialist Medical Doctors		
Midwives		√
Nurses		√
Laboratory Scientists	√	√
Pharmacists	√	
Community Health Nurses		
IEC materials	√	√
Guidelines /Protocols		
Registers	√	√
Continuous education and training in postnatal care		
Supervision	√	√
Number of Doctors (O&G)		46
Doctor patient ratio (Average)		1:8
Total score	22 (66.7%)	11 (33.3%)

observation on both the wards and the clinic was 4 weeks.

The mothers were selected for an exit interview and each respondent's questionnaire was marked and their phone numbers obtained to facilitate a follow up in the postnatal clinic. The mothers were followed up to their clinic appointment date, consent was obtained again and they were administered their individual questionnaires to complete on their exit from the postnatal clinic. Quantitative data obtained was analyzed using the Statistical package for social sciences (SPSS) version 22 and all results were presented using descriptive statistics, t-test, ANOVA and Chi square test.

RESULTS

Facility assessment (structure)

The result that only 66.7% of the required resources were available in the study setting, which is an indication of poor adherence to the WHO recommendation for postnatal care facility. The facility provides 24 h services and emergency preparedness alongside the availability of basic equipment needed to meet the health needs of postnatal women (Table 1). However, electricity supply, regular water supply, bathrooms and toilets are inadequate for the care of the postnatal women. The numbers of functional bathrooms and toilets on the wards and in the clinic appear insufficient in comparison to the population of the women. There are a total of 50 beds in the postnatal wards with an average of 25 patients on each ward including antenatal patients on admission, postnatal patients who had normal delivery and those who had complicated deliveries. In each ward and the clinic, there are two functional bathrooms and toilets with no regular water supply. On the average, 25 patients are seen in the postnatal clinic every clinic day. The available specialist medical doctors, midwives are insufficient with an average midwife to patient ratio of 1:8 per shift. There are no standardized postnatal guidelines and protocols used in the provision of care to the postnatal women in the facility. Although there are various in-service trainings organized in the institution on life saving skills, evaluation of nursing care, pain management, documentation, geriatrics, care of placenta, essential care of the newborn, advancement of health care, basic trauma care and cardio pulmonary resuscitation; continuing education and training on postnatal care is lacking.

Assessment of postnatal care (process)

From the findings, only 42.9% of the required postnatal care was observed to be provided on the wards (Table 2) and 42.3% in the postnatal clinic (Table 3). This depicts poor adherence to the WHO practice guideline for postnatal care in the postnatal unit of the study setting. All women with uncomplicated vaginal delivery received care for at least 24 h after delivery in the study setting. On the wards, the initial assessment within the first 24 h after birth were conducted except checking for excessive bleeding which was not visually assessed, although the women were verbally asked if bleeding was normal or excess of 25% of the observation period. Meanwhile urine voiding resumption, frequency and characteristics were not assessed throughout the observation period. During the physical assessment beyond 24 h after birth bladder and bowel function, lochia, healing of perineal wound and breast were assessed about 30% of the observation period. Midwives were observed not to assess mothers for complaints such as headache, fatigue, back pain, and perineal hygiene during the period under investigation. Prophylactic antibiotics were prescribed for patients with perineal tears. Mothers were not provided with discharge counseling on the physiology of puerperium and danger signs. However, midwives (30%) provided counseling on family planning, maternal nutrition, breast care and follow up. Documentation was done in all cases and emotional support was observed in 16.7% of the observation period. While the only prescribed routine postnatal visit is from 6 weeks after birth and there is no provision for home visits within the first week of childbirth. A physical examination that was observed being conducted in the postnatal clinic was; blood pressure check, pallor, lochia, and uterine involution, while temperature, inspection of perineum for healing, and breasts were not assessed. Assessment of emotional and psychological wellbeing, resumption of sexual intercourse and dyspareunia were not observed in all the visits to the clinic.

Socio-demography of mothers

Table 4 illustrates the analysis of the demographic data of the postnatal women (mothers). A total of 57 mothers were sampled between the age of 20 and 40 with mean ±SD = 31±1.58. The majority (49.1%) were first time mothers. Reasons for choosing the facility included availability of modern facilities (15.4%), quality care (42.3%), convenience (11.5), and availability of good doctors (21.8%).

Mothers' level of satisfaction

Satisfaction on the postnatal ward

Findings indicated that 36.5% of the mothers were not satisfied and 28.4% were fairly satisfied with the care received on admission after delivery. The majority (94%) of the women expressed satisfaction with routine vital signs monitoring and drug administration, but were not satisfied with the inadequate water and electricity, inadequate toilet and bathroom facilities, lack of individualized care (Table 5a). The analysis of variance revealed a significant difference ($p<0.05$) between the level of mothers' satisfaction on the postnatal wards and the number of deliveries, the numbers of days they were on admission as well as the maternal age.

Satisfaction at the clinic

Majority (82.5%) of the mothers expressed good satisfaction with care received in the postnatal clinic. Specific areas of satisfaction were the attitude of the staff

Table 2. Assessment of postnatal care on the ward.

Provision of postnatal care	Done (%)	Not done (%)
After an uncomplicated vaginal birth in a health facility, healthy mothers receive care at the facility for at least 24 h after birth	12 (100)	0 (0)
Assessment within the first 24 h after birth		
Check for excessive bleeding	3 (25)	9 (75)
Check uterine contraction	8 (66.6)	4 (33.4)
Check fundal height	8 (66.6)	4 (33.4)
Check temperature	12 (100)	0 (0)
Check blood pressure within 6hours after birth)	12 (100)	0 (0)
Check blood pressure after 6 h	12 (100)	0 (0)
Check urine void in 6 h	0 (0)	12 (100)
Physical assessment beyond 24 h after birth		
Micturition and urinary continence	3 (25)	9 (75)
Bowel function	3 (25)	9 (75)
Healing of perineal wound	3 (25)	9 (75)
Headache	0 (0)	12 (100)
Fatigue	0 (0)	12 (100)
Back pain	0 (0)	12 (100)
Perineal hygiene	0 (0)	12 (100)
Breast pain, swelling or tenderness	4 (33.4)	8 (66.6)
Uterine tenderness	6 (50)	6 (50)
Lochia	3 (25)	9 (75)
Use of prophylactic antibiotics in perineal tear to prevent infection	12 (100)	0 (0)
Discharge counseling on		
Physiology of pueperium	0 (0)	12 (100)
Healthy timing and spacing of pregnancies	3 (25)	9 (75)
Family planning including LAM /transition	4 (33.4)	8 (66.6)
Maternal nutrition	4 (33.4)	8 (66.6)
Breast care and personal hygiene	3 (25)	9 (75)
Danger signs	0 (0)	12 (100)
Follow up appointment	12 (100)	0 (0)
Emotional support	2 (16.7)	10 (83.3)
Documentation	12 (100)	0 (0)
Total	141 (41.9)	195 (58.1)
Average score	**12 (42.9)**	**16 (57.1)**

at the clinic, information provided and healthcare received. However, poor satisfaction was reported in the clinical environment (waiting area, toilet and bathroom) and cumbersome registration and payment procedures in the hospital (Table 5b). Additionally, the women in this study verbalized areas of dissatisfaction which include the following: bureaucracy, poor counseling, cumbersome registration and payment processes, inadequate provider-client relationship, admissions for days more than necessary, the assumption that patient knows everything, inadequate toilet and bathroom facilities, lack of regular water supply, waiting time, much cold at night on the wards, poor attention, lack of individualized care, lack of patient specific counseling and care by inexperienced doctors at the postnatal clinic. The analysis of variance revealed that there is a significant difference ($p<0.05$) between the mothers' level of satisfaction with PNC at the clinic and the maternal age.

DISCUSSION

The findings of this study suggest that there is an insufficient human resources and infrastructure in

Table 3. Assessment of postnatal care in the clinic.

Provision of postnatal care	Done (%)	Not done (%)
Postnatal visit on day 3 (48-72 h)	0 (0)	4 (100)
Between days 7–14 after birth	0 (0)	4 (100)
Six weeks after birth	4 (100)	0 (0)
Home visits within the first week of birth	0 (0)	4 (100)
History taking	2 (50)	2 (50)
Physical examination		
Blood pressure	4 (100)	0 (0)
Temperature	1 (25)	3 (75)
Pallor	4 (100)	0 (0)
Lochia	4 (100)	0 (0)
Perineum	0 (0)	4 (100)
Involution of the uterus	4 (100)	0 (0)
Vaginal discharge	2 (50)	2 (50)
Breasts	0 (0)	4 (100)
Assessment of emotional wellbeing (mood, social support and coping strategies)	0 (0)	4 (100)
Assessment of psychological wellbeing	0 (0)	4 (100)
Resumption of sexual intercourse and dispareunia	0 (0)	4 (100)
Counseling on/ Information given to client		
Physiology of pueperium	0 (0)	4 (100)
Danger signs	2(50)	2 (50)
Healthy timing and spacing of pregnancies	2 (50)	2 (50)
Family planning including LAM /transition	4 (100)	0 (0)
Maternal nutrition	2 (50)	2 (50)
Breast care and personal hygiene	2 (50)	2 (50)
Assessment of client's understanding	2 (50)	2 (50)
Emotional support	1 (25)	3 (75)
Interpersonal care/rapport	1 (25)	3 (75)
Documentation	4 (100)	0 (0)
Total	45	59
Average score	**11 (42.3)**	**15 (56.7)**

accordance with the recommendations of the WHO. As explained by Donabedian (1988), poor structural quality will affect the provision of postnatal services to mothers and eventual outcome of postnatal care in this facility. Lotto (2015) also linked inadequate postnatal facility for the quality postnatal care to eventual decrease in the quality of postnatal services.

The facility is deficient in the staffing of Midwives and Doctors who are central to the provision of postnatal care to mothers. The average midwife: patient ratio in this study setting is 1:8 on the postnatal wards which is below the recommended standards and what is peculiar in more developed economies. Adelani et al. (2015) also observed a nurse/midwife to patient ratio ranging from ratio1:9 in a general hospital in Osun state, Nigeria. The NICE postulated for the Australian Nursing and Midwifery Federation a midwife/nurse to patient ratio of 1:4 plus a charge nurse in the morning and afternoon shift and 1:6 on the night shift (ANMF, 2015). The British Columbia Nurses Union (2016) on the other hand, recommended a range of midwife to patient ratio of 1:4 to 1:6 in an inpatient unit.

There are 46 Obstetrics/Gynecology specialists in this facility which are insufficient as opined by Agboghoroma and Gharoro (2015) in their study. They submitted that the number of Obstetrics/Gynecologists in Nigeria is inadequate in view of the population size, when computed this suggest a ratio of 1:181458 patients. When compared with the WHO (2010) recommendation of a ratio of one obstetric/Gynecologist to one thousand patients (1:1000), this is a far cry and may contribute to the poor maternal care services. In line with this majority of the women in a study in Nigeria submitted that the health providers are burdened with heavy workloads in

Table 4. Socio-demographic Variables of Mothers.

Variables	Frequency	Percentage (%)	
Age (In years)			
20-24	5	8.8	**Mean age = 31 year**
25-29	14	24.6	**SD** = 1.58
30-34	31	54.4	
35-40	7	12.2	
Marital status			
Single	5	8.8	
Married	52	91.2	
State of origin	45	78.9	
Western state	8	14.1	
Eastern state	4	7	
Northern state	14	0	
Southern state	14	0	
Level of education			
No formal education	14	0	
Primary school	6	10.5	
Secondary school	10	17.6	
Diploma	41	71.9	
Degree	14	0	
Others	24	42.1	
Occupation			
Civil servant	9	15.8	
Private institution employee	9	15.8	
Trading	10	17.6	
Self-employed	5	8.8	
Unemployed	14	0	
Others	24	42.1	
Number of pregnancies			
1	19	33.3	
2	9	15.8	
3	3	5.3	
4	2	3.5	
>4	28	49.1	
Number of deliveries			
1	16	28.1	
2	9	15.8	
3	2	3.5	
4	2	3.5	
>4	39	68.4	
Number of deliveries in UCH?			
1	12	21.1	
2	2	3.5	
3	2	3.5	
4	2	3.5	

Table 4. Contd.

>4	14	0
Number of days spent on admission in the last delivery		
1	6	10.5
2	27	47.4
3	15	26.3
4	9	15.8
>4	12	15.4
Reason for choosing UCH		
Modern facilities	33	42.3
Quality care	7	9
Referral	9	11.5
Convenience	17	21.8
Availability of good doctors	0	0
Others		

Table 5. Mothers' level of satisfaction.

Variable	Fully satisfactory (%)	Fairly satisfactory (%)	Not satisfactory (%)
		(a) On the ward	
Orientation to the hospital and ward	14.2 (24.9)	18.3 (32.2)	24.5 (42.9)
Informed consent	20 (35.1)	23 (40.3)	14 (24.6)
Attitude of care providers	23 (40.3)	21.7 (38.1)	12.3 (21.6)
Quality of ward environment	10 (17.5)	20 (35.1)	27 (47.4)
Postnatal care received	20 (35.1)	16.2 (28.4)	20.8 (36.5)
Professionalism of care providers	28 (49.1)	21 (36.8)	8 (14.1)
Health education and counseling	7.5 (13.2)	11.5 (20.2)	38 (66.6)
Overall assessment of the ward	18 (31.6)	19 (33.3)	20 (35.1)
		(b) In the clinic	
Waiting time	16 (28)	20 (35.2)	21 (36.8)
Registration process	14 (24.6)	19.5 (34.2)	23.5 (41.2)
Attitude of clerical staff	30 (52.6)	13 (22.8)	14 (24.6)
Quality of clinic environment	10 (17.5)	19 (33.3)	28 (49.2)
Attitude of postnatal care providers	26.7 (46.8)	26 (45.7)	4.3 (7.5)
Postnatal care received	22 (38.6)	20 (35.1)	15 (26.3)
Overall assessment of the postnatal clinic	24 (42.1)	23 (40.4)	10 (17.5)

the provision of maternal health care and linked the burden to the low quality of care (Ogu et al., 2017).

The high patient ratio to each of the postnatal care providers may be a contributing factor to the suboptimal quality of postnatal care offered at this facility. Empirical evidences suggest the number of patients allocated to a health provider on a shift is directly related to patient safety, patient satisfaction, mortality and quality of care (ANMF 2015). It is therefore imperative for the Nursing and Midwifery Council of NIGERIA and the National Association of Nigerian Nurses to collaborate to design a standard nurse: patient ration that is suitable to Nigerian health need which should also apply to the Nigerian medical association.

Consequently, the legislation of standard ratio would serve as a baseline for employment in all government hospitals in the country, reduce waiting time, improve the quality of care, improve retention of health providers as a result of better and safer working environment, increase capability of hospitals to meet patient demands, and improves the economic performance of hospitals. Inadequate in-service training was also observed in this study, as none of the 50 postnatal care providers who had continuous education in the last 2 years had any training on postnatal care. Continuous training and education is an essential pre-requisite for quality improvement in the provision of services and also contributes to quality of inpatient and outpatient care (Chaghari et al., 2017). Staff shortages and inadequate in-service training were also observed in China (Chen et al., 2014) while Chimtembo et al. (2013) in addition to inadequate facility, identified poor postnatal counseling in their study in Malawi.

There is non-availability of a guideline or protocol for the postnatal care of mothers in the study setting, as such there is no laid down standard for care givers in providing their services. Some healthcare providers in Tanzania also perceived that postnatal care was suboptimal in their facilities resulting from care being based on clinical experiences due to lack of guidelines and inadequate health personnels (Pallangyo et al., 2016). Kopp (2011) opined that use of clinical guidelines is an indispensable part of a professional quality system, and is an important tool to improve the knowledge, processes and outcomes in healthcare. They also provide a foundation for assessing and evaluating the effectiveness of healthcare.

The findings in this study suggest that the routine postnatal care provided in both the postnatal clinic and the wards of the facility are below the standard in accordance with WHO practice guidelines. This finding is supported by Chimtembo et al. (2013) whose study in Malawi revealed that the contents of postnatal services were below reproductive health standards. A sub-standard process component of postnatal care was also observed by Lotto (2015) in Tanzania. Luegmair et al. (2018) identified shortcomings in puerperal care and counseling in their study in Austria. Assessment is the second recommendation on the WHO (2014) practice guideline for postnatal care which was found to be poorly adhered to in this setting. Routine assessments are important for early identification of complications, prompt treatment or referral as needed. The majority of the assessment within the first 24 h after birth was done while the majority of the assessment beyond 24 h after birth was not done. Assessment of the psychological and emotional wellbeing of the mothers was not given much attention. Kanyunyuzi et al. (2017) study in Uganda revealed that assessment of the mothers after admission to the postnatal ward was found to be low.

Poor adherence to practical guidelines identified in this study can be attributed to the non-availability of a standard guideline in this facility, inadequate human resources and infrastructure amongst others. To achieve this vision of "every pregnant woman receives quality care throughout pregnancy, childbirth and the postnatal period", six strategic areas have been identified by the WHO (2016) for improving the quality of maternal care namely; clinical guidelines, standards of care, effective interventions, quality measures, and the relevant research and capability building. The results of the evaluation of this study revealed that mothers received postnatal services that were below the WHO standard of quality postnatal care an indication of poor compliance with the guideline. In this study, 36.5% of the mothers were not satisfied and 28.4% were fairly satisfied with the overall postnatal care received on the postnatal wards. This was also the findings of Okonufua et al. (2017) who evaluated 8 secondary and tertiary hospitals in Nigeria. Many of the mothers had areas of dissatisfaction, or were not satisfied at all with the quality of care in antenatal, intra-partum and postnatal period. Reasons for dissatisfaction with postnatal care included poor staff attitude, long waiting time, high cost of services, and sub-standard facilities.

Most of the participants in a Pakistan study verbalized low quality of maternity care, disrespect and impolite behavior of health professionals (Munawar et al., 2017). On the other hand, Sacks et al., (2017) submitted that a large proportion of their participants reported positive postnatal experiences with more satisfaction among the Zambian than the Ugandan women. The third hypothesis tested in this study found a relationship between maternal satisfaction on the wards and the age and parity of the mother out of all the other selected maternal socio-demographic characteristics tested. While the fourth hypothesis revealed the absence of a significant difference between maternal satisfaction on the ward and in the clinic. Therefore, it is important for postnatal care providers to provide individualized, age and parity appropriate care to mothers in order to be able to meet their various health needs and yield satisfaction.

It was observed that this facility does not have any system in place for measuring outcomes of postnatal care. Measuring the quality of health care provided is an important evaluation that leads to improved care and accountability among care providers. Patient satisfaction in one of the indicators of quality care and it requires the provision of patient-centered care (including health education and counseling). Patient-centered care is health care that is respectful of, and responsive to, the preferences, needs and values of patients and consumers. Therefore, the quality of PNC in this facility can be greatly improved by the provision of individualized care and regular evaluation of patients through various feedback mechanisms. There should be awareness of feedback mechanisms among patients followed by inquiry through feedback questionnaires and other platforms (interviews, group discussions, online reviews etc) for expressing their complaints, satisfaction and suggestions on exit from the facility. There should be record keeping and analysis of degree of patients' satisfaction through which gaps in care can be identified and resolved. Regular feedback evaluation will also promote accountability among the health care givers.

Additionally, hospital managers should ensure availability and adherence to guidelines and protocols in all the hospital department and wards. The hospital should also have a unit in charge of formulating protocols from recent evidences, from research and guidelines. In-service training of health workers should be specific to their units and specialties within the hospital.

Conclusion

The findings of this study have shown a poor adherence to the international practice guideline for postnatal care in the study setting in the structural, process and outcome aspects of postnatal care. Maternal satisfaction was good on exit from postnatal clinic and poor on exit from the postnatal wards. There is a need to strengthen the facility by availability of recommended resources and also need to have a standard guideline that will serve as a framework for provision of quality postnatal care.

CONFLICT OF INTERESTS

The authors have not declared any conflict of interests.

REFERENCES

Agboghoroma CO, Gharoro EP (2015). Coverage and Distribution of Obstetricians and Gynecologists in Nigeria. International Journal of Gynecology andObstetrics 129(1):50-53.

African Population and Health Research Center (APHR) 2017. Maternal Health in Nigeria Facts and Figures. APHRC facts sheet June 2017. Available @ www.aphrc.org/wp. accessed June 23, 2018

Australian Nursing & Midwifery Federation (2015). Nurse/Midwife: Patient Ratios. It"s a matter of saving lives publication. ANMF Victoria Branch.

Blencowe H, Cousens S, Oestergaard MZ, Chou D, Moller AB, Narwal R, Adler A, Vera Garcia C, Rhode S, Say L, Lawn JE (2012). National, regional and worldwide estimates of preterm birth rates in the year 2010 with time trends since 1990 for selected countries: a systematic analysis and implications. The Lancet 379(9832):2162-2172.

Carvajal-Aguirre L, Amouzou A, Mehra V, Ziqi M, Zaka N, Newby H (2017). Gap between contact and content in maternal and newborn care: An analysis of data from 20 countries in sub–Saharan Africa. Journal of Global Health 7(2).

Chaghari M, Saffari M, Edabi A, Ameryoun A (2017). Empowering Educataion: A new Model for In-service Training of Nursing Staff. Journal of Advances in Medical Education and Professionalism 5(1):26.

Chen L, Qiong W, Velthoven M, Yanfeng Z, Shuyi Z, Ye L, Wei W, Xiaozhen D, Ting Z (2014). Coverage, quality of and barriers to postnatal care in rural Hebei, China: a mixed method study. BMC Pregnancy and Childbirth 14(1):31.

Chimtembo L, Maluwa A, Chimwaza A, Chirwa E, Pindani M (2013). Assessment of quality of postnatal care services offered to mothers in Dedza district, Malawi. Open Journal of Nursing 3(04):343.

Donabedian A (1988). The quality of care. How can it be assessed? JAMA 260(12):174-1748

Kanyunyuzi AE, Ekong EN, Namukwaya RE, Namala AL, Mudondo L, Mwebaza E, Smyth R (2017). A criteria-based audit to improve early postnatal care in Jinja, Uganda. African Journal of Midwifery and Women's Health 11(2):78-83.

Kearns AD, Caglia JM, Hoope-Bender P, Langer A (2016). Antenatal and postnatal care: a review of innovative models for improving availability, accessibility, acceptability and quality of services in low-resource settings. BJOG: An International Journal of Obstetrics & Gynaecology 123(4):540-548.

Khanal V, Adhikari M, Karkee R, Gavidia T (2014). Factors associated with the utilization of postnatal care services among the mothers of Nepal: analysis of Nepal Demographic and Health Survey 2011. BMC Women's Health 14(1):19.

Kinney M, Kerber K, Black R, Cohen B, Nkrumah F, Coovadia H, Nampala P, Lawn J, Axelson H, Bergh A, Chopra M, Diab R, Friberg I, Odubanjo O, Walker N, Weissman E (2010). Sub-Saharan Africa's mothers, newborns, and children: where and why do they die? PLoS Medicine 7(6): e1000294.

Kopp IB (2011). From Clinical Practice Guidelines towards Quality Assurance. Bundesgesundheitsblatt, Gesundheitsforschung, Gesundheitsschutz 54(2):160-165.

Lotto TD (2015). Assessment of the quality of postnatal Care services (Doctoral dissertation, Mzumbe University).

Luegmair K, Zenzmaier C, Oblasser C, Konig-Bachmann M (2018). Women's satisfaction with care at the birthplace in Austria: Evaluation of the babies born better survey national dataset. Midwifery 59:130-140.

Munawar A , Hassan Z, Ayub A , Shaikh BT , Buriro NA, Ahmed F, Kumar R (2017). Women's perceptions about quality of maternity care at tertiary care hospital Karachi, Pakistan. Pakistan Journal of Public Health 7(2):109-112.

Nigeria Demographic and Health Survey (NDHS) (2013). Nigeria Demographic and Health Survey by National Population Commission Federal Republic of Nigeria.

Ogu RN, Ntoimo LFC, Okonofua FE (2017). Perceptions of women on workloads in health facilities and its effect on maternal health care: A multi-site qualitative study in Nigeria. Midwifery 55:1-6.

Okonofua F, Ogu R, Agholor K, Okike O, Abdus-salam R, Randawa A, Abe E, Durodola A, Galadanci, The WHARC WHO FMOH MNCH Implementation Research Study Team (2017). Qualitative assessment of women's satisfaction with maternal health care in referral hospitals in Nigeria. Reproductive Health 14(1):44.

Pallangyo E, Mbekenga C, Olsson P, Källestål C (2017). A baseline mixed-methods study on postpartum care among health professionals in Tanzania. African Journal of Midwifery and Women's Health 11(3):115-122.

Pallangyo EN, Mbekenga C, Källestål C, Rubertsson C, Olsson P (2016). Healthcare provides' perceptions of postpartum care and its potential for improvement in low-income suburbs in Dar es Salaam, Tanzania. Sexual & Reproductive Healthcare 11:7-12.

Sacks E, Masvawure TB, Atuyambe LM, Neema S, Macwan'gi M, Simbaya J, Kruk M (2017). Postnatal care experiences and barriers to care utilization for home and facility delivered newborns in Uganda and Zambia. Maternal and Child Health Journal 21(3):599-606.

World Health Organization (2014). Trends in Maternal Mortality: 1990-2013, Estimates by WHO, UNICEF, UNFPA, The World Bank and the United Nation"s Population Division, Geneva.

World Health Organization (WHO) (2014). WHO recommendations on postnatal care of the mother and the newborn. WHO Library Cataloguing-in- Publication Data. ISBN 978 92 4 1506649.

World Health Organization (WHO) (2010). WHO Technical Consultation on Postpartum and Postnatal Care. Geneva, Switzerland.

World Health Organization (WHO) (2016). Standards for improving quality of maternal and newborn care in health facilities. ISBN: 9789241511216.

Permissions

All chapters in this book were first published in IJNM, by Academic Journals; hereby published with permission under the Creative Commons Attribution License or equivalent. Every chapter published in this book has been scrutinized by our experts. Their significance has been extensively debated. The topics covered herein carry significant findings which will fuel the growth of the discipline. They may even be implemented as practical applications or may be referred to as a beginning point for another development.

The contributors of this book come from diverse backgrounds, making this book a truly international effort. This book will bring forth new frontiers with its revolutionizing research information and detailed analysis of the nascent developments around the world.

We would like to thank all the contributing authors for lending their expertise to make the book truly unique. They have played a crucial role in the development of this book. Without their invaluable contributions this book wouldn't have been possible. They have made vital efforts to compile up to date information on the varied aspects of this subject to make this book a valuable addition to the collection of many professionals and students.

This book was conceptualized with the vision of imparting up-to-date information and advanced data in this field. To ensure the same, a matchless editorial board was set up. Every individual on the board went through rigorous rounds of assessment to prove their worth. After which they invested a large part of their time researching and compiling the most relevant data for our readers.

The editorial board has been involved in producing this book since its inception. They have spent rigorous hours researching and exploring the diverse topics which have resulted in the successful publishing of this book. They have passed on their knowledge of decades through this book. To expedite this challenging task, the publisher supported the team at every step. A small team of assistant editors was also appointed to further simplify the editing procedure and attain best results for the readers.

Apart from the editorial board, the designing team has also invested a significant amount of their time in understanding the subject and creating the most relevant covers. They scrutinized every image to scout for the most suitable representation of the subject and create an appropriate cover for the book.

The publishing team has been an ardent support to the editorial, designing and production team. Their endless efforts to recruit the best for this project, has resulted in the accomplishment of this book. They are a veteran in the field of academics and their pool of knowledge is as vast as their experience in printing. Their expertise and guidance has proved useful at every step. Their uncompromising quality standards have made this book an exceptional effort. Their encouragement from time to time has been an inspiration for everyone.

The publisher and the editorial board hope that this book will prove to be a valuable piece of knowledge for researchers, students, practitioners and scholars across the globe.

List of Contributors

Martha Assefa Sahile
Department of Nursing, College of Health Science, Arsi University, Assela, Ethiopia

Mesfin Tafa Segni
Department of Public Health, College of Health Science, Arsi University, Assela, Ethiopia

Tadese Awoke
Department of Epidemiology and Biostatistics, Institute of Public Health, University of Gondar, Gondar, Ethiopia

Dessalegn Bekele
Department of Psychiatry, Amanuel Specialized Hospital, Addis Ababa, Ethiopia

Tsehay Terefe and Abraham Irena
Tikur Anbessa Specialized Hospital, College of Health Sciences, Addis Ababa University, Ethiopia

Yohannes Tekalegn
Gobba Referral Hospital, College of Health Sciences, Madda Walabu University, Ethiopia

Zaid Altawil
Department of Emergency Medicine, Boston Medical Center, Boston, MA 02118, USA

Zaid Altawil, Emily de Redon, Hao Dinh, Daniela Suarez-Rebling and Thomas F. Burke
Division of Global Health and Human Rights, Department of Emergency Medicine, assachusetts General Hospital, Boston, MA 02114, USA

Thomas F. Burke
Harvard Medical School, Boston, MA 02115, USA
Harvard T.H. Chan School of Public Health, Boston, MA, 02115, USA

Daisy Andal Vcencio, Bandar Saad Albagawi and Farhan Alshammari
College of Nursing, University of Ha'il, Kingdom of Saudi Arabia

Hatim Ali Elsheikh
Department of Clinical Pharmacology, College of Medicine, Taif University, Kingdom of Saudi Arabia

Gebeyaw Molla
Amara Regional Private Health Facility and Professional Association, Bahirdar, Ethiopia

Alemayehu Gonie
College of Medicine and Health Sciences; Maddawalabu University, Robe, Ethiopia

Tefera Belachew and Bitiya Admasu
College of Medicine and Health Sciences; Jimma University, Jimma, Ethiopia

Yuko Uemura, Reiko Sakae and Keiko Matsumura
Department of Nursing, Kagawa Prefectural College of Health Sciences, Kagawa, Japan

Yuko Uemura
Tokushima University Graduate School, Tokushima, Japan

Toshiyuki Yasui
Department of Reproductive and Menopausal Medicine, Institute of Biomedical Sciences, Tokushima University Graduate School, Tokushima, Japan

Kimiyo Horike and Kazuhisa Maeda
Shikoku Medical Center for Children and Adults, Kagawa, Japan

Hirokazu Uemura
Department of Preventive Medicine, Institute of Biomedical Sciences, Tokushima University Graduate School, Tokushima, Japan

Mari Haku
Department of Midwifery, Institute of Biomedical Sciences, Tokushima University Graduate School, Tokushima, Japan

Dessalegn Tamiru
College of Public Health and Medical Science, Arba Minch University, Ethiopia

Hunduma Jisha
College of Health Science, Jimma University, Ethiopia

Patricia Obiajulu Onianwa
Department of Clinical Nursing, University College Hospital Ibadan, Ibadan, Nigeria

Temitope O. Alonge, Jesse A. Otegbayo, Elizabeth U. Ike, Felicia O. Chukura, Olufunke O. Are, Folashade O. M. Akanbi and Mary O. Ayorinde Iyanuoluwa O. Adubi
Department of Medicine, University College Hospital Ibadan, Ibadan, Nigeria

Olaoluwa S. Yaya
Department of Statistics, University of Ibadan, Ibadan, Nigeria

Christiana Nsiah-Asamoah
Department of Health Sciences Education, University of Cape Coast, Cape Coast, Ghana

Evelyn Asamoah Ampofo
School of Nursing and Midwifery, University of Cape Coast, Cape Coast, Ghana

T. Ebunoluwa Oshinyemi
Department of Nursing Science, College of Medicine, University of Lagos, Nigeria

J. Ojo Aluko and O. Abimbola Oluwatosin
Department of Nursing, College of Medicine, University of Ibadan, Oyo State, Nigeria

Zelalem Tenaw
School of Nursing and Midwifery, College of Medicine and Health sciences, Hawassa University, Ethiopia

Mikyas Arega
School of Nursing and Midwifery, College of Medicine and Health sciences, Debre Berhan University, Ethiopia

Erdaw Tachbele
School of Nursing and Midwifery, College of Medicine and Health sciences, Addis Ababa University, Ethiopia

Awoleye Abayomi F, Victor Chima and Alawode Oluwatobi A
Department of Demography and Social Statistics. Obafemi Awolowo University, Ile-Ife, Nigeria

Priscar Sakala Mukonka, Patricia Katowa Mukwato, Concepta Namukolo Kwaleyela and Margaret Maimbolwa
School of Nursing Sciences, University of Zambia, Zambia

Dereje Tsegaye, Muluneh Shuremu and Kebebe Bidira
Department of Public Health, Faculty of Public Health and Medical Sciences, Mettu University, Mettu, Ethiopia

Dawit Hoyiso
Department of Nursing College of Health Science Hawassa University, Ethiopia

Abinet Arega
Department of Health Education and Behavioral Sciences, Jimma University, Jimma, Ethiopia

Terefe Markos
Department of Epidemiology, Jimma University, Jimma, Ethiopia

Veronica Millicent Dzomeku
Department of Nursing, Kwame Nkrumah University of Science and Technology, Kumasi, Ghana

Brian van Wyk
School of Public Health, University of the Western Cape, South Africa

Lucia Knight
School of Public Health, University of the Western Cape, South Africa

Jody Rae Lori
School of Nursing, University of Michigan, USA

Oluwakemi Ajike Kolade
Department of Nursing, Ladoke Akintola University of Technology, Ogbomoso, Oyo State, Nigeria

Hanson Victoria Funmilayo
Ras AL Khaimah Medical and Health Science University, RAKCON, United Arab Emirate

Salisu Abubakar, Sanusi R. Adejumoke and Adelani Tijani
Department of Nursing Sciences, Bayero University, Kano State, Nigeria

Ada Carol Nwaneri, Ifeoma Ndubuisi, Ijeoma Lewechi Okoronkwo, Okwudili Ezike and Umebuani Nkiruka
Nursing Sciences Department, Faculty of Health Sciences and Technology, College of Medicine, University of Nigeria, Enugu Campus, Enugu State, Nigeria

Legesse Tadesse Wodajo, Solomon Tejineh Mengesha and Teresa Kisi Beyen
Department of Public Health, College of Health Sciences, Arsi University, Ethiopia

Gebresilasea Gendisha Ukke and Mekdes Kondale Gurara
Department of Midwifery, College of Medicine and Health Sciences, Arba Minch University, Arba Minch, Ethiopia

Temesgen Worku Gudayu
Department of Midwifery, College of Medicine and Health Sciences, University of Gondar, Gondar, Ethiopia

Negash Wakgari Amanta
School of Nursing and Midwifery, College of Medicine and Health Sciences, Hawassa University, Hawassa, Ethiopia

Mulugeta Shegaze Shimbre
Department of Nursing, College of Medicine and Health Sciences, Arba Minch University, Arba Minch, Ethiopia

Michele Rocha Kadri
Oswaldo Cruz Foundation - Amazonia, Leonidas e Maria Deane Institute, Rua Terezina, 476 - Adrianópolis, 69057-070, Manaus, Amazonas, Brazil

Debra Rose Wilson
Walden University, USA

Julio Cesar Schweickardt
Oswaldo Cruz Foundation - Amazonia, Leonidas e Maria Deane Institute, Brazil

James G. Linn
University of Valparaiso, Chile

Lisandra N. Guimarães Farias
Municipal Health Department of Borba, Brazil

Adriana Moreira
Secretaria Estadual de Saúde do Amazonas, Brazil

Rodrigo Tobias Lima
Oswaldo Cruz Foundation - Amazonia, Leonidas e Maria Deane Institute, Brazil

Iyare C. O., Uzoigwe J., Okorie P. O., Ugwu P. I., Ezeh C. O. and Iyare E. E.
Reproductive and Developmental Programming research Group, Department of Physiology, Faculty of Basic Medical Sciences, University of Nigeria, Enugu Campus, Enugu, Nigeria

Isabella Neri
Department of Mother-Infant, University of Modena, Italy

Maria Cristina Gemmi and Elisabetta Romei
Territorial Service, Reggio Emilia, Italy

Alba Ricchi
Department of Mother-Infant, University of Modena and Reggio Emilia, Italy

Hayelom Abadi Mesele
Department of Sociology, College of Social Sciences and Humanities, Wollo University, Dessie, Ethiopia

Miwa Fukuoka and Toshiyuki Yasui
Department of Reproductive and Menopausal Medicine, Graduate School of Biomedical Sciences, Tokushima University, Tokushima, Japan

Yuna Hamada
Tokushima Red Cross Hospital, Irinokuchi-103 Komatsushimacho, Komatsushima, Tokushima Prefecture 773-8502, Japan

Mari Fujikawa
Takamatsu Public Health Center, Kagawa Prefecture, Shikoku, Japan

Sayuri Hatanaka
Kitano Hospital, 2 Chome-4-20 Ogimachi, Kita Ward, Osaka, Osaka Prefecture 530-8480, Japan

Mekiya Ediris and Kidest Getu
Department of Midwifery, College of Health Sciences and Medicine, Wolaita Sodo University, Wolaita Sodo, Ethiopia

Tefera Belachew
Department of Population and Family Health, College of Health Sciences, Jimma University, Jimma, Ethiopia

Fekadu Yadassa and Kidest Getu
Department of Nursing and Midwifery, College of Health Sciences, Jimma University Jimma, Ethiopia

Sima Kermanshahi
Department of Nursing, Tarbiat Modarres University, Tehran, Iran

Rose Ekama Ilesanmi and Janet Atinuke Akinmeye
Department of Nursing, College of Medicine, University of Ibadan, Ibadan, Oyo State, Nigeria

Index